Management of psychiatric disorders in pregnancy

Management of psychiatric disorders in pregnancy

Edited by

KIMBERLY A. YONKERS MD
Associate Professor, Department of Psychiatry, Yale
University School of Medicine, New Haven, Connecticut,
USA

BERTIS B. LITTLE PhD
Associate Vice President for Academic Research and
Grants, Office of Sponsored Projects, Tarleton State
University, Stephenville, Texas, USA

A member of the Hodder Headline Group
LONDON

First published in Great Britain 2001 by
Arnold, a member of the Hodder Headline Group,
338 Euston Road, London NWI 3BH

http://www.arnoldpublishers.com

Whilst the advice and information in this book is believed to be true and
accurate at the date of going to press, neither the authors nor the publisher
can accept any legal responsibility or liability for any errors or omissions
that may be made. In particular (but without limiting the generality of the
preceding disclaimer) every effort has been made to check drug dosages;
however, it is still possible that errors have been missed. Furthermore,
dosage schedules are constantly being revised and new side-effects
recognized. For these reasons the reader is strongly urged to consult the
drug companies' printed instructions before administering any of the drugs
recommended in this book.

British Library Cataloguing in Publication Data
A catalogue record for this book is available from the British Library

Library of Congress Cataloging-in-Publication Data
A catalog record for this book is available from the Library of Congress

ISBN 0 340 76126 1

1 2 3 4 5 6 7 8 9 10

Commissioning Editor: Joanna Koster
Development Editor: Paula O'Connell
Production Editor: Lauren McAllister
Production Controller: Iain McWilliams

Typeset in 10/12 pt Minion by
Scribe Design, Gillingham, Kent, UK
Printed and bound in Great Britain by
MPG Books Limited, Bodmin, Cornwall

What do you think about this book? Or any other Arnold title?
Please send your comments to feedback.arnold@hodder.co.uk

Contents

Contributors

Margaret Altemus MD
Weill Medical College, Cornell University, Department of Psychiatry, New York, USA

Lori L. Davis MD
Coordinator of Research and Development, Assistant Professor of Psychiatry, University of Alabama at Birmingham, VA Medical Center, Tuscaloosa, Alabama, USA

Roger G. Drake Pharm D
Boyce Hospital, Tuscaloosa, Alabama, USA

Tana A. Grady-Weliky MD
Associate Professor of Psychiatry, Department of Psychiatry, University of Rochester School of Medicine and Dentistry, Rochester, New York, USA

Shelly F. Greenfield MD MPH
Assistant Professor of Psychiatry, Harvard Medical School and Medical Director, Alcohol and Drug Abuse Ambulatory Treatment Program, McLean Hospital, Belmont, Massachusetts, USA

A. Chris Heath MD
UT Southwestern Medical Center, Departments of Psychiatry and Obstetrics and Gynecology, Dallas, Texas, USA

Marie Kelly MD
Fort Worth, Texas, USA

Bertis B. Little PhD
Assistant Vice President for Academic Research and Grants, Office of Sponsored Projects, Tarleton State University, Stephenville, Texas, USA

Dana March
Clinical Research Assistant, Yale University, New Haven, Connecticut, USA

Frederick Petty PhD MD
University of Texas Southwestern Medical Center, Dallas, Texas, USA

Stacy Shannon Pharm D
Broughton Hospital, Morganton, N.C., USA

Margaret G. Spinelli MD
Columbia University/New York State Psychiatric Institute, Assistant Professor of Clinical Psychiatry, Director, Maternal Mental Health Program, New York, USA

Dawn E. Sugarman BA
Clinical Research Assistant, McLean Hospital, Belmont, Massachusetts, USA

Janet L. Tekell MD
Assistant Professor, VA North Texas Health Care System, UT Southwestern Medical Center, Department of Psychiatry, Dallas, Texas, USA

Jennifer C. Yolles MD
Assistant Professor, Department of Psychiatry, SUNY-Upstate Medical University, Syracuse, New York, USA

Kimberly A. Yonkers MD
Associate Professor, Department of Psychiatry, Yale University School of Medicine, New Haven, Connecticut, USA

Preface

The intent of assembling this volume was to address what we perceived to be an area of need for clinicians. The notion of writing a book on the treatment of psychiatric disorders during pregnancy was conceived while we, Drs. Yonkers and Little, worked together in a maternal-fetal medicine clinic assessing, counseling and devising diagnostic and treatment plans for pregnant psychiatric patients. The need for a book which pulled together information in this area became abundantly clear. For the next several years we collaborated on writing a book to address these unmet requirements of physicians providing care for pregnant psychiatric patients.

The selection of topics covered was guided by our own clinical experiences and the experiences of others who have treated pregnant psychiatric patients. We have ordered the book's chapters to provide an overview of treatment paradoxes and options, beginning with the dilemma of whether or not to treat disorders pharmacologically during gestation. We then address obstetrical issues that may complicate pregnancies of psychiatric patients, and present an overview of the potential complications that may arise from ingestion of medication during gestation. The leading psychiatric disorders encountered in practice are discussed in the ensuing chapters focusing specifically on the course of the disease during pregnancy, management issues and treatment options (pharmacologic versus psychotherapeutic).

It is our intent to provide information that is as accurate as possible, but we are aware that treatment regimens change and improve over time. Therefore, it is important to consult contemporary prescribing and indication guidelines prior to treating individual patients. In addition, the disorders discussed in this volume do not comprise an exhaustive listing. As need is identified for treatment of other disorders, coverage will be expanded.

K.A. Yonkers, M.D.
B.B. Little, M.A., Ph.D

Dedicated to our spouses,
Charles Landau, M.D. and Beverly A. Del'Homme, J.D.

Introduction

EPIDEMIOLOGY OF PSYCHIATRIC DISORDERS AND THE IMPORTANCE OF GENDER

An understudied area of medical investigation is that of the pregnant woman with a psychiatric disorder. Few textbooks have been published on the topic, and only limited literature is available in a synthesized form. Gender-related biological and psychological factors are recognized as important factors in the etiology, persistence and treatment of mental disorders. Mental disorders are major sources of disease-related disability. The Global Burden of Disease report identified major depressive disorder, bipolar disorder, schizoprenia and obsessive-compulsive disorder among the 10 leading sources of disease-related disability in women worldwide.[1] The magnitude of this is highlighted by the fact that major depressive disorder is projected to be the second leading cause of disability worldwide in the next decade. The majority of serious mental disorders have an onset in adolescence or early adulthood and show a recurrent or chronic course (DSM-IV, American Psychiatric Association).[2] Thus, the social impact of mental disorders falls disproportionately on women during the childbearing and childrearing years, suggesting the need for more intervention research including women who are pregnant or lactating.

Epidemiological studies show that women are more likely to have experienced certain kinds of stress (e.g. childhood and adult sexual abuse) which are risk factors for mental disorders.[3,4] Research also indicates that women are twice as likely as men to develop stress-related disorders and depression following exposure to traumatic events.[5-7]

Menarche coincides with the onset of gender disparities in the incidence of depression, many anxiety disorders and eating disorders.[8-10] Menstruation is associated with severe mood variations in a small percentage of women.[11,12] Since variation in hormonal levels *per se* does not correlate with mood or mood change in human research, there is a need for studies of the interaction between multiple biological, clinical and environmental factors.[11] Recent childbearing may be associated with higher rates of depressive disorders.[13,14] This association, as well as the fact that psychotropic drugs are commonly prescribed for women of childbearing age, raises special gender-related clinical and treatment considerations. Importantly, the safety of specific regimens for use during pregnancy remains largely unexplored.

It is critical to present, study, evaluate and implement changes derived from gender-based research. Depression is one of the most common psychiatric problems encountered in primary care, including primary care obstetrics and gynecology practices. An estimated 7.5 million Americans suffer from depression, and 10% of patients in primary care settings present with that diagnosis.[15] In addition, anxiety disorders are present in 25–60% of the medically ill.[14,16] On average, one in four patients seen in primary care settings is suffering from a mental disorder.[17] Women have prevalences of psychiatric disorders that are equal to or higher than those in men for all categories except substance abuse.[18] Of all the demographic variables in epidemiological research, gender is the single strongest correlate of risk for different types of mental disorders. Depressive disorders and most anxiety disorders are, on average, two to three times more common in females than in males.[19] Eating disorders are eight to ten times more common in females.[18] Males are more likely to be affected by developmental disorders such as autism and attention deficit disorder, substance and alcohol abuse, and conduct disorders. For all disorders, including those that are more common in males than in females and those in which gender prevalence is equal (e.g. schizophrenia, bipolar disorder), gender-related differences may occur in etiological risk factors or in clinical aspects.[18] Gender differences in such features as neuropsychological profiles, risk for onset or recurrence, and symptom severity or disabilities have important practical significance for treatment and services needs. In general, women are the primary consumers of treatments and services for mental disorders, yet there has been little consideration of epidemiological and clinical findings with regard to gender differences applied to public mental health policy and service delivery systems.

The finding of a large national study was that the prevalence of mental illness and substance abuse is far higher than was previously thought, and that these disorders are underdiagnosed and undertreated. Americans between the ages of 25 and 34 years are more likely than any other age group to have suffered a psychiatric disorder at some time in their lives. This is partly because modern young people are more stressed and have easier access to alcohol and drugs.[18] In total, 30% of respondents reported a psychiatric disorder of some kind in the year before the survey, but only 40% of these individuals sought treatment. Serious mental illness (i.e. three or more episodes of major depression, manic-depression, schizophrenia or substance abuse) is concentrated among 14% of the nation's population. In a given year, this group accounts for 89% of all cases of the most severe psychiatric disorders (e.g. schizophrenia and manic-depressive psychosis). The largest subgroup in this 14% patient group consists of low-income, low-educated, city-dwelling white women in their twenties or thirties. Only 6 in 10 people in this group ever receive treatment, and only 1 in 3 individuals had received treatment for psychotic episodes in the year before the survey.

Women have higher prevalences than men of affective disorders (with the exception of mania, for which there is no sex difference) and anxiety disorders. Men have higher rates than women of substance abuse disorders and antisocial personality disorder (ASPD). Furthermore, women have higher prevalences than men of both lifetime and 12–month comorbidity of three or more disorders.[9,18]

The highest prevalences are generally in the group aged 25–34 years, with declining prevalences at later ages.[18] Twelve–month disorders are consistently most prevalent in the youngest cohort (15–24 years) and generally decrease monotonically with age. Furthermore, the rates of almost all disorders decline monotonically with increasing income and level of education.

In summary, investigators consistently report finding more affective disorders and anxiety disorders among women, more substance abuse disorders and ASPD among men, and declining rates of most disorders with age and higher socio-economic status.

TYPES OF PSYCHIATRIC DISORDERS AMONG WOMEN

Depression

It is estimated that the lion's share (> 80%) of unipolar major depression occurs in women between the ages of 15 and 44 years.[9] During this age span, women are students, workers, partners in family relationships and mothers. Because women of childrearing age represent the largest proportion of individuals with depression, the maintenance of their mental health during pregnancy is of paramount importance.

Bipolar disorder

Bipolar disorder occurs with the same frequency in men and women, although women are more likely to experience rapid cycling and the depressed phase of the illness.[20] This disorder takes a substantial toll on a person's life, and nearly all patients will require life-long pharmacological and psychological therapy. Furthermore, since it typically strikes an individual in late adolescence or early adulthood, it can truncate psychosocial development in a number of realms. Bipolar women do not have a less severe course of bipolar illness than bipolar men. It has been suggested that reproductive risks play an important role in the clinical course of bipolar illness in women, and that these influences can be pronounced even in the context of high genetic propensity for the illness. Reproductive transitions are high-risk periods and highlight the need for new treatment strategies for childbearing women with bipolar disorder.[21]

Anxiety disorders

Anxiety disorders are the most common psychiatric disorders and they occur more frequently among women, approximately two-thirds of individuals who are treated for anxiety disorders being females. Anxiety disorders commonly coexist with other anxiety disorders as well as with other psychiatric disorders, including major depressive disorder.[22] Not only is the risk of selected anxiety disorders greater in women, but the likelihood that a woman will have a chronic course is higher among women with panic disorder and post-traumatic stress disorder compared to their male counterparts.[3,23] This increases the likelihood that a woman who conceives will have an anxiety disorder. It is also suggested that the biological changes which occur during pregnancy promote some anxiety disorders, specifically obsessive-compulsive disorder.[9] This further increases the need for clinicians to have a thorough knowledge of the management of psychiatric illness during pregnancy.

Schizophrenia

Schizophrenia is another severe and persistent mental disorder that has a similar prevalence in men and women.[18] However, women develop the illness at a later age (on average) than men,[24] increasing the likelihood that they will have found a partner and be in a stable relationship before they are fully symptomatic. Thus, women with schizophrenia may become pregnant and require management of their illness during this time.

Eating disorders

Eating disorders are a serious public health concern in the USA. An estimated 2–4% of teenagers and young women are affected by anorexia or bulimia. When eating disorders become chronic they frequently have serious psychological and medical consequences. When they occur in a pregnant woman, the patient's offspring can be seriously at risk. Clinical depression and anxiety disorders commonly coexist with eating disorders and treatment approaches include therapy for the comorbid conditions.

The majority of women with an eating disorder have had or currently have major depression as well as at least one anxiety disorder when they are first seen by clinicians. These patients typically participate in a variety of treatments, primarily individual therapy, but also group therapy, family therapy, pharmacotherapy and nutritional counseling.[25]

Special obstetric issue: depression in infertile women

Unsuccessful attempts to conceive are accompanied by significant psychological distress according to clinical descriptions, anecdotal accounts in the medical literature, and the lay press.[26] It is clear that coupling psychological interventions with fertility treatment can enhance patient well-being, and this may also translate into improved fertility rates.

EFFECTS OF PREGNANCY ON DISEASE COURSE

Conditions may worsen, improve or remain unchanged during pregnancy. Pharmacokinetic changes during gestation may affect the disease course during pregnancy, but other factors (e.g. hormonal changes, emotional stress) are also involved. Thus the natural history of specific diseases must be considered in the treatment plan because no general guidelines can be formulated.

TREATMENT OF DISORDERS WITH MEDICATION DURING PREGNANCY

Frequently, psychiatric disorders that occur during pregnancy require medications. Mood stabilizers are a class of psychotropics that are known to pose significant risks to embryofetal development, and their use should be closely scrutinized. For other medication classes, the data either suggest no or minimal risk, or else no information on their use during pregnancy is available. Importantly, the absence of information on pregnancy risk should not be regarded as evidence of the absence of risk for the pregnancy.

PHARMACOLOGICAL TREATMENT

Psychiatric treatment is often multimodal, incorporating both psychopharmacological and psychotherapeutic treatment of psychiatric disorders in the medically ill.

The term *pharmacokinetics* describes the action of drugs in the body over time, and refers to the processes of absorption, distribution, metabolism and elimination. A drug's pharmacokinetic properties are affected by the patient's age, genetics, gender and medical illness(es). Pregnancy also affects pharmacokinetics profoundly.[27] For psychotropic medications, the dose generally needs to be increased during the third trimester to maintain therapeutic drug levels. However, no clear pattern exists (see Table 1) even among medications in the same class.[27] Therefore, dosing regimens need to be managed for each specific medication.

CONCLUSION

Contemporary women are delaying childbearing in increasing numbers. Consequently, the window of opportunity for planning and preparing for pregnancy will become wider. Initia-

Table 1 *Qualitative analysis of pharmacokinetics in pregnancy*

Index	n	Studies reporting pharmacokinetic data: Changes associated with pregnancy			Studies not reporting pharmacokinetic data
		Decrease	No change	Increase	
AUC	17	7	5	5	44 (72.1%)
Vd	23	3	11	9	38 (62.3%)
C_{max}	30	10	17	3	31 (50.8%)
C_{ss}	42	19	4	19	19 (31.1%)
$T_{1/2}$	39	16	17	6	22 (36.1%)
T_{max}	9	3	4	2	52 (85.2%)
Cl	44	5	15	24	17 (27.9%)
PPB	7	6	1	0	54 (88.5%)

AUC, area under the curve;
Vd, volume of distribution;
C_{max}, peak plasma concentration;
C_{ss}, steady-state concentration
$T_{1/2}$, half-life;
T_{max}, = time to peak plasma concentration;
Cl, clearance;
PPB plasma protein binding.
Adapted from Little.[27]

tion of treatment in women of reproductive age and gravidas relies on an appropriate psychiatric diagnosis, the selection of a safe psychopharmacologic agent for use during pregnancy, employing knowledge of pharmacokinetics, drug–drug interactions and side-effect profiles. This volume addresses all of these issues.

Bertis B. Little PhD
Kimberly A. Yonkers MD

REFERENCES

1. Murray CJ, Lopez AD. *The global burden of disease.* Cambridge, MA: Harvard University Press, 1996.
2. American Psychiatric Association. *Diagnostic and statistical manual of mental disorders,* 4th edn. Washington, DC: American Psychiatric Association, 1994.
3. Breslau N, Davis G. Post-traumatic stress disorder in an urban population of young adults: risk factors for chronicity. *American Journal of Psychiatry* 1992; **149:** 671–5.
4. Brown GW, Harris TO. *Social origins of depression: a study of psychiatric disorder in women.* New York: Free Press, 1978.
5. Breslau N, Davis GC, Andreski P. Traumatic events and traumatic stress disorder in an urban population of young adults. *Archives of General Psychiatry* 1991; **48:** 218–22.
6. McGrath E, Keita GP, Strickland BR *et al. Women and depression* Washington, DC: American Psychological Association,1990.
7. Weiss EL, Longhurst JG, Mazure CM. Childhood sexual abuse as a risk factor for depression in women: psychosocial and neurobiological correlates. *American Journal of Psychiatry* 1999; **156:** 816–28.

8. Eaton WW, Kramer M, Anthony JC *et al*. The incidence of specific DIS/DSM-III mental disorders: data from the NIMH Epidemiologic Catchment Area Program. *Acta Psychiatrica Scandinavica* 1989; **79**: 163–78.

9. Kessler RC, McGonagle KA, Swartz M *et al*. Sex and depression in the National Comorbidity Survey I. Lifetime prevalence, chronicity and recurrence. *Journal of Affective Disorders* 1993; **29**: 85–96.

10. Yonkers KA. Panic disorder in women. *Journal of Women's Health* 1994; **3**: 481–6.

11. Steiner M. Premenstrual syndromes. *Annual Review of Medicine* 1997; **48**: 447-55.

12. Yonkers KA. Medical management of premenstrual dysphoric disorder. *Journal of Gender Specific Medicine* 1999; **2**: 40–44.

13. O'Hara MW. *Postpartum depression: causes and consequences* New York: Springer-Verlag, 1995.

14. Sherbourne CD, Wells KB, Meredith LS *et al*. Comorbid anxiety disorder and the functioning and well-being of chronically ill patients of general medical providers. *Archives of General Psychiatry* 1996; **53**: 889–95.

15 Kaplan HI, Sadock BJ (eds) *Kaplan and Sadock's synopsis of psychiatry: behavioral sciences/clinical psychiatry*. Baltimore, MD: Lippincott, Williams & Wilkins, 1997.

16. Sherbourne CD, Jackson CA, Meredith LS *et al*., Prevalence of comorbid anxiety disorders in primary care outpatients. *Archives of Family Medicine* 1997; **5**: 27–34.

17. Steffens D. When to make an adult psychiatric referral. *Primary Psychiatry* 1997; **4**: 8–40.

18 Kessler RC, McGonagle KA, Zhao S *et al*. Lifetime and 12-month prevalence of DSM-III-R psychiatric disorders in the United States. Results from the National Comorbidity Survey. *Archives of General Psychiatry* 1994; 51: 25–37.

19. Yonkers KA, Ellison JM. Anxiety disorders in women and their pharmacological treatment. In: Jensvold MF, Halbreich U, Hamilton JA, *Psychopharmacology and women. Sex, gender, and hormones*. Washington, DC: American Psychiatric Press, 1996: 262–85.

20. Leibenluft E. Women with bipolar illness: clinical and research issues. *American Journal of Psychiatry* 1996; **153**: 163–73.

21. Blehar MC, DePaulo JR, Gershon ES, Reich T, Simpson SG, Nurnberger JI. Women with bipolar disorder: findings from the NIMH genetics initiative sample. *Psychopharmacology Bulletin* 1998; **34**: 239–43.

22. Yonkers KA, Gurguis G. Gender differences in the prevalence and expression of anxiety disorders. In: Seeman MV (ed.) *Gender psychopathology*. Washington DC: American Psychiatric Press, 1995; 113–30.

23. Yonkers KA, Zlotnick C, Allsworth J *et al*. Is the course of panic disorder the same in women and men? *American Journal of Psychiatry* 1998; **155**: 596–602.

24. Goldstein JM, Tsuang MT. Gender and schizophrenia: an introduction and synthesis of findings. *Schizophrenia Bulletin* 1990; **16**: 179–83.

25. Herzog DB, Nussbaum K, Marmor A. Comorbidity and outcome in disorders. *Psychiatric Clinics of North America* 1996; **19**: 843–59.

26. Yonkers KA, Bradshaw KD. Psychological factors and infertility. Causal or consequential. In: Baniewicz C, *Infertility and reproductive medicine. Clinics of North America. Controversies in infertility management*. Philadelphia, PA: W.B. Saunders Co, 1997: 305–19.

27. Little BB. Pharmacokinetics during pregnancy: evidence-based maternal dose formulation. *Obstetrics and Gynecology* 1999; **93**: 858–68.

Psychotropics versus psychotherapy: an individualized treatment plan for the pregnant patient

JENNIFER C. YOLLES

INTRODUCTION

Pregnancy is one of the landmark events in a woman's life. Few life events are as complex or far-reaching in their impact, particularly the first pregnancy. In the course of a completed pregnancy a woman undergoes enormous changes in her physical, emotional, intrapsychic, interpersonal and social functioning. The majority of women regard pregnancy as an exciting time, with joyful anticipation overshadowing the discomforts and worries that most experience at least sporadically throughout the months of gestation. This is the image that is generally called to mind when we think about pregnancy. However, for most women the months of pregnancy are an emotionally turbulent time, and for some they are a time of real distress. Mental health professionals are often called upon to evaluate psychiatric and emotional problems that arise during pregnancy. These may be problems directly related to the pregnancy itself, or they may be pre-existing mental health problems exacerbated by – or merely coincident with – the pregnancy. Data on the actual incidence of major mental illnesses during pregnancy are conflicting and are complicated by a number of methodological factors. Symptoms of anxiety, depression and emotional instability are common during pregnancy, and have been shown to occur more frequently than in age-matched non-childbearing women.[1-3] In general practice, women of reproductive age represent a sizable percentage of the patients who receive mental health care. Mood and anxiety disorders are highly prevalent in this population. Substance abuse, eating disorders, personality disorders and schizophrenia are all common disorders of young and middle adulthood as well. Since pregnancy does not confer a protective effect against any of these disorders,[4-8] and because it is a major life stressor in its own right, it is to be expected that many women will experience symptoms of emotional or psychological distress during the course of their pregnancy. Obstetricians and patients alike may turn to mental health providers for guidance in determining which individuals require treatment, and what form of treatment is most appropriate.

Psychiatry has been slow to address specifically the question of how to identify and best meet the mental health needs of pregnant women. Many clinicians feel uncomfortable when faced with a gravid patient in distress. Until relatively recently, the only guidance available in standard texts about managing mental illness during pregnancy focused primarily on the risks and potential teratogenicity of psychotropic medications.[9] The importance of minimizing fetal exposure to medications – especially when the absolute risk of exposure cannot be determined with any degree of certainty – does make this an issue of paramount importance. However, the full range of psychiatric treatments is quite broad and treatment planning should be more comprehensive than deciding which treatments to withhold. Reflexive and universal recommendations to discontinue psychotropic medications for the sake of the developing fetus sound reasonable on the surface, but minimize the importance of maternal well-being as a priority in treatment. A more reasoned approach to clinical decision-making attempts to balance the needs of both mother and child by finding the most benign treatment strategy that will effectively support the health and functioning of both.

In this chapter we shall look briefly at some of the factors which contribute to making pregnancy such a powerful and at times emotionally destabilizing life event. We shall then elaborate the issues involved in assessing a pregnant patient's treatment needs and the process of balancing the risks and benefits of various treatment modalities. The specifics of treating various psychiatric disorders are addressed elsewhere in this book. The focus here will be on the evaluation process itself and the factors which influence clinical decision-making. Because there is a paucity of literature addressing this issue, much of this chapter reflects the author's opinions derived from experience of working with pregnant women and their partners in both mental health and primary care settings. The last section of this chapter describe a number of clinical cases which demonstrate some of the complexities outlined previously.

PREGNANCY – A TIME OF CHANGE

Pregnancy is a time of monumental life change. No other routine life event so profoundly alters a person's world in so many different spheres simultaneously. In less than a year a pregnant woman has to incorporate major changes in her physical, psychological, interpersonal and social functioning. Conflict triggered by the disruption of any of these realms may lead to emotional distress, including anxiety and depressive symptoms. Such emotional turbulence is to be expected during any period of rapid growth or change. In some cases, the turmoil may reach to pathologic proportions or may interfere with the woman's ability to function, requiring specific treatment.

The physical changes of pregnancy begin almost immediately after conception. Massive alterations in the reproductive hormones alter the woman's internal milieu. The hormonal manifestations of early pregnancy are experienced by many women prior to the first missed menstrual period in the form of breast tenderness and swelling, fatigue and, in some cases, mood symptoms. These hormonal changes continue throughout the pregnancy and the postpartum period. For women who are sensitive to the neuropsychiatric effects of reproductive hormones, the physical state of pregnancy can induce unfamiliar and unpredicted emotional reactions. Because the hormonal and physiologic phenomena do not occur in isolation, it is not possible to pinpoint precisely which affective symptoms are attributable specifically to these factors. Anecdotally, however, clinicians working with pregnant patients report that some individuals with a history of mood instability feel more stable during the months of pregnancy. This has been demonstrated in several studies of women with bipolar disorder.[10,11] A number of authors have noted that symptoms of panic disorder may diminish during pregnancy,[12–14] although the data on this subject remain controversial.[4] Some neurohormonal hypotheses have been offered as an explanation for these phenomena.[14,15] Alternatively, some individuals experience pregnancy as a time of increased emotional volatility and affective dysregulation, presumably also of a hormonal origin.

The hormonal changes represent only a small part of the physical changes of pregnancy. Every aspect of a pregnant woman's body is affected by the pregnancy, and the changes continue inexorably from early in the first trimester through the early postpartum months and beyond. Although these changes are often greeted with excitement and pride, the loss of control over one's body shape and the unfamiliarity of some of the bodily experiences can be disturbing and unsettling. At the same time, these physical changes are very public and obvious, causing some women to feel exposed and scrutinized in a manner that makes them feel uncomfortable. Women with pre-existing conflicts related to body image or sexuality may be particularly discomfited by physical changes and the public evidence of their sexuality as the pregnancy progresses.[16]

The psychological work of becoming a mother is quite considerable. The shift in identification from 'adult woman' to 'mother' is a deep and irreversible process. This has been called a 'developmental crisis',[17] akin to the period of adolescence during which physical and psychological phenomena propel the young adult to reorganize much of their self-concept in the process of moving towards a new level of development. At such maturational turning points there is a degree of psychological upheaval, during which earlier conflicts tend to re-emerge and are reworked in a manner that fits the new intrapsychic equilibrium which is being established.[18] During adolescence, the resolution of the crisis involves settling into an adult identity. During pregnancy, the resolution involves the psychological transition to being – and accepting the role of – a mother.

This developmental process tends to evolve in predictable stages.[19–21] Early in the pregnancy the main task is to adapt to the idea of pregnancy and its impact on the individual's life. As the pregnancy progresses, and particularly after fetal movements are detected, maternal attachment to the baby increases, often with some accompanying psychological withdrawal from others. An intense dyadic connection to the fetus usually develops, and expectant mothers typically assign 'personalities' and unique characteristics to the unseen child. During the last months of pregnancy the beginnings of differentiation from the future baby emerge. There is a greater focus on and preparation for life after delivery, involving caring for an infant who is separate from the mother herself. Preparatory or 'nesting' behaviors are a typical and important sign that the mother is progressing through this stage of development.

For most women, pregnancy is a time when they psychologically rework their own mother–daughter relationship.[22,23] The mother to be begins to identify in a new way with her own mother and her own conception of motherhood. Earlier conflicts regarding dependency, nurturance and issues in the woman's own relationship with her mother are typically reawakened as the pregnant woman moves towards motherhood. This can be an opportunity for further personal growth and resolution, or it can be experienced as a trigger for emotional regression and turmoil.

Accompanying these developmental steps, there are common, predictable emotional responses which the clinician should anticipate.[19,20] The immediate reaction to learning that one is pregnant is typically an amalgam – or series – of diverse responses. Even when the pregnancy is planned and desired there is invariably some degree of ambivalence, anxiety and fear as one begins to contemplate the enormity of the life changes ahead. Later in the pregnancy the ambivalence generally diminishes, but it may be replaced by significant worry and anxiety about the health and well-being of the baby, and about the parents' ability to parent and care for it.[24] A heightened level of anxiety, particularly when the anxiety is focused on the fetus and not on the mother herself, is not necessarily a sign of pathology, and may in fact correlate with a high level of maternal attachment to the unborn child.[25] Fears about labor and delivery, and sadness about the end of the 'special' period of pregnancy are frequent towards the end of the third trimester, and may coincide with apparent contradictory feelings of impatience with the physical discomforts, and a growing readiness for pregnancy to 'be over.' These 'normal' reactions are fluid and transitory and should be differentiated from more severe emotional distress which may be indicative of an obstacle to the psychological adaptation process.

In addition to being a time of physical and psychological changes, pregnancy and child-birth lead to major changes in a woman's social roles and relationships.[16] In a first pregnancy, the dyadic relationship between the woman and her partner – if such a partner is present – must adapt sufficiently to accommodate a third person whose demands and needs are unlike any that previously existed in the relationship. Either or both of the parents may struggle with the anticipated loss of autonomy and the heightened responsibilities associated with caring for a new child. If there have been previous pregnancies, there are older children whose relationship with their mother will be irrevocably altered by an addition to the family. The woman's relationship with her parents and with her partner's parents also changes with the addition of a new generation. Conflicts may flare over childrearing and parenting issues or there may be a new measure of closeness and empathic connection between a new mother and her own mother.

Pregnancy and motherhood affect the way in which a woman functions in her other social roles as well. Choices must be made about how best to meet her occupational and financial responsibilities and the baby's childrearing needs. Frequently this requires a readjustment of the woman's professional or educational goals, and a reordering of the priority assigned to her other personal pursuits. Becoming a parent alters one's status within many cultural and religious institutions and is associated with many societal expectations about behavior and responsibility.

Having reviewed the enormous range of stresses associated with pregnancy, it seems to be a miracle that any woman can navigate such a treacherous process and survive unscathed! In fact, not only do the vast majority of women manage the process successfully, but most do not consider pregnancy to be a problematic or difficult experience. What makes some women more vulnerable to mental and emotional difficulties during pregnancy? Several psychological risk factors have been identified.[3,26,27] The cumulative impact of any combination of these vulnerability factors should raise clinicians' concern about the likelihood that an individual will experience emotional or psychiatric complications.

Women become pregnant in widely differing life circumstances. Some situations clearly increase the emotional demands on a woman, while others mitigate the potential for crisis. Age is a major risk factor predictive of many complications of pregnancy, including antena-tal depression.[28–30] Teenagers are less likely than older women to be in a supportive relation-ship with a spouse, to be economically self-sufficient, or to have planned the pregnancy, all of which are stressors associated with increased risk for depressive symptoms during pregnancy.[3,26,27] Psychologically, adolescents are still in the midst of another and earlier devel-opmental process. As they have not completed the transition to adulthood, adolescents are poorly prepared to manage an additional, simultaneous maturational process and they may require a great deal of adult guidance and support in order to cope well with pregnancy and new motherhood.

Marital status, as well as the quality of the relationship between partners and the degree of instrumental support available to the expectant woman, have been repeatedly shown to correlate with maternal adjustment during and after pregnancy.[5,31] The presence of other coincidental negative life events and ongoing psychosocial and economic stressors have all been linked to increased rates of depression, anxiety disorders and psychological symptoms during pregnancy.[3,26,27,32]

Many pregnancies are planned, but up to 50% are not.[33,34] Reacting to the news of an unexpected pregnancy adds to the normal emotional turmoil of the early months of pregnancy as the woman and her partner wrestle with feelings of surprise and ambivalence and make plans about how to respond to the pregnancy. A related issue is whether the pregnancy, intended or not, is initially regarded as a positive or negative event.[16] For example, a woman who finds herself pregnant after a period of disappointing infertility is in a vastly different situation to one who realizes that she has become pregnant while in the throes of separation or divorce from her spouse, or who has been impregnated by a rape or within an abusive relationship. A crisis in adjustment to an unwanted pregnancy is one of the factors associated with depression and suicide in early pregnancy.[35] Individual circumstances and the meaning of the pregnancy to the individuals involved play a major role in the mother's emotional responses to the pregnancy.

Obstetric factors can also increase the risk of emotional disturbance during pregnancy. A woman's previous experience of pregnancy, abortion, miscarriage or infertility can profoundly affect her ability to accept fully the current pregnancy.[5] It is not uncommon for women who have suffered miscarriage or stillbirth to experience enormous anxiety throughout subsequent pregnancies and to experience low levels of attachment to the developing fetus. Coping with a high-risk pregnancy carries its own unique psychological burden for expectant mothers who may feel angry about their situation, guilty and inadequate for having 'caused' the pregnancy complication and/or constantly worried about the outcome of the pregnancy.[36] The level of depressive symptoms in women with high-risk pregnancies has been shown to be significantly higher during late pregnancy than the rate in low-risk controls.[37]

The most important predictors of psychiatric problems during pregnancy are the woman's past history of psychiatric disturbance and her level of emotional adjustment and personality organization. A woman who has experienced difficulty in adapting to previous life changes, who responds to stress by adopting regressive or immature coping strategies, or who has particular conflicts related to dependence, nurturing or motherhood, is at higher risk for difficulties during pregnancy. There are no systematic data on the experience of pregnancy in women with personality disorders, but one can anticipate that for individuals who struggle with separation – individuation conflicts, interpersonal boundary difficulties and unresolved developmental issues, pregnancy may activate or intensify pre-existing difficulties.[38]

Previous experience of psychiatric illness is the factor most strongly predictive of psychiatric illness during pregnancy.[5,8,39] A personal history or significant genetic loading for depression, anxiety disorder or psychosis puts one at risk during any significant life event. As outlined above, pregnancy constitutes a profound multifactorial stressor. It is not surprising, therefore, that women with a past history of illness are more likely to experience difficulties at this time of life. Thorough preventative obstetric care should include a brief review of the woman's past psychiatric history.[28,40] Once a woman has been identified as being at increased risk for emotional complications during pregnancy, her response to the pregnancy can be monitored more carefully and her possible treatment needs can be anticipated.

ASSESSMENT OF THE PREGNANT PATIENT

Difficulties facing the clinician

What makes treating a pregnant patient different from treating a non-pregnant woman? As a physician or mental health caregiver, the primary commitment is to providing safe and effective care for one's patient. In the case of treating an expectant mother, there are actually two individuals whose welfare must be considered. Almost any illness or distress which affects the mother has the potential to affect the fetus as well. Likewise, treatments given to the mother may have a direct impact on the fetus. In many situations, clinicians experience a conflict between being an advocate for the perceived needs of the fetus (who presumably has no psychiatric illness and does not require treatment!) and their more comfortable role of addressing the needs of the adult patient. In situations where the father of the fetus is involved, discussions about treatment and clinical decision-making may involve more parties than usual. This may cause the clinician to feel that the customary limits of confidentiality are being stretched. It can be unclear what the father's rights are to advocate for his child if there is a conflict between the partners. Clinicians may also be concerned about poorly defined legal issues concerning fetal rights, and about their potential exposure for malpractice allegations if there is a negative outcome of the pregnancy, or if the child has subsequent developmental difficulties which could be ascribed to the medications and treatment that are prescribed – or withheld – during the pregnancy.

For all of the above reasons it is important to articulate guidelines to help clinicians to make reasoned and appropriate decisions about treatment for pregnant patients. As is true throughout the practice of medicine, no standard protocol can replace careful, thoughtful consideration of the individual patient and the unique circumstances of a given clinical situation. However, it is helpful to have a rationale and a plan for how to approach this common situation.

The traditional dictum which guides medical practice – *prima non nocere* (first do no harm) applies equally well to the treatment of pregnant patients. However, it can be difficult to tease apart exactly what constitutes 'harm'. Harm can be caused from several directions. Patients and clinicians alike tend to think first about the potential for harm that can arise from exposure of a fetus to psychotropic medications. The issue of specific medications and the risk that they pose to fetal development, obstetric complications and issues associated with behavioral teratogenesis will be the focus of other chapters of this book. Overall, there are very limited data available on the safety of most medications for use during pregnancy.[41] New medications are not tested in pregnant women prior to their release, and epidemiological studies of the teratogenic risk associated with various medications take time to complete. In the absence of clear data, an important guiding principle is that exposure of a fetus to medications of any kind should be kept to a minimum[41,42] This is particularly important during the early months of gestation when organogenesis occurs, but it remains true throughout pregnancy. When treating pregnant women, non-pharmacologic treatment options should always be employed to their maximum potential, each and every medication prescribed should be evaluated with regard to its necessity during the pregnancy, and dose reduction of those medications that are deemed to be crucial should be carefully considered. Although many psychiatrists and non-psychiatric physicians turn readily to the use of newer-generation antidepressants, antipsychotics and anxiolytic agents in their routine practice, the necessity of exposing a 'second' patient to these medications when treating a pregnant woman should be cause for the practitioner to pause and evaluate all of the options before writing a prescription. Is this a condition that might be responsive to psychotherapy? Are there particular forms of therapy with demonstrated utility in this condition? Would increased contact and support from the caregiver, coupled with psychoeducation or additional support by social services or others, ameliorate the symptoms sufficiently? Are there alternative treatments (e.g. acupuncture or hypnosis) that are relevant to the individual's condition? In many cases, even if pharmacologic treatment may be the quickest or most potent 'bullet', other approaches may yield an acceptable result.

Returning to the injunction to 'do no harm', one must also assess the potential for harm from not treating – or undertreating – the basic mental health problem which brought the patient for treatment. A mother who is psychotic and agitated, delusional about the meaning of the bodily changes she is experiencing or too paranoid to tolerate the necessary prenatal care clearly presents a risk to her unborn child. Similarly, a depressed woman who is not eating or who is actively suicidal needs urgent and aggressive psychiatric attention. Other conditions may be more subtle but also require treatment for the well-being of both mother and child. There are many reports about the negative effects of maternal anxiety on neonatal outcome. Although the data are not conclusive,[43] numerous studies have linked maternal anxiety to obstetrical complications (including preterm delivery), intrapartum complications (including prolonged or precipitous labor), forceps delivery, abruptio placenta and reduced Apgar scores in the neonate.[44-49] Depressive symptoms during pregnancy have been correlated with poor health behaviors, including the increased use of cigarettes, alcohol and illicit drugs,[50] all of which can impact negatively on fetal outcome. Depression during pregnancy is also associated with an increased risk of postpartum depression,[3,51] and behavioral difficulties in the neonate.[52] Substance abuse is very frequently comorbid with other psychiatric illness, and the level of use often correlates with the degree of psychiatric symptoms that the patient is experiencing. Thus symptom reduction may reduce an individual's intake of agents which are known to affect the incidence of preterm delivery, low-birth-weight babies and complications such as fetal alcohol syndrome. In many situations medications are required in order to manage a patient's psychiatric condition as safely and effectively as possible. Not treating, or undertreating, mental disorders by withholding *necessary* psychotropic medication is not a benign course of action.

PREGNANCY-RELATED FACTORS

The starting point of any clinical assessment is a thorough biopsychosocial evaluation that is attentive to the specific issues associated with pregnancy. By definition, the pregnant woman is in the midst of a significant life-changing process. Any clinical assessment that does not address the issues involved in that process is unlikely to lead to a clear understanding of the patient and her request for help. Careful inquiry into the meaning of the pregnancy, the individual's wishes and hopes for herself and her family, and the onset of her difficulty in relation to the developmental stages of pregnancy is likely to be more informative than a strictly phenomenological cataloging of signs and symptoms.[20] Exploration of the impact of the pregnancy on the patient's life circumstances and relationships, her degree of interest in and attachment to the fetus, and how she is preparing for life as a mother will provide information about how successfully this woman is accomplishing the emotional and psychological tasks of pregnancy. In this way one can assess to what degree her symptoms may be related to conflicts or 'arrests' in the expected adaptation process.

Understanding what is difficult about the pregnancy for a given individual may well clarify what intervention is most likely to be useful for treating the resulting emotional symptoms. For example, consider the example of a patient we shall call Janet, whose panic and anxiety symptoms emerge at the point in her pregnancy when she must make a decision about returning to her job after delivery. Until now she has derived much self-esteem and personal satisfaction from her occupational performance. None the less, she and her husband both feel that it is important for their child to have the kind of upbringing they had – being cared for at home by mother. Janet is excited about becoming a mother, but is uncertain about how she will adjust to the relative isolation and slower pace of life associated with staying at home with an infant. She has been reluctant to express her concerns to her husband, as she is worried that her misgivings suggest that she will be in some way deficient as a mother. Over the past few weeks she has started to awaken in the middle of the night with feelings of suffocation, anxiety and dread. During the day her heart sometimes races and she becomes dizzy and weak for periods of 10 minutes or so. In this rather straightforward case it is clear that the first approach to treatment of Janet's anxiety symptoms would be to help her to focus on the conflict she is experiencing with regard to her changing social role, her parenting expectations and her difficulty in communicating about these issues with her husband.

Sarah, pregnant with her first child, sought help for depression early in her third trimester. She and her husband both love children and were thrilled at the news of her pregnancy. Sarah describes herself as an outgoing, active woman, and someone on whom 'everyone' relies for her optimism, energy and 'big heart'. However, during the weeks prior to her presentation for treatment, she has become withdrawn, tearful, anergic and unremittingly sad. She has been unable to buy furniture for the baby's room because of the stabbing pain she feels in her 'heart' when she envisions herself with her baby. She and her husband find this particularly strange, as she delighted in caring for her younger siblings as they grew up, and has been very involved in rearing several young nieces and nephews. As she begins to explore her thoughts about motherhood, Sarah is flooded with long-suppressed memories of her mother's protracted illness during her own early childhood, and with the feelings of loneliness which she never allowed herself to recall. In this case, as in the previous one, aspects of the pregnancy itself triggered the psychiatric symptoms, and a short course of psychotherapy helped to ease the transition to motherhood. Issues related to marital stress, previous pregnancy or fertility experiences, dynamic issues associated with parenting and the woman's relationship with her own parents are some of the themes which can be addressed specifically in psychotherapy, often leading to resolution of depressive or anxiety symptoms without the use of medications.[53]

SEVERITY

Another dimension along which an individual's symptoms must be assessed is their severity, and the degree to which they lead to incapacity or functional impairment. In the examples described above the women were in significant distress but able to function well enough to manage their daily lives. They both felt that their symptoms were tolerable in the short term while psychological issues were being addressed. Other situations may be so extreme as to present a clinical emergency that requires much more aggressive and immediate intervention, including somatic therapies. Acute psychosis during pregnancy – either arising *de novo* or in the context of a recurrent or chronic disorder – can present a grave risk. Unpredictable behavior, poor judgement and distorted reality testing may jeopardize both the mother and the fetus. Paranoia may impede prenatal obstetrical care, and delusions about the fetus, or psychotic denial of pregnancy are not uncommon.[54] Psychiatric hospitalization may be imperative in order to ensure safety and compliance with treatment, and antipsychotic medication is almost invariably necessary.

Severe depression can become an emergency that requires rapid intervention as well. Although the actual rate of suicide during pregnancy is reduced relative to that in the general population,[9] the risk of suicide is real, and suicidal patients may require hospitalization and medication for their own safety. A woman who is so depressed that she is not eating and is neglecting her self-care, or who is unable to function, must be treated rapidly with a combination of psychosocial and somatic therapies. In such circumstances electroconvulsive therapy (ECT) is an important modality to consider. Many studies have confirmed the safety and efficacy of ECT during pregnancy.[55,56]

In less extreme situations the assessment of severity is more complicated. In order to avoid unnecessary medications, most patients and their doctors will tolerate a higher degree of symptoms than they would if the patient were not pregnant. The goal of treatment during this time may be to ameliorate symptoms, rather than to eliminate them altogether. For example, a young woman whose panic disorder has in the past remitted completely on antidepressants may be willing to tolerate occasional panic attacks of moderate severity, rather than restart medication during her pregnancy. Alternatively, one could recommend the use of a benzodiazepine on an 'as-needed' basis, rather than the daily use of an antidepressant to control panic symptoms, in order to minimize the patient's total medication consumption during pregnancy. The use of cognitive therapy, which is known to be an effective treatment for panic disorder, would be an appropriate recommendation as well.

When the severity of distress is in the mild to moderate range, one can often begin by introducing or increasing the intensity of psychosocial interventions. These include psychotherapy, psychoeducation, relaxation training, parenting and/or support programs. Recent work with interpersonal therapy during pregnancy suggests that this can be a useful modality of treatment for antenatal depression.[57] Clinical experience demonstrates that such interventions may enable the use of psychotropic medication to be avoided or reduced. However, it is crucial that the patient's condition is monitored closely for any worsening of symptoms that may suggest the need for a revised treatment plan.

COURSE OF ILLNESS

In addition to severity, it is necessary to consider the individual patient's illness course when making a treatment plan to manage pre-existing psychiatric problems during pregnancy. What has been this individual's previous pattern of illness and response to treatment? Before recommending any changes in the medication that an individual has been taking, it is imperative to understand what the response has been when this has been attempted in the past. Even though the symptoms may be in remission at present, if a patient has been unable to discontinue antidepressant medication without relapsing into severe depression, it may be decided that the relapse risk outweighs that of continuing the medication through the pregnancy. In other circumstances, if the patient is – by history – very likely to relapse only after several months off medication, one may decide that it is worth discontinuing medication for the first few months of the pregnancy, while watching carefully for evidence of relapse, and then reinstituting the medication later on, after the period of greatest teratogenic risk.

Schizophrenia is a chronic illness in which the likelihood of relapse while off maintenance medication is extremely high. Schizophrenic women are also likely to have multiple psychosocial stressors associated with difficulty during pregnancy, including impoverishment, poor social support, unplanned pregnancy and single parenthood, all of which further increase their likelihood of relapse or worsening of symptoms.[32] Many schizophrenic patients require significantly higher doses of medication or multiple medications to treat an acute exacerbation, compared to lower maintenance dose requirements. These factors ought to be considered prior to routinely discontinuing medications when a pregnancy is diagnosed.

The risk/benefit analysis becomes particularly challenging when working with patients with bipolar disorders. All of the standard mood-stabilizing agents have demonstrated teratogenic potential.[41] Furthermore, the data suggest that the rapid withdrawal of lithium can – in and of itself – have a destabilizing impact on vulnerable patients, possibly triggering an episode of illness.[58] The specifics of an individual's history, including the number and severity of affective episodes, the individual's ability to recognize signs of early relapse, and the responsiveness of the individual's illness to treatment need to be reviewed carefully in order to make an appropriate recommendation. For some women with severe illness, the risk of relapse while off medication constitutes a far greater threat than does the relatively low actual incidence of fetal malformation associated with continuing medication. Generic algorithms cannot adequately address the unique issues of any given patient.

STAGE OF PREGNANCY

Decision-making about psychiatric treatment options is influenced considerably by the stage of pregnancy the patient is in when she presents for care. This factor has been addressed implicitly in earlier comments, but is worth noting further. The impact of teratogens on fetal development is greatest during the early months of pregnancy, when the major organ systems are being formed. If the diagnosis of pregnancy is delayed for several months, the woman may have already passed the period of highest risk. This situation occurs with unfortunate frequency among chronically mentally ill women.[59] Adolescents represent another group in which there is often a delay in recognizing or admitting to a pregnancy.[30] This leads to delay in receiving prenatal medical care, and the potential for unnecessary first-trimester exposure to medications that the young woman may be taking. Some medications which one tries to avoid early in pregnancy are less problematic if added later, during the second or third trimester.

Many of the medications used to treat psychiatric illness are associated with a low risk of fetal malformation.[60] Much less clear is the potential for such medications to impact on neuronal development and the morphology and functioning of the developing brain. The developing brain is shaped through complex mechanisms of cell migration, differentiation and programmed cell reduction and 'pruning'.[61] These processes continue throughout intrauterine development and long afterwards. Our understanding of how these processes are regulated is still in its infancy. The possible impact on these processes from exposure to medications which alter brain neurotransmitter levels – or in fact from illnesses characterized by alterations in brain chemistry – is unknown.

Medications that are started early in pregnancy and continued through to term lead to greater overall drug exposure, a fact that is unclear in its exact implication, but which raises concern, particularly about the impact on the fetal central nervous system. The physician should be reminded to reassess on a regular basis the ongoing need for all drugs prescribed. Medications that have the potential to cause withdrawal reactions or other postnatal complications in the newborn should be specifically re-evaluated during the third trimester for discontinuation, if appropriate, prior to delivery.

PATIENT PREFERENCES

The final thread to weave into the clinical decision-making process concerns the wishes of the patient herself. It is critically important that, whenever possible, the final decision about how to treat an individual's mental or emotional difficulties lies in the hands of the pregnant woman herself, preferably with the involvement of the baby's father. It is the clinician's role to make a careful assessment of the woman's condition, her relevant past history, and medical, psychiatric and obstetrical considerations, and to provide a coherent statement of recommendations, including the risks and benefits of alternative courses of action. Patients should be helped to understand the known risks and benefits of various treatments, as well as those of the illness for which treatment is being sought.[41] It is the right of any competent patient to choose their own course of treatment. It is also the responsibility of the pregnant woman to make her own decisions about matters that affect her unborn child. As clinicians, it is often difficult to watch patients make decisions with which we disagree, or which we believe are not in their best interests. When there is a future life involved, emotions and opinions can be much more intense. Nevertheless, it is most important that the pregnant woman is encouraged to act in a way that she feels is most appropriate for herself and her family. In some situations, individuals will adamantly reject any treatment plan that includes the use of medications during pregnancy. Despite the possibility – and in some cases near certainty – of relapse or an increase in symptoms without medications, some women will choose to use any other interventions that are available, tolerating whatever is necessary in order to avoid exposing their fetus to foreign substances. Such a decision, if it is a competent and informed one, is the patient's right, and it is the role of the treater to follow expectantly, in case there should be a need to alter plans at a later time. Quite the opposite situation occurs with some frequency as well, where women who have achieved stability on medication may be reluctant to discontinue it in the absence of compelling data to suggest that the medication is harmful. Again, the physician's duty is to inform, advise and respond to the patient's individual needs. In the majority of situations there are multiple reasonable decisions that can be made. It is rarer for there to be only one defensible course of action. In cases where there is more than the usual degree of uncertainty about what course to pursue, or where the physician and patient cannot reach a decision with which they can both work comfortably, clinical consultation with one of the growing number of specialists in the field of reproductive psychiatry is appropriate.

What if the woman is too impaired to make informed choices? When a pregnant woman's mental condition renders her incapable of making competent treatment decisions, the psychiatrist is bound by the legal restrictions of the state in which he or she is practicing governing the provision of treatment without consent. Typically this involves the judicial system and representatives who are assigned to advocate for each of the involved parties. Sometimes rapid decisions must be made about continuation of the pregnancy or involuntary hospitalization of the mother in order to ensure the safety of the fetus. In such cases the legal and ethical complexities of dealing with an incompetent patient far exceed the medical ones. The psychiatrist may be called upon to advise legal advocates for both the mother and the unborn child regarding the potential risks to each.

A few closing words on the somber subject of malpractice litigation are unfortunately in order. The possibility of becoming the target of a malpractice allegation is one of the risks assumed the moment one enters clinical practice. There are individuals who will seek to place blame whenever an unexpected or unfortunate outcome occurs. Few situations in life are as emotionally charged as childbirth, and few events are as emotionally devastating as an unanticipated complication affecting the health or life of one's baby. Some parents respond irrationally by blaming clinicians for events that were not preventable. Obstetricians have to deal with this reality on a daily basis, and psychiatrists, when dealing with pregnant and postpartum patients, need to be attentive to this situation as well. Some physicians respond to the implicit threat of suit by declining to be responsible for the care of pregnant women. Others adhere to the position of never prescribing medications to pregnant patients, as though that were a defensible position. A more sound clinical response is to be diligent in one's efforts to work closely with patients in order to minimize the risks to both the mother and her baby in the manner outlined above. A finding of malpractice is based largely on demonstrating that a caregiver was negligent in the performance of his or her duties. Clear and open communication with the woman and her partner about all aspects of treatment, a collaborative therapeutic relationship, and documentation of the same are generally sufficient to prevent legal entanglements. In those relatively rare cases where an individual still makes an allegation of malpractice on the basis of the outcome of her pregnancy, documentation of one's discussions with the patient about the risks of her illness, the possible complications of treatment and the reasoning behind one's treatment recommendations is ample evidence that negligence was not the cause of the negative outcome.

Let us now turn to some clinical examples which will illustrate several of the issues that have been addressed.

Case 1: Denise

Denise is a 28-year-old, married woman with a past history of depression associated with anxiety and panic symptoms. She was treated 3 years ago with a combination of individual psychotherapy and fluoxetine, with good results. The medication alleviated her symptoms quickly with few side-effects. In therapy, she focused on difficulties she has experienced in relation to her family of origin, specifically addressing the ways in which she felt that her needs were not adequately attended to by others, and her pattern of subordinating her wishes to the needs of her parents. She did well and terminated therapy confidently 1 year ago. However, each time she attempted to discontinue the fluoxetine, her anxiety flared, accompanied by irritability and worsening mood. Each time she restabilized quickly with the resumption of fluoxetine.

Denise has returned to treatment shortly after learning that she is pregnant. She reports that she discontinued her medication 2 months earlier when she and her husband decided to try to conceive. Although she has felt quite anxious and has had several panic attacks, she has decided that she does not want to take medication while she is pregnant. She has come to talk over how she is feeling and to elicit her psychiatrist's 'permission' to continue the pregnancy without medication.

During this consultation, the facts that are known about the use of fluoxetine during pregnancy are reviewed with Denise. She continues to be very clear in her wish to avoid medication, although she is uncomfortably anxious and experiencing difficulty in falling asleep. Further inquiry about the pregnancy and how she is feeling about it has afforded Denise the opportunity to talk about one of her 'hidden' reasons for coming back to her psychiatrist. Although she is generally quite excited about having a baby, she finds herself having occasional second thoughts about having embarked on this step, and is worried that her anxiety and panic symptoms reflect more deep-seated ambivalence that will interfere with her ability to be a good mother. This does not appear to be the case. After some discussion it appears that her misgivings are those typical of a woman who is newly pregnant, and her anxiety symptoms are no different to those she experienced when she had stopped fluoxetine previously. Denise felt relieved to hear this opinion. She met on two further occasions to refresh her relaxation skills, and she accepted referral to a mothers-to-be peer discussion group.

Six months later, Denise's husband telephones. Denise is becoming increasingly depressed, but does not want to come in because she still does not want to take medication and feels reluctant to admit this to her psychiatrist. On urging, she returns for evaluation. Although she is feeling very depressed she is functioning adequately at work and appears to be caring for herself well. The affectionate manner with which she pats her abdomen and speaks about her 'little guy' suggests an appropriate degree of attachment and interest in her baby's welfare. Denise asks to resume therapy because of an increasing sense that the 'old family stuff' is bothering her again, and she is unsure about her ability to be a mother without replicating her own mother's behavior. At this visit she and her doctor outline the criteria that will indicate to both of them that her depression is worsening to a degree that medication intervention is warranted.

Denise eventually delivered a healthy baby at term and resumed taking fluoxetine postpartum.

Case 2: Ellen

Ellen is a 24-year-old who was referred by her primary care doctor for treatment of severe depression. By her report, shortly after the birth of her son 2 years earlier she became depressed. Her condition has steadily worsened over time. Her slightly disheveled appearance is 'the best I can do'; she had her first shower in several days just prior to coming to the appointment. She spends her days lying on the couch and dozing while watching her toddler play in the living room. Tearfully, she admits to knowing that she is not taking good care of him, but she does pride herself on keeping him 'out of harm' by putting him to bed before her alcoholic husband returns home in the evening. Prior to her pregnancy Ellen had a good job which she enjoyed, but she gave this up to care for her son. Since being at home she has lost her drive and her ability to stand up to her husband's violent behavior. On several occasions he has pushed her down, slapped her and pulled her hair viciously, but he has not inflicted more serious injury.

Ellen began weekly therapy with a social worker and was started on sertraline. Within several weeks she became more animated and involved in her surroundings, and she began attending a playgroup/mothers' support group twice a week. The following week, when her husband raised his voice in his typical threatening manner, Ellen gathered her son and spent the night with a friend.

Just as she was beginning to explore other options for getting out of her house and becoming more involved in the community, Ellen discovered that she was pregnant. Her first reaction was shock. After considering her situation for a day, she decided that she wanted to have the baby, even though another child would put even further strain on the difficult marriage. She called her doctor the next day to discuss what to do about her medication.

Reviewing her life over the preceding few years and thinking about the stresses that another pregnancy would add, it was clear to Ellen, her therapist and her psychiatrist that stopping her antidepressant so soon after she had begun to feel better constituted a grave risk. Ellen understood that there was only limited experience of the use of sertraline during pregnancy, but was clear that there would be risks to the baby if she were to revert to her previous level of depression and passivity. She continued the medication throughout her pregnancy and the following year.

REFERENCES

1. Gotlib LA, Whiffen VE, Mount JH *et al*. Prevalence rates and demographic characteristics associated with pregnancy and postpartum. *Journal of Consulting Clinical Psychology* 1989; **57**: 269–74.
2. Coble PA, Day NL. Epidemiology of disorders during pregnancy and postpartum. In: Cohen R (ed.) *Psychiatric consultation in childbirth settings*. New York: Plenum, 1988: 37–47.
3. O'Hara MW. *Postpartum depression: causes and consequences*. New York: Springer-Verlag, 1995.
4. Cohen LS, Sichel DA, Faraone SV *et al*. Course of panic disorder during pregnancy and the purperium: a preliminary study. *Biological Psychiatry* 1996; **39**: 950–4.
5. Kumar R, Robson KM. A prospective study of emotional disorders in childbearing women. *British Journal of Psychiatry* 1984; **144**: 35–48.
6. O'Hara MW, Zekoski EM, Philipps LH *et al*. Controlled prospective study of postpartum mood disorders: comparison of childbearing and nonchildbearing women. *Journal of Abnormal Psychology* 1990; **1**: 3–15.

7. Spielvogel A, Wile J. Treatment of the psychotic pregnant patient. *Psychosomatics* 1986; **27**: 487–92.

8. Watson JP, Elliott SA, Rugg AJ, Brough DI. Psychiatric disorders in pregnancy and the first postnatal year. *British Journal of Psychiatry* 1984; **144**: 453–62.

9. Talbott JA, Hales RE, Yudofsky SC (eds) *Textbook of psychiatry*. Washington, DC: American Psychiatric Press, Inc., 1988.

10. McNeil TF, Malmquist-Larsson A. Women with nonorganic psychosis: mental disturbance during pregnancy. *Acta Psychiatrica Scandinavica* 1984; **70**: 127–39.

11. Sharma V, Persad E. Effect of pregnancy on three patients with bipolar disorder. *Annals of Clinical Psychiatry* 1995; **7**: 39–42.

12. Villeponteaux VA, Lydiard RD, Laraia MT *et al*. The effects of pregnancy on pre-existing panic disorder. *Journal of Clinical Psychiatry* 1992; **53**: 201–3.

13. Cowley DS, Roy-Byrne RP. Panic disorder during pregnancy. *Journal of Psychosomatic Obstetrics and Gynaecology* 1989; **10**: 193–210.

14. Klein DF, Skrobala AM, Garfinkel RS. Preliminary look at the effects of pregnancy on the course of panic disorder. *Anxiety* 1994/1995; **1**: 227–32.

15. George DT, Ladenheim JA, Nutt DJ. Effect of pregnancy on panic attacks. *American Journal of Psychiatry* 1987; **144**: 1078–9.

16. Brockington I. *Motherhood and mental illness*. Oxford: Oxford University Press, 1996.

17. Bibring G. Some considerations of the psychological processes in pregnancy. *Psychoanalytic Study of the Child* 1959; **14**: 113–21.

18. Bibring GL, Valenstein AF. Psychological aspects of pregnancy. *Clinical Obstetrics and Gynecology* 1976; **19**: 357–71.

19. Nadelson CL. 'Normal' and 'Special' aspects of pregnancy: a psychological approach. In: Notman M, Nadelson C (eds) *The woman patient*. New York: Plenum, 1978: 73–86.

20. Cohen RL. Developmental tasks of pregnancy and transition to parenthood. In: Cohen R (ed.) *Psychiatric consultation in childbirth settings*. New York: Plenum, 1988: 51–70.

21. Robinson GE, Stewart DE. Motivation for motherhood and the experience of pregnancy. *Canadian Journal of Psychiatry* 1989; **34**: 861–5.

22. Bibring GL, Dwyer TF, Huntington DS, Valenstein AF. A study of the psychological processes in pregnancy and of the earliest mother-child relationship. *Psychoanalytic Study of the Child* 1961; **16**: 9–72.

23. Lester EP, Notman MT. Pregnancy, developmental crisis and object relations: psychoanalytic considerations. *International Journal of Psycho-analysis* 1986; **67**: 357–66.

24. Lubin B, Gardener SH, Roth A. Mood and somatic symptoms during pregnancy. *Psychosomatic Medicine* 1975; **37**: 136–46.

25. Leifer M. Psychological changes accompanying pregnancy and motherhood. *Genetic Psychology Monographs* 1977; **95**: 55–96.

26. Kitamura T, Shima S, Sugawara M, Toda MA. Clinical and psychosocial correlates of antenatal depression: a review. *Psychotherapy and Psychosomatics* 1996; **65**: 117–23.

27. Seguin L, Potvin L, St-Denis M, Loiselle J. Chronic stressors, social support and depression during pregnancy. *Obstetrics and Gynecology* 1995; **85**: 583–9.

28. Gise LH. Psychiatric implications of pregnancy. In: Cherry S, Berkowitz R, Kase N (eds) *Rovinsky and Guttmacher's medical, surgical and gynecological complications of pregnancy*. 3rd edn. Baltimore, MD: Williams and Wilkins, 1985: 614–47.

29. Cohen RL. Emotional disorders and mental illness associated with pregnancy and the postpartum period. In: Cohen R (ed.) *Psychiatric consultation in childbirth settings*. New York: Plenum, 1988: 71–84.

30. MacFarlane RM. Adolescent pregnancy. In: O'Hara M, Reiter R, Johnson S, Milburn A, Engeldinger J (eds) *Psychological aspects of women's reproductive health*. New York: Springer, 1995: 248–64.

31. O'Hara MW. Social support, life events and depression during pregnancy and the puerperium. *Archives of General Psychiatry* 1986; **43**: 569–73.
32. McNeil TF, Malmquist-Larsson A. Pregnant women with nonorganic psychosis: life situation and the experience of pregnancy. *Acta Psychiatrica Scandinavica* 1983; **68**: 445–57.
33. Jones EF, Forrest JD, Henshaw SK, Silverman J, Torres A. *Pregnancy, contraception and family planning services in industrialized countries*. New Haven, CT: Yale University Press, 1986.
34. Cartwright A. Unintended pregnancies that lead to babies. *Social Science and Medicine* 1988; **27**: 249–54.
35. Weir JG. Suicide during pregnancy in London 1943–1962. In: Kleiner G, Greston W (eds) *Suicide in pregnancy*. Boston, MA: Wright, 1984: 41–62.
36. Wohlreich MM. Psychiatric aspects of high-risk pregnancy. *Psychiatric Clinics of North America* 1986; **10**: 53–68.
37. Gorman LL. High-risk pregnancy. In: O'Hara M, Reiter R, Johnson S, Milburn A, Engeldinger J (eds) *Psychological aspects of women's reproductive health*. New York: Springer, 1995: 224–47.
38. Miller LJ. Psychiatric disorders during pregnancy. In: Stewart D, Stotland N (eds) *Psychological aspects of women's health care*. Washington, DC: American Psychiatric Press, Inc., 1993: 55–70.
39. O'Hara MW, Neunaber DJ, Zekoski EM. Prospective study of postpartum depression: prevalence, course and predictive factors. *Journal of Abnormal Psychology* 1984; **93**: 158–61.
40. Carnes JW. Psychosocial disturbances during and after pregnancy. *Postgraduate Medicine* 1983; **73**: 135–45.
41. Koren G, Pastuszak A, Ito S. Drugs in pregnancy. *New England Journal of Medicine* 1998; **338**: 1128–37.
42. Berkowitz RL, Coustan DR, Mochizuki TK. *Handbook for prescribing medications during pregnancy*, 2nd edn. Boston, MA: Little, Brown and Co., 1986.
43. Istvan J. Stress, anxiety and birth outcomes: a critical review of the literature. *Psychological Bulletin* 1986; **100**: 331–48.
44. Davids A, DeVault S. Maternal anxiety during pregnancy and childbith abnormalities. *Psychosomatic Medicine* 1962; **24**: 464–70.
45. Crandon AJ. Maternal anxiety and neonatal wellbeing. *Journal of Psychosomatic Research* 1979; **23**: 113–15.
46. Crandon AJ. Maternal anxiety and childbirth complications. *Journal of Psychosomatic Research* 1979; **23**: 109–11.
47. Gorsuch RL, Key MK. Abnormalities of pregnancy as a function of anxiety and life stress. *Journal of Psychosomatic Research* 1974; **36**: 352–62.
48. Cohen LS, Rosenbaum JF, Heller VL. Panic attack-associated placental abruption: a case report. *Journal of Clinical Psychiatry* 1989; **50**: 266–67.
49. Berkowitz GS, Kasl SV. The role of psychosocial factors in spontaneous preterm delivery. *Journal of Psychosomatic Research* 1983; **27**: 283–90.
50. Zuckerman B, Amaro H, Bauchner H, Cabral H. Depressive symptoms during pregnancy: relationship to poor health behaviors. *American Journal of Obstetrics and Gynecology* 1989; **160**: 1107–11.
51. Appleby L. Suicide during pregnancy and in the first postnatal year. *British Medical Journal* 1991; **302**: 137–40.
52. Zuckerman B, Bauchner H, Parker S, Cabral H. Maternal depressive symptoms during pregnancy and newborn irritability. *Journal of Development of Behavioral Pediatrics* 1990; **11**: 190–4.
53. Misri S. *Shouldn't I be happy? Emotional problems of pregnant and postpartum women*. New York: The Free Press, 1995.
54. Miller LJ. Psychotic denial of pregnancy: phenomenological and clinical management. *Hospital and Community Psychiatry* 1990; **41**: 1233–7.

55. Miller LJ. Use of electroconvulsive therapy during pregnancy. *Hospital and Community Psychiatry* 1994; **45**: 444–50.
56. Walker R, Swarz CM. Electroconvulsive therapy during high-risk pregnancy. *General Hospital Psychiatry* 1994; **16**: 348–53.
57. Spinelli M. Interpersonal therapy for depressed antepartum women: a pilot study. *American Journal of Psychiatry* 1997; **154**: 1028–30.
58. Suppes T, Baldessarini RJ, Faedda GL *et al*. Risk of recurrence following discontinuation of lithium treatment in bipolar disorder. *Archives of General Psychiatry* 1991; **48**: 1082–8.
59. Apfel RJ, Handel MH. *Madness and loss of motherhood: sexuality, reproduction and long-term mental illness*. Washington, DC: American Psychiatric Press, Inc., 1993.
60. Altshuler LL, Cohen L, Szuba MP, Burt VK, Gitlin M, Mintz Journal of pharmacological management of psychiatric illness during pregnancy: dilemmas and guidelines. *American Journal of Psychiatry* 1996; **153**: 592–606.
61. Cowan WM. Development of the nervous system. In: Asbury A, McKhann G, McDonald W (eds) *Diseases of the nervous system. Clinical neurobiology*. Philadelphia, PA: WB Saunders Co., 1992: 5–23.

2

Obstetrics for the non-obstetrician

MARIE KELLY AND BERTIS B. LITTLE

INTRODUCTION

Mood and anxiety disorders occur more frequently among women than men, and women of reproductive age comprise the majority of patients who are diagnosed and treated. On average, 10% of women of reproductive age are pregnant at any point in time. Consequently, there is a relatively high likelihood that psychiatric treatment, including medication, will be needed during gestation in some women. Treatment of depression results not only in improved quality of life for the woman concerned, but may also prevent the neurobehavioral and other complications that occur in infants born to anxious and depressed mothers.[1] Typically, psychiatrists are not trained in obstetrics, and conversely obstetricians are not trained in psychiatry. Similarly, internists and family practitioners are not specialists in either obstetrics or psychiatry, but are often the first physicians to be consulted by pregnant patients, and will therefore find this chapter to be of value. The objective of the chapter is to provide an overview of normal pregnancy for psychiatrists, internists and family physicians that is adequate to enable them to understand the physiological changes that occur during pregnancy, and the relevance of these always to the treatment and management of psychiatric disorders. Complications of pregnancy and conception problems are also discussed, because they are likely to exacerbate underlying conditions of anxiety and depression.

The birth rate in the USA is 15–16 per 1000 members of the total population. The majority of pregnancies are unplanned. In the USA, 27% of pregnancies are aborted. Of live births, 25% are unwanted and 15% are mistimed. In 1991, 30% of births were to unmarried women. The teenage pregnancy rates are 1 pregnancy per 1000 girls aged 10–14 years, and 62 pregnancies per 1000 girls aged 15–19 years. The majority of births are to women aged 20–29 years, with a fertility rate of 117 per 1000 women aged 20–29 years.[2,3]

Human gestation lasts for 266 days (± 14 days). Delivery dates are calculated at 280 days (40 weeks) from the first day of the last menstrual period (LMP), as the first day of the last menstrual period is more frequently known than the date of conception, which is estimated to occur 2 weeks after the LMP. By 12 weeks postpartum, unless she is breastfeeding the mother's physiology has returned to the non-pregnant status. Maternal mortality statistics include the first 6 months after delivery.

The most common pre-existing psychiatric conditions are depression and anxiety disorders. Other common psychiatric conditions in women of childbearing age include eating disorders, substance abuse and adjustment disorders (e.g. from breakup of a relationship). In addition, women with schizophrenia and bipolar illness often become pregnant. Adjustment disorders and bereavement are often seen after miscarriage and pregnancy losses. The rate of spontaneous miscarriage is 15%, although miscarriage rates as high as 60% have been reported based on weekly positive pregnancy tests followed by normal menstrual periods.[4]

Like other illnesses, psychiatric illnesses may worsen, improve or remain the same during the pregnancy. The stress of pregnancy may cause a woman with dysthymia or minor depression to go into a major depressive episode. On the other hand, a woman who is dealing with bereavement or an adjustment disorder may be able to recover and progress forward because of her new pregnancy. Obstetric difficulties arise more frequently in patients with psychiatric illnesses, but not in any specific pattern. Some of the difficulties are associated with behavior inherent to the illnesses (e.g. substance abuse, lack of medical care, improper nutrition).

Antidepressant treatment does not significantly affect the course of pregnancy. Initial studies have shown no significant effect of sertraline, fluvoxamine or paroxetine on congenital anomalies, stillbirths, premature labor or neonatal problems.[5] One study of fluoxetine did show a higher rate of prematurity and neonatal problems (e.g. jitteriness, respiratory difficulties) for infants exposed to fluoxetine in the third trimester, although the matched controls were not depressed women.[6]

Depression is associated with social isolation and loss of sexual interest, so pregnancy is less likely in severely depressed women. A severe emotional upset may disrupt the cycle and cause anovulation or complete amenorrhea, thus preventing pregnancy. On the other hand, the poor concentration and lack of initiative that are typical of depression may prevent a woman from seeking contraception, and her low self-esteem may then place her in situations where she has unprotected sex. Antidepressants and antipsychotics may disrupt the menstrual cycle. Psychotropic medications that act on the dopamine and prolactin receptors are more likely to disrupt the cycle. Thus tricyclic antidepressants and most antipsychotics disrupt the cycle, whereas the selective serotonin reuptake inhibitors and the atypical antipsychotic clozapine are less likely to disrupt the menstrual cycle.

Depression may interfere with prenatal care. Depression saps both energy and initiative, and pregnancy causes additional tiredness. This low energy state may prevent a mother from seeking prenatal care, eating properly, attending childbirth classes and arranging for a supportive partner to be with her during labor. Agitated depressions may be associated with increased vomiting, anorexia and poor weight gain. In addition, the impaired insight that occurs with depression may prevent the mother from following her physician's advice, may place her at risk of suicide or overdose, and may result in her making decisions which she may later regret – such as separation, divorce, or releasing the infant for adoption.

Bipolar illness in the manic phase is associated with hypersexuality and impulsive behavior, placing the woman at risk not only of pregnancy, but also of sexually transmitted diseases which might affect the fetus (e.g. syphilis, HIV, chlamydia). Untreated mania during pregnancy is associated with lack of prenatal care, missed appointments, not eating properly, and the mother placing herself in dangerous situations that might result in injury to herself or her fetus.

Schizophrenia is associated with social isolation and poor judgement, which may affect sexual behavior. However, schizophrenic women are more likely than men to be married, and pregnancies do occur. In treated schizophrenia, fecundity is decreased because the dopamine-blocking properties of the antipsychotics cause a rise in prolactin levels. The elevated prolactin levels result in amenorrhea and anovulation.

Eating disorders include anorexia nervosa, bulimia nervosa and binge-eating disorder. Fecundity is decreased in eating disorders, particularly anorexia, in which amenorrhea often precedes weight loss. Fetal outcome is poor if the eating disorder continues throughout the pregnancy. The incidence of low birth weight is increased, prematurity is increased by twofold, and perinatal deaths are increased by sixfold.[7] Problems with infant feeding occur during the first year.[8] Pregnancy is a strong motivator for some women to control their eating disorders, as normal eating and weight gain are associated with normal fetal outcome.[9] However, some women with eating disorders do not attempt to alleviate hyperemesis. In fact, they may deliberately eat foods that they discover will perpetuate vomiting.[10] Some women binge-eat during pregnancy and gain in excess of the recommended 25–30 pounds weight gain. Excessive maternal weight gain is associated with gestational diabetes, hypertension and a slightly increased Cesarean-section rate.

The effects of post-traumatic stress disorder depend on the nature and severity of the trauma. Reactions vary from being isolated and untrusting of caregivers, to being clingy and overly dependent.

Physical abuse continues during pregnancy. There is disagreement as to whether pregnancy is a risk factor for abuse. However, the overall prevalence of abuse is high, and pregnancy does not protect against physical or sexual abuse. Over 15% of pregnant women report physical and sexual abuse during pregnancy.[11,12] Physical injury during pregnancy is associated with higher rates of prematurity and fetal death. Abuse is more common at younger ages in both pregnant and non-pregnant women. Abuse will often go unrecognized unless the woman is specifically asked about it. An over-involved husband who will not leave his wife's side may be intimidating her into not telling her obstetrician about the abuse.

Alcohol abuse and substance abuse cause both fetal and maternal problems. Fecundity may be decreased in case of heavy abuse of substances. Substance abusers make fewer visits for prenatal care and are less likely to follow their doctor's advice. Pregnancy complications, fetal growth retardation and congenital anomalies are common.

A bereavement reaction is normal after losing a pregnancy. However, becoming pregnant immediately afterwards does not resolve the grief. Waiting 3 months after a first trimester loss and 6 months after a loss in the third trimester or neonatal period allows enough time for most women to grieve. Anxiety levels during the next pregnancy are high, and extra visits and reassurance are needed during a pregnancy that follows a loss. Grieving may be complicated and require psychotherapy or antidepressants if the mother is unable to take care of herself and eat properly during the pregnancy.

Women with personality disorders have patterns of perception and behavior that impair their social or occupational functioning. They often have dysfunctional social interactions, poor impulse control, labile emotions and altered ways of perceiving people and events. Such perceptions and behaviors interfere with establishing good rapport and receiving care from the obstetrician, office staff and delivery-room personnel. Someone with a paranoid personality disorder will find it difficult to trust others, while an individual, with schizoid personality disorder will appear indifferent. Antisocial personality disorder, which is more often diagnosed in men, is characterized by lack of remorse for irresponsible behavior, and does not lead to good relationships with one's care providers. Individuals with borderline personality disorder or histrionic personality disorder can be very dramatic – they tend to idealize relationships at the beginning of the relationship, including their relationship with their physician. Women with avoidant personality disorder will obviously avoid interactions, whereas women with dependent personality disorder will have difficulty in making decisions and will need directed counseling in decision-making both for themselves and for their infants. Those with obsessive–compulsive personality disorder will be preoccupied with details, rules and lists, making it difficult to accomplish a task or even discuss the matter at hand, and in such cases obtaining their informed consent can be challenging.[13]

Somatization disorder occurs five times more frequently in women than in men, and pregnancy does not protect against the symptoms of this disorder. The obstetrician must evaluate the symptoms but manage them as conservatively as possible.

STRESS AND REPRODUCTION

Stress – that is, any physical or psychological condition that causes an increase in the stress hormones cortisol, epinephrine, norepinephrine or beta-endorphins – affects reproduction in many ways. Purely psychological cases of infertility are not known.[14] However, reproduction in both humans and animals is adversely affected by stress, and the rates of infertility, pregnancy loss, prematurity and infanticide are increased. Such stressors range from severe conditions such as war and famine to depression and 'miscellaneous psychological conflicts'.[1,15–17]

Reduced stress has been associated with improved reproduction in a few studies. Improved psychological functioning and success in *in-vitro* fertilization (IVF) programs are positively correlated.[18,19]

Psychotherapy is associated with higher fertility rates in some cases.[20,21] The myth that couples will conceive if they just relax is untrue. However, 25% of couples conceived within 6 months of completing Domar's group sessions for relaxation training – a program designed to deal with the grief and anxiety of being unable to conceive.[22]

Approximately 10% of women are pregnant at the time when they adopt, and about one-third of mothers conceive naturally after they have adopted a child.[23] Stress-induced anovulation is the best-documented association between emotional factors and reproduction.

Additional evidence for the interplay between hormones and mood is provided by pseudo-cyesis, a rare condition that is a state of amenorrhea, with swollen breasts and abdomen and sometimes also galactorrhea. The patient is convinced that she is pregnant, often feels fetal movements and may have experienced this state for as long as 9 months. Psychological evaluation indicates that pseudocyesis patients have suffered infertility, social rejection or loss of a pregnancy in the recent past. Pseudocyesis has also been reported in animals, which display swollen abdomens and nesting behavior.[24,25]

RELATIONSHIP BETWEEN PHYSICIAN AND PATIENT

A good relationship with one's physician is an important component of positive obstetrical experience, with the incidence of postpartum depression being higher if the delivery staff is unsupportive.[26,27] Some women neglect prenatal care because of poor relationships with obstetrical staff. In the USA, approximately 2% of women do not receive prenatal care for a variety of reasons.[28] A positive relationship between a pregnant woman and her obstetrician allows the woman to feel more comfortable discussing the following:

- marital and premarital relationships;
- traumatic events (e.g. adjustment disorder, relationship abuse or breakup, rape, incest, sexually transmitted disease, abortion, infertility, infertility treatments and miscarriage);
- chronic physical symptoms (e.g. pelvic pain, dyspareunia, vulvodynia, vaginismus, functional bowel pain, irritable bowel syndrome and tension headaches); and
- hormonally related mood changes, especially premenstrual symptoms and perimenopausal symptoms.[29,30]

Lack of preconception planning and lack of prenatal care are common.[31] Patients often cite financial barriers and discomfort relating to an obstetrician. Embarrassment and lack of trust cause some patients to withhold information about a previous pregnancy, a sexually transmitted disease or a psychiatric disorder. Such failure to tell the truth is common, and obstetricians offer care without inviting women to reveal their secrets. Obstetricians test rhesus (Rh)-negative women for isoimmunization, even if the husband is Rh-negative. Rh immune globulin is offered to all Rh-negative women because the patient is often too embarrassed to admit that the father of the baby is someone other than her Rh-negative husband.

RELATIONSHIP BETWEEN OBSTETRICIAN AND PSYCHIATRIST

Obstetricians may be comfortable undertaking brief psychological counseling, but most are not at ease dealing with such issues as personality disorders, chronic suicidal threats, sexual abuse or self-mutilation. Therefore a psychiatrist is frequently consulted about these (see Box 2.1). The obstetrician may seek a consultation after noticing depressive, psychotic or dissociative symptoms, or the patient may request a psychiatric consultation. Patients under a psychiatrist's care for primary psychiatric disorders (e.g. schizophrenia, depression, panic attacks or anxiety) remain under the care of both the psychiatrist and the obstetrician during the pregnancy. Psychiatrists may also be consulted to help manage refractory hyperemesis or unexplained physical symptoms, and they may be consulted about medication management and to provide supportive counseling or therapy during periods of acute stress (e.g. associated with bereavement, pregnancy loss, fetal surgery or fetal reduction). In

---

Box 2.1 *Issues about which psychiatrists may be consulted by obstetricians*

Primary psychiatric illness
- Patient displays bizarre behavior or thoughts
- Patient has pre-existing schizophrenia, bipolar disorder, chronic depression or anxiety
- Patient is abusing drugs and/or alcohol
- Patient requests a psychiatric consultation

Pregnancy-related illnesses
- New onset of primary psychiatric illness (e.g. depression, anxiety or obsessive-compulsive disorder)
- Postpartum depression or psychosis
- Obsessive worries or fears of the mother about her own or her baby's health
- Psychiatric illness in the mother's partner

Collaborate on management of medical illness
- Rule out a psychiatric cause of symptoms prior to hospital discharge
- Hyperemesis not responding to usual measures
- Evaluate for somatoform illnesses
- Pain out of proportion to physical findings
- Hypochondriasis
- Conversion symptoms
- Somatization disorder
- Malingering
- Factitious illness

Supportive counseling and evaluation for medication
- Bereavement (miscarriage, stillbirth, loss of a child)
- Genetic counseling
- Infertility treatment
- Stressful 'high-tech' procedures (e.g. fetal surgery, fetal reduction)
- Fetal/neonatal problems
- Prematurity
- Birth defect
- Stay in neonatal intensive-care unit
- Chronic pain and other chronic physical symptoms

Legal and ethical issues (assessments of competency)
- Ability of mother to parent adequately
- Ability of patient to understand procedure and then give informed consent
- Agreeing to medical procedure for herself and her fetus or newborn
- Releasing the infant for adoption or a medical procedure
- Deciding whether to abort a pregnancy

---

addition, psychiatrists may be asked to assist in difficult legal and ethical decisions, such as patient refusal for Cesarean-section or cancer treatment during pregnancy.[32]

Collaborative obstetrical and psychiatric management is the best approach. An obstetrician may ask a psychiatrist to treat the patient during a period of 1–2 h. However, few psychiatric issues can be resolved within such a short time. The first hour of psychiatric consultation may involve convincing the patient that the psychiatrist is there to help her rather than to label her with a mental illness that the patient fears might cause her to lose custody of her child. Once rapport has been established, the patient may ask the psychiatrist for advice during the pregnancy. It is important to avoid conflicting advice being given by the obstetrician and the psychiatrist, and it is therefore important that the psychiatrist has a basic understanding of common pregnancy problems.

PRECONCEPTION COUNSELING

Prenatal care should begin before conception. All women of childbearing age should be asked about the possibility and desirability of pregnancy. Education is an important part of prepregnancy planning. Contraceptive practices often do not reflect a woman's conscious thoughts about becoming pregnant – some women who want to become pregnant use contraception, and other women who do not want a pregnancy fail to use contraception.

Contraception should be encouraged until a woman is prepared to assume the role of motherhood. Fertility and normal menstrual cycles usually return within 3 months following cessation of oral contraceptives, within 12 months after stopping Depo Provera (depot medroxyprogesterone), and immediately after removal of an intrauterine device (IUD) or Norplant (levonorgestrel) implants.

Anticonvulsants may inactivate oral contraceptives by accelerating with liver metabolism. For this reason, women with bipolar disorder need special contraceptive counseling if they are using anticonvulsants as a mood stabilizer.

LIFESTYLE CHANGES RECOMMENDED PRIOR TO PREGNANCY

Healthy habits should be developed before conception (see Box 2.2). Pregnancy is often a time when one is highly motivated to change one's behavior.[33] Chronic illness and chronic

---

Box 2.2 *Check-list for women who may become pregnant*

Diet
- Healthy diet, including adequate amounts of iron, calcium and folic acid
- Folic acid supplementation, 0.4 mg daily

Healthy lifestyle
- Use seat belt
- Exercise in moderation; avoid overheating and exhaustion

Avoid unnecessary exposure to known teratogens
- Avoid cigarettes
- Avoid alcohol and illicit drugs
- Avoid excessive heat (e.g. hot tubs, exercising to the point of exhaustion)
- Avoid antineoplastic drugs, including isotretinoin (Accutane®)

Avoid unnecessary exposure to potential or unknown teratogens
- Over-the-counter medications (unless essential)
- Avoid prescription medications (unless essential)
- Use a lead shield over the abdomen when X-rays are taken

Avoid workplace hazards
- Avoid excessive standing or long hours
- Avoid teratogenic substances; review workplace chemicals with physician

Medical review with physician
- Review family history and perform genetic testing if indicated (e.g. Tay Sachs' disease)
- Treat all medical conditions before conception
- Ensure optimal control of chronic medical conditions

Prepare a plan for medication changes during pregnancy
- Educate the patient about early diagnosis of pregnancy
- Ensure that the patient is familiar with medications
- Decide which medications can be continued during pregnancy
- Decide which medications must be stopped or substituted

medication can affect both fertility and pregnancy, and these should be discussed before conception is attempted.

Lifestyle changes in anticipation of pregnancy include moderate exercise, a healthy diet and the avoidance of teratogenic substances at home and in the workplace. Exercise is associated with improved stamina during labor. A healthy diet and iron supplement prevent maternal anemia. High iron stores prior to pregnancy reduce the need for iron supplementation during pregnancy, when nausea or constipation limit iron intake. Avoiding excessive sugar and fat intake helps to prevent excessive weight gain and gestational diabetes. Folic acid supplementation, 0.4 mg daily, is recommended by the Centers for Disease Control (CDC) to prevent neural-tube defects. Women who are taking anticonvulsants, or those who have had a previous child with a neural-tube defect, should take 4 mg of folic acid daily.[34] Another health-related habit is the regular use of seat-belts, because in the pregnant individual, seat-belts can protect both the mother and the fetus from injury.

The toxicity of many medications and chemicals is unknown, and often it is many years after the pregnancy that a birth defect is traced back to a particular chemical.[35] Therefore a good rule of thumb is to avoid all medications and chemicals unless they are essential. Although most drugs and chemicals are not teratogenic or fetotoxic, some substances are highly teratogenic. Isotretinoin (Accutane), a common acne medication, causes severe facial and brain abnormalities. Other substances, such as marijuana, do not cause malformations during pregnancy, but do cause problems in infancy and childhood (disturbed sleep cycles and tremulousness in infancy, followed by lowered performance on standardized tests given in grade school).[36]

Alcohol, cigarettes and street drugs should be avoided. Cigarette smoking is associated with an increased risk of tubal pregnancy, spontaneous abortion, placenta previa, placental abruption, hydramnios, premature rupture of membranes, preterm labor and low-birth-weight infants.[37] Fetal alcohol syndrome occurs in 50% of babies whose mothers drink the equivalent of 3 ounces of absolute alcohol or 6 drinks a day. The syndrome is characterized by a small head, characteristic facial changes, poorer growth and lower IQ in childhood.[38] Cocaine is associated with a number of malformations, predominant of the urinary tract, together with pregnancy complications of premature labor, placental abruption, hypertension and fetal growth retardation. Some patients take a larger than normal dose of cocaine in order to induce labor.[39] Amphetamines taken in supervised doses have not yet been associated with fetal problems. The illicit use of amphetamines in pregnancy is not associated with fetal anomalies,[40] but few data are available. Abuse of inhalants, especially toluene, is associated with premature labor and renal problems in both the mother and the infant. Opiate abuse is associated with preterm labor, abruptions, prematurity and neonatal withdrawal.

Physically demanding work, especially that involving heavy lifting or shift work, is associated with a lower birth weight. Exposure to lead, toluene and certain other chemicals is associated with a higher rate of birth defects. Medical workers handling antineoplastic drugs have a higher incidence of birth defects unless precautions are taken (the use of gloves, and drug handling under a hood with a strong exhaust fan).

High doses of irradiation are associated with miscarriage, but normal diagnostic radiology is not. The average chest X-ray exposes the mother to 1 rad and the fetus to 0.01 rads. The risk of fetal birth defects correlates with doses of more than 10 rads to the fetus. Diagnostic radiology may be associated with an increased incidence of childhood leukemia, so the use of a lead shield over the abdomen is recommended for pregnant women for whom X-ray is a medical necessity.

TREATING MEDICAL CONDITIONS BEFORE PREGNANCY

Medical illnesses should be treated prior to conception (see Box 2.3). Collagen vascular illness, major depression, psychosis, mania, hypertension, cardiac disease, anemia, alcoholism,

---

Box 2.3 *Medical conditions that should be treated before conception*

Alcohol and substance abuse
Anemia
Inflammatory bowel disease
Cancer
Cardiac illness
Collagen vascular disease
• Lupus erythematosus
• Rheumatoid arthritis
Diabetes
Hypertension
Infection
• Acute and chronic infections
• Sexually transmitted diseases
• HIV
• Tuberculosis
• Hepatitis
Neurologic diseases and disorders
• Epilepsy
• Myasthenia
• Multiple sclerosis
Organ transplantation
Psychiatric Illness
• Anorexia, bulimia
• Depression
• Mania
• Psychosis
• Anxiety disorders
• Schizophrenia
• Obsessive-compulsive disorder
Pulmonary disease
• Asthma
Renal disease
Thyroid disorders

---

anorexia, bulimia, major depression, hyperthyroidism, infections and renal disease all place the mother and fetus at increased risk of adverse outcomes. If the disease is chronic, it should be under optimal control, and the prescribed medications should be those with the least teratogenic potential that will still maintain control of the illness.

Medical advances have enabled more women than ever before in history to live to child-bearing years and be healthy enough to reproduce. Victims of severe trauma, valvular heart disease, diabetes, HIV, cancer and organ failure survive to potentially reproduce. Pregnancies occur after kidney, liver, heart and pancreas transplants. Many pregnancies progress normally after organ transplantation, but the rates of pregnancy complications, prematurity and organ rejection are markedly increased (by 15–40%). Some patients find themselves unexpectedly pregnant after years of anovulatory infertility caused by their disease, and are surprised to learn that they should have used contraception after the organ transplant. Other patients choose to take the risk of pregnancy, and even undergo infertility treatments. An ethical dilemma is posed for some physicians if they feel that a woman should not conceive unless she is in sufficiently good health to raise the child for 18 years.

Pregnancy in diabetics is common. Previously, insulin-dependent diabetes mellitus was associated with a high incidence of abortions, birth defects and fetal deaths. Now, if diabetes is mild and glucose levels are strictly controlled, complications are markedly reduced. However, advanced cases of diabetes are still associated with maternal and fetal complications.

Compensated cardiac disease prior to pregnancy may progress to cardiac failure during pregnancy or delivery if the heart does not have the reserve to deal with the additional hemodynamic demands and increased blood volume. Valvular heart surgery and cardiac bypasses have been necessary in pregnancy, resulting in a fetal death rate of 17%. Of those who tolerated the surgery, about half developed cardiac failure postpartum.[41]

Patients in remission from cancer are at risk of recurrence but may, because of advancing maternal age, not want to wait 5 years before conceiving. Cancer survivors are more likely to request fertility treatments because there is an increased incidence of infertility after chemotherapy and radiation.[42]

Pregnancies after spinal cord injury generally have good outcomes, but require close monitoring for urinary tract infection, during pregnancy to prevent pyelonephritis. During labor, blood pressure is monitored closely for autonomic hyperreflexia, a condition in spinal cord injuries which causes marked fluctuations in blood pressure.[43]

The prevalence of HIV in pregnant women in 1995 was 1–2 in 1000. The leading cause of HIV in children is maternal transmission. Approximately 25% of the infants will be HIV-positive from infection transmitted transplacentally, at delivery or during breastfeeding. Zidovudine is recommended during pregnancy to reduce the rate of perinatal transmission. This drug is not teratogenic, nor are the systemic medications for candidiasis, toxoplasmosis or pneumocystis.[44] Protease inhibitors are also used during pregnancy.

TREATMENT PLAN – FORMULATION CONSIDERATIONS

The patient should be educated as to when to take a pregnancy test and what actions to take if it is positive. Having a pregnancy test on the second day of the missed menses allows detection the week before organ systems start to develop. If medications are to be stopped during the first trimester, the patient should already be aware of the plan for doing this. For instance, patients with depression may want to stop an antidepressant while pregnant, or patients with bipolar disorder may want to switch from mood stabilizers to an antipsychotic. Mood stabilizers (e.g. lithium, carbamazepine, valproate) are teratogenic. Lithium causes Ebstein's anomoly in 0.1% of cases, and carbamazepine and valproate cause spinal cord defects in 1–2% of cases.[45] Overall, the risk of congenital anomalies in epileptic women taking anticonvulsants is 5–6%. If a teratogenic medicine must be continued, a discussion of the woman's feelings about prenatal testing, birth defects and late abortion will help her to make a decision about pregnancy. Some women choose to stay on medication because of the severity of the illness. Early detection will help the mother to begin prenatal care early, and to schedule accurately any diagnostic tests (e.g. chorionic villus sampling, alpha-fetoprotein, and sonogram for fetal anomalies or amniocentesis). If anomalies are detected, the woman has the option of considering pregnancy termination or of being prepared at the time of delivery for whatever defect might be present.

BASIC EMBRYOLOGY

Embryonic dating is 2 weeks discrepant from gestational dating. The weeks of gestation date from the first day of the last menstrual period, but embryonic age is based on the date of

Table 2.1 *Embryology chart*

	Embryonic age (weeks)	Menstrual age (weeks)
Limbs	4–12	6–14
Heart	3–8	5–10
Brain and spinal column	3–5 (38 for minor anomalies)	5–40
Eyes	4–38	6–40
Palate	6–12	
Genitalia	6–12 (6–38)	8–14

conception. By 7 weeks from the last menstrual period, or 5 weeks' embryonic age, the heart is already beating and the face and limbs are forming (see Table 2.1). The embryo is most sensitive to teratogens between 3 and 8 weeks after conception (5–10 weeks' gestational age), when the limbs and major organs form. Between 8 and 12 weeks of embryonic life (10–14 weeks' gestational age) the palate and genitalia continue to form, and some systems (e.g. the eyes and nervous system) remain vulnerable throughout pregnancy.

Toxic substances affect the fetus in three ways:

1. The embryo may fail to develop and a miscarriage may occur.
2. Exposure during the critical period of organ formation (3 to 10 weeks of embryonic life) may cause major anomalies of the arms, legs, heart, brain, spinal column and other organs.
3. Toxic effects after the major organs are formed include minor organ defects, poor fetal growth, prematurity or neonatal withdrawal, and neonatal toxicity.

ASSISTED REPRODUCTIVE TECHNOLOGY

Many pregnancies are now conceived with assisted reproductive technology (ART) (see Table 2.2).[46] Ovarian hyperstimulation is indicated if eggs are not being produced, or if eggs are being produced but not fertilizing. The easiest method of stimulation is clomiphene citrate therapy. This involves administering an oral estrogen antagonist that stimulates gonadotropin production and is taken for 5 days early in the cycle. If this is unsuccessful, then follicle-stimulating hormone (FSH) is given. FSH, which is more effective in stimulating ovaries than clomiphene citrate, is considerably more expensive and requires intramuscular injections 1–2 times daily for 5–14 days. Intramuscular human chorionic gonadotropin (HCG) is added to the regimen to mimic the luteinizing hormone (LH) surge, which causes ovulation to occur 36–48 h later. Eggs are harvested after HCG administration but before release from the follicle. If it is necessary to suppress endogenous estrogen and FSH production, subcutaneous gonadotropin-releasing hormone agonist is given subcutaneously for several weeks prior to FSH. Following ovulation, progesterone may be given to maintain the pregnancy until the placenta produces sufficient hormones to maintain the pregnancy (see Table 2.3).

FSH-stimulated cycles carry a small risk of ovarian hyperstimulation syndrome. The syndrome consists of massive enlargement of the ovaries, ascites, and hypovolemia. It is potentially fatal, but is rare with careful monitoring. Stopping FSH shots before the estradiol levels rise too high, or even stopping a cycle instead of proceeding with HCG injection, may prevent such hyperstimulation. The monitoring consists of frequent serum estradiol levels and frequent vaginal sonograms to measure follicular size. It was recently speculated that

Table 2.2 *Methods of assisted reproduction*

Method	Description
Ovarian hyperstimulation	Clomid® or FSH given. Increased number of eggs improves likelihood of pregnancy, but also increases risk of multiple gestations
IVF - ET (*in-vitro* fertilization and embryo transfer)	Eggs harvested after hyperstimulation Fertilization in petri dish Zygote placed in uterus at 48 h
ZIFT (zygote intrafallopian tube transfer)	Eggs harvested after hyperstimulation Fertilization in petri dish Zygote placed in fallopian tube
GIFT (gamete intrafallopian tube transfer)	Eggs harvested after hyperstimulation Washed sperm and ova mixed in petri dish Sperm – egg mixture placed in fallopian tube
ICSI (intracytoplasmic sperm injection)	Eggs harvested after hyperstimulation Spermatozoa inserted directly into egg Zygote placed in uterus at 48 h
IUI (intrauterine insemination)	Washed sperm is inserted directly into uterine cavity
Donated gametes	Sperm donation – used instead of partner's sperm Donated ova – donor undergoes ovarian hyperstimulation Cycles of donor and recipient are synchronized with hormones

Table 2.3 *Drugs used in fertility treatments*

Drug	Route	Physiologic effect

Clomiphene citrate
    Clomid®
    Serophene®
	Oral	Stimulates ovulation

Follicle-stimulating hormone (FSH)
    Pergonal® (FSH+LH)
    Metrodin® (pure FSH)
    Follistim® (subQ) (follitropin beta)
	IM	Stimulates multiple follicles to develop eggs

Gonadotropin-releasing hormone
    GnRH analog
    Lupron®
    Nasarelin®
    Synarel®
	Intranasal,
	subcutaneous
		Reduces endogenous estrogen and FSH production

Oral contraceptives		Reduces endogenous estrogen and FSH production
HCG Profasi®		Mimics surge of LH causing ovulation in 36–48 h
Progesterone Crinolone®		Supports pregnancy until placenta produces sufficient hormones IM, po, vaginal cream

fertility drugs may increase the risk of ovarian cancer. No conclusive evidence exists that they do so, but this speculation is compounded because women with infertility problems may be predisposed to an increased risk of ovarian cancer.[47] Hormonally stimulated cycles are described by couples as emotional roller-coasters. Some report discomfort from the decreased mood changes that may result from hormones therapy. Others report a great sense of hope and relief because an active medical therapy is being used.[48]

After hyperstimulation, eggs may be fertilized during coitus or by intrauterine insemination, or the eggs may be retrieved surgically and fertilized in a petri dish in-vitro. In cases of severe male factor problems, the sperm is placed directly inside the ovum.

ART procedures that involve removing the ova from the body include: in-vitro fertilization and embryo transfer (IVF-ET), gamete intrafallopian tube transfer (GIFT), zygote intrafallopian tube transfer (ZIFT), and intracytoplasmic sperm insertion (ICSI). Traditional IVF (in-vitro fertilization and embryo transfer) involves harvesting the woman's ova, washing the partner's sperm, and allowing the ova and sperm to fertilize in a petri dish. The embryo is then gently inserted into the woman's uterus approximately 48 h later. GIFT (gamete intrafallopian tube transfer) involves retrieving eggs, mixing them with washed sperm and inserting the mixture of sperm and ova into the fallopian tube, where fertilization occurs naturally. ZIFT (zygote intrafallopian tube transfer) is a combination of IVF and GIFT. The ova and sperm are allowed to fertilize in a petri dish, but the embryo is then inserted into the fallopian tube rather than the uterus. In zona drilling (also called intracytoplasmic sperm insertion or ICSI), the cumulous oophorous is washed off the egg and, under microscopic visualization, the egg is punctured with a thin needle and a single sperm is inserted directly into the egg. Traditionally these procedures needed one or more laparoscopic operations, but now it is common to retrieve ova transvaginally using ultrasonic guidance. Either a general anesthetic or intravenous sedation is used.

Once the egg is implanted, the pregnancy progresses normally. Any problems that arise are usually related to the advanced age of the mother or prematurity typically associated with multiple fetuses. About 20–35% of FSH-stimulated cycles will result in two or more fetuses.[49] Emotionally, it may be difficult for the mother to bond to the fetus, due to her fear that she will be disappointed again by not becoming a mother. However, the overall psychological adjustment and bonding to such babies are normal.[50]

Success rates of IVF are highest for women under 35 years of age, resulting in 24 deliveries for every 100–treatment cycle started. Over the age of 40 years, the success rate is 7% deliveries per treatment cycle started. In 1995, 36 035 cycles were started, ova were retrieved in 30 223 cycles, and embryo transfers occurred in 27 125 cycles.[51]

Women over the age of 40 years are often advised to use a donated egg. The egg donors are usually young women who are both altruistically motivated and in need of the several thousand dollars they are reimbursed for each cycle.

The embryo needs a receptive uterus in which to grow. Uterine and vaginal anomalies, a previous hysterectomy, and certain medical conditions (e.g. hypertension, multiple sclerosis, collagen vascular disease) are indications for using the uterus of another woman to gestate the pregnancy. Either a gestational carrier or a surrogate is used. A gestational carrier is a woman who provides a hormonally primed uterus. She is treated with hormones so that her menstrual cycle is synchronized with the cycle of the egg donor and the endometrial bed will be receptive. The genetic material (ovum and sperm) may be provided by the parents, by a sperm donor or by an egg donor. A surrogate mother is inseminated with the father's sperm, but ovulation and fertilization occur in the normal way in her body.

Lawsuits do occur, but the majority of such pregnancies are free of legal complications. Couples work out on an individual basis what to tell their friends, relatives and children about the pregnancy. Infertility counseling may be helpful prior to accepting donated gametes or freezing gametes or embryos. Instructions for disposition of the gametes or embryos in the event of death or divorce should be decided before starting the process.

DIAGNOSIS OF PREGNANCY

Pregnancy is diagnosed conclusively when a fetal heartbeat is detected or when an embryo is seen on a sonogram (see Table 2.4). Pregnancy is assumed when a blood or urine test detects the presence of HCG (the β-subunit of human chorionic gonadotropin). β-HCG is highly specific for pregnancy, but is also produced in embryonic or placental-type tumors (e.g. hydatidiform mole), and is occasionally measurable in extremely low titers in men and non-pregnant women. Home urine tests detect 50 mIU/nL of HCG. Serum tests can detect as low a concentration as 5 mIU/nL. β-HCG is detectable 7 days after conception, and the level of HCG doubles every 2–3 days during the first 2 months after conception. An β-HCG serum level of 6500 mIU/nL is typical at 6 weeks' gestation.

Some women who are taking teratogenic agents do not use reliable contraception, and the question then arises of how often one should perform a pregnancy test. A reasonable solution is to not test as long as the menses remain regular. However, if there is *any* change at all in the menstrual cycle (interval or flow), a pregnancy test can be performed on the second day of the missed or abnormal menses. Many pregnant women have a light menstrual period at 4 weeks, sometimes referred to as 'implantation bleeding'. Early detection of pregnancy

Table 2.4 *Methods of detecting pregnancy*

Methods	Earliest menstrual age (weeks)	False-positive causes
Urinary β-HCG	4–6	Ovarian tumor, hydatidiform mole, choriocarcinoma, HCG-producing bronchial carcinoma. False-negative from dilute urine
Serum β-HCG	2.5–3	Ovarian tumor, hydatidiform mole, choriocarcinoma, HCG-producing bronchial carcinoma
Fetal movement	18–20	Gas, pseudocyesis, pedunculated fibroid
Enlarged abdomen	12–14	Obesity, tumors, ascites, gas, pseudocyesis
Enlarged uterine size	5–6	Fibroids, adenomyosis, uterine tumors
Detection of fetal heart with fetoscope	18–20	Rapid maternal pulse
Detection of fetal heart with handheld Doppler	8–14	Rapid maternal pulse
Detection of fetal heart on ultrasound	5–6	Operator error
Fetal image on sonogram	6	None
Fetal image on X-ray	16–18	None

requires that a pregnancy test be performed during this lighter menses. Knowledge of a pregnancy detected this early – at 4 weeks' gestational age or 2 weeks' embryonic life, before major organ formation has started – enables the woman to stop any medication that may be harmful to the developing fetus.

EMOTIONAL CHANGES OF NORMAL PREGNANCY

Pregnancy and delivery of a newborn child represent a major developmental change for the couple. Like any developmental stage in life, they can lead to personal growth or to conflict.[52] In the first trimester, a woman sometimes finds herself to be emotionally labile. Many physical symptoms develop, some of which are uncomfortable. Abdominal fullness, urinary frequency, nausea, breast tenderness and breast enlargement begin in the first trimester. As the pregnancy progresses, the woman's body image changes. Stretch marks appear, and fatigue and weight gain occur. These physical changes, together with the fear of labor and delivery, can give rise to ambivalence about the pregnancy. Marital changes may occur, with differences in sexuality and anxiety about the parents' new responsibilities. A woman's role in society associates pregnancy with a sense of accomplishment and pride, and the anticipation of becoming a mother and producing an heir. Pregnancy changes a woman's role in the family system. In addition, a special maternal bond with the fetus begins long before birth for most women. For some, it may begin with the first feelings of fetal movement at around 18–20 weeks. For others, it occurs when a heartbeat is first seen on the sonogram, or at a special moment such as when the fetus waves its hand during a sonogram. Fear of losing the fetus or the presence of physical discomfort may delay bonding. Women may worry more than they ever have before, and in some individuals this worry takes on an obsessive quality. Obsessive-compulsive disorder is often noted retrospectively to have its onset during pregnancy, although at the time the symptoms were attributed to normal worries about pregnancy. Unresolved conflicts about her relationship with a parent or about dependency may surface during pregnancy as the mother anticipates the childhood of her unborn child.

SEXUALITY IN PREGNANCY

Sexual activity decreases as the pregnancy advances, from an average of 10–15 acts per month prior to pregnancy to 2–4 acts in the ninth month. Coital and non-coital activities decrease, and orgasms tend to be less frequent and less intense. Many men report a decreased desire for intercourse during their partners' pregnancies, especially during the third trimester.[53] Rear entry (vaginal) and side-by-side positions are more common in the third trimester. Older reports of increased sexual desire in the second trimester have not been confirmed.[54] Pregnancy-associated decreases in sexual activity do not correlate with socio-economic status. Commonly cited reasons for decreased sexual activity include physical discomfort (46%) and fear of injuring the baby (27%). Very few women reported receiving advice from their physicians about coitus, and only 8% reported stopping coitus because of their physicians' advice.[55]

Sexual activity does not precipitate premature labor in a normal pregnancy, but in cases of bleeding, premature labor or premature rupture of membranes, coital activity is contraindicated.

Prior sexual adjustment is the best predictor of sexual activity after pregnancy.[56] However, sex occurs less frequently during the first year postpartum, with 57% of women reporting a reduced frequency.[57] By 6 weeks, one-third of parturients have resumed sexual activity, and by 3 months 90% of women have resumed sexual activity. Despite early reports that some women who breastfeed experience a more rapid return of sexual desire and sometimes more intense sexual feelings than before, most breastfeeding mothers report a decreased sexual desire and less frequent sex.[58,59] Factors contributing to decreased sexual interest include vaginal atrophy resulting from the hypoestrogenic state of lactation, breast tenderness, and embarrassment about milk letdown (triggered by orgasm). Reduced sexual desire also correlates with episiotomy pain, maternal depression and lowered levels of serum testosterone.[56] Glazner reported that 7–13% of women experience postpartum sexual problems.[60]

Table 2.5 *Physiologic changes during pregnancy*

System	Symptom	Trimester
Endocrine	Elevated levels of most hormones, but glandular functions remain normal	Highest in third trimester
Gastrointestinal	Nausea and vomiting	Usually first trimester
	Constipation	First, second and third trimester
	Heartburn	Mostly third trimester
	Hemorrhoids	First, second and third trimester
Cardiovascular	Blood volume increases to 145%	Increases over 3 trimesters
	Heart rate increases by 10–15 beats/min	Increases over 3 trimesters
	Cardiac output increases by 150%	Increases over 3 trimesters
	Palpitations, PVCs*, PACs**	Increases over 3 trimesters
	Syncope (may also be a warning sign of internal bleeding)	First and second trimester
Hematologic	Hb decreases to 10, hematocrit to 30% (vol)	Lowest in second trimester
	Fibrinogen levels increase	Second and third trimester
	Leukocytosis	Marked during labor
Pulmonary	Increased awareness of breathing	First, second and third trimester
	Increased tidal volume	First, second and third trimester
	No change in respiratory rate	First, second and third trimester
Breasts	Mastalgia	First trimester
	Increased size	All 3 trimesters
	Galactorrhea	Third trimester
Musculoskeletal	Lordosis causes back pain	Second and third trimester
	Hand tingling and burning	Second and third trimester
	Laxity of pelvic ligaments	Second and third trimester
	Edema of hands and feet	Second and third trimester
Dermatologic	Hyperpigmentation of face, linea nigra	First, second and third trimester
	Spider angiomata	First, second and third trimester
	Palmar erythema	First, second and third trimester
	Increased sweat gland activity	First, second and third trimester
Renal	Increased glomerular filtration	First, second and third trimester
	Increased renal blood flow	First, second and third trimester
	Lowered blood urea nitrogen and creatinine	First, second and third trimester
	Dilatation and stasis of ureters	Second and third trimester
Neurologic	No significant changes	–
Ocular	Decreased corneal thickness	–
Genitourinary	Increased vaginal discharge	First, second and third trimester
	Increased urinary frequency	First and third trimester

*PVC, premature ventricular contraction; **PAC, premature atrial contraction.

PHYSIOLOGICAL CHANGES OF NORMAL PREGNANCY

Hormone levels

Circulating hormone levels rise markedly during pregnancy. Hormones are produced by the mother, fetus and placenta, with the placenta producing the majority of estrogen and progesterone (see Table 2.5). After 10 weeks' gestation, the ovaries are no longer needed to maintain a pregnancy because the placenta is producing sufficient progesterone. Estrogen and progesterone production increase more than a 1000-fold. Aldosterone, deoxycorticosterone (DOC), androstenedione and testosterone levels are also increased. Cortisol production does not increase, but serum levels are higher because of the increased production of cortisol-binding globulin (see Table 2.6). Corticotropin-releasing hormone levels increase. Prolactin levels increase during gestation steadily until term, when the concentration is 10 times higher than non-pregnant levels.[61]

Both the pituitary and thyroid glands enlarge during pregnancy.[61] The changes in thyroid measurements during pregnancy are similar to the changes that occur with estrogen replacement therapy or with oral contraceptives. Total serum thyroxine levels are increased, because of increased levels of thyroxine-binding globulin, and T_3 uptake is decreased (see Table 2.7). Free thyroxine and thyroid-stimulating hormone (TSH) levels do not change, although there

Table 2.6 Hormone changes in pregnancy

Hormone	Laboratory values	
	Non-pregnant	Pregnant (third trimester)
Aldosterone (µg/100 mL)	12.01 ± 0.98	121–148
Androstenedione (µg/mL)	201 ± 42	306 ± 79
Cortisol (ng/mL)	78–150	268–365
Corticobinding globulin (µg/dL)	1.6–2.1	5.5–7.0
DOC (deoxycorticosterone) (pg/mL)	112 ± 20	1309 ± 155
Estradiol (ng/mL)	0–14	10.5–16.0
Estriol (ng/mL)	< 2	80–350
Growth hormone (µg/mL)	< 10	< 10
Progesterone (plasma) ng/mL	0.02–0.9	136–158
Prolactin (ng/mL)	5–23	99–559
Testosterone (total) (ng/mL)	0.3	104

Adapted from Cherry SH, Merkatz IR (eds) *Complications of pregnancy: medical, surgical, gynecologic, psychosocial and perinatal*, 4th edn. New York: Williams & Wilkins, 1991: 1233–42.

Table 2.7 Thyroid changes in pregnancy

Test	Laboratory values	
	Non-pregnant	Pregnant (third trimester)
Thyroid hormones	Normal	Normal
Free T_4 (ng/dL)	0.8–2.4	0.8–2.4
Total T_4 total (µg/dL)	5.8–6.8	8.6–9.9
FTI (free thyroxine index)	5.5–10.0	7.26±1.25
T_3	Normal	Normal
T_3 reuptake	Normal	Decreased
TSH	Normal	Normal
Thyroid-binding globulin (µg/mL)	18–25	56.2±3.0

is a slight rise in free T_4 levels during the first trimester when HCG levels are high. β-HCG may stimulate the thyroid and hyperthyroidism may occur with hydatidiform moles, which produce very high levels of HCG. Thyroid function abnormalities are common postpartum.

Endorphin levels are increased in the third trimester, and they rise even more during labor. The analgesic effect of β-endorphin helps parturients to tolerate labor. Following delivery of the placenta, hormone levels fall precipitously to low levels, below non-pregnant baseline values.[62]

Laboratory values

Several laboratory values are altered during pregnancy and there are further variations depending on the stage of the pregnancy (see Table 2.8). Alkaline phosphatase levels double because of increased placental production. Hematocrit levels decrease from 37–42% to 30–37%, and they rise again slightly at term. Plasma albumin levels drop from 4.3 to 3.0 g/dL. Levels of calcium, which is bound to albumin, also drop slightly. Blood gases show a mild respiratory alkalosis with lowered pCO_2 and bicarbonate. Creatinine clearance is increased, resulting in lower serum creatinine and blood urea nitrogen. Fibrinogen is increased.

Table 2.8 *Laboratory values in pregnancy*

	Laboratory values	
Laboratory analysis	**Non-pregnant**	**Pregnant**
Complete blood count		
White blood count/mm³)	4400	10 500
Hemoglobin (g/dL)	12–16	10.9 - 12.4
Platelets (µ/L)	150–400 000	Slight decrease
Fibrinogen (g/dL)	300	450
Bleeding time (min)	3–10	3–10
Blood urea nitrogen (mg/dL)	12	8
Creatinine level (mg/dL)	0.8	0.5
Creatinine clearance (mL/min)	88–128	Increased
Plasma osmolality (mOsm/kg H_2O)	280–290	270–280
Alkaline phosphatase (U/L)	32–92	Increased
HCO_3 (mEq/L)	26	23
Calcium (mg/dL)	8.4–10.2	Decreased in second and third trimester
Albumin (g/dL)	3.6–4.6	2.4–3.7

Gastrointestinal changes

Gastric motility is decreased due to the effects of progesterone. Constipation is common, and is often exacerbated by iron supplements, and hemorrhoids are a frequent sequela. Nausea and vomiting are common in the first trimester. Although frequently referred to as 'morning sickness', symptoms often persist throughout the day. Heartburn is common in the third trimester. Gallbladder function is sluggish, but liver enzyme levels remain unchanged. Gastric acid is decreased in the first and second trimesters.

Cardiovascular changes

Blood volume steadily increases to 145% of non-pregnant values by the ninth month. Red blood cell counts increase, but less so than blood volume – hence the lowered hematocrit values of pregnancy. Edema is common, especially of the ankles. The heart rate increases by 10–15 beats/min during pregnancy, and cardiac output is increased. Blood pressure drops during the second trimester and then rises to normal levels in the third trimester. Premature ventricular contractions, premature atrial contractions and palpitations are common during pregnancy. Syncope may occur from postural hypotension, but it always requires evaluation for other causes.

Pulmonary changes

Oxygen consumption at rest is increased by 15–20%. Although many women become aware of a need to breathe more deeply, the respiratory rate does not change during pregnancy. Such awareness of breathing may cause women to complain of shortness of breath.[63] Approximately 15% of pregnant women complain of dyspnea in the first trimester, and 75% at term. In late pregnancy, diaphragmatic discomfort may occur. Total lung capacity in pregnancy remains unchanged, but the tidal volume is increased by 40–50%. Thus the minute volume (tidal volume × respiratory rate) is increased by 50%. Residual volume is decreased by 20% during pregnancy.[64] Nasal mucosa hypertrophy occurs during pregnancy, and complaints of congestion are common.[65] This amplifies the parturient's sensation of being unable to breathe adequately.

Renal changes

Renal plasma flow and glomerular filtration are both increased during pregnancy. Hydronephrosis results from relaxation of the ureters. Urinary tract infections, even asymptomatic bacteriuria, should be treated promptly during pregnancy because of the increased risk of pyelonephritis during pregnancy. Pyelonephritis is a cause of premature labor.

Genitourinary changes

Urinary frequency is common, especially during the first and third trimesters when the uterus is resting on the bladder and incontinence may occur. The amount of vaginal discharge is increased.

Neurological changes

The neurological system remains intact during pregnancy. Mild headaches are common in the first trimester, but pregnant women do not become clumsy or lose their fine motor skills. However, the center of gravity does shift with the pregnancy, and the increased size of the abdomen may make a pregnant woman feel awkward.

Musculoskeletal changes

Increased lordosis occurs during pregnancy and backache is common. Standing with one foot on a 6-inch stool will often relieve the backache. Ligament laxity occurs in the third trimester and may cause pain in the ischial-sacral joints or the symphysis pubis. Lordosis and ligament laxity may cause previously asymptomatic knee or spinal conditions to become painful.[66]

Burning, numbness and tingling of the hands occur in 25% of pregnant women. Carpal tunnel syndrome, which is one cause of numbness, can be treated conservatively. Edema of the hands and feet can often be managed by rest and elevation. Facial edema is not normal and may be a sign of incipient pre-eclampsia. Leg cramps, especially in the lower legs, are common and may respond to calf-stretching exercises.

Separation of the abdominal muscles (diastasis recti) may occur, but this is mainly a cosmetic concern.

Ocular changes

Intraocular pressure increases slightly and a decrease in corneal thickness occurs during pregnancy. Pregnancy and lactation are accompanied by a transient blurring of vision due to loss of accommodation. This may be exacerbated if the patient is taking tricyclic antidepressants or other anticholinergic medications.

Dermatologic changes

Melasma (hyperpigmented blotches on the face), spider angioma and palma erythema occur in 60–70% of pregnant women.[67] Stretch marks also occur, especially if the skin is stretched rapidly by weight gain or polyhydramnios.

Sleep changes

Sleep complaints are common during pregnancy. Physical discomfort (due to urinary frequency, heartburn and lack of a comfortable position) frequently awakens the mother. Sleep changes are also present on EEG monitoring, probably reflecting hormonal changes.[68–70]

Nutritional needs

Despite the popular notion of 'eating for two', caloric needs only increase by 300 kcal a day during pregnancy. Folate and iron requirements double, and usually need to be supplemented, but increases in other vitamins and protein can be met by eating a well-balanced diet (see Table 2.9). Total vitamin intake from all sources should be considered, reviewing the patient's diet, supplemented foods (as cereal) and other vitamin or mineral supplements. Folic acid (400 µg/day), and ferrous iron (30 mg/day of elemental iron or 200 mg ferrous fumarate) should be prescribed. Folic acid reduces the incidence of neural-tube defects. Patients at high risk, such as those with a history of previous pregnancy with neural-tube defect or those taking certain anticonvulsants (e.g. carbamazepine or valproic acid), are advised to consume 4.0 mg folic acid daily. The calcium requirement remains unchanged at 1200 mg/day.[71,72]

The Centers for Disease Control recommend 800–1000 µg (8000–10 000 IU) of vitamin A daily during pregnancy. Vitamin A is teratogenic in high doses. Serum levels of vitamin A are higher in the fetus than in the mother, and doses above 10 000 IU should not be consumed. Increasing the dosage of vitamin A fourfold causes a more than fourfold increase in the likelihood of fetal malformations. The teratogenic effects of vitamin A are similar to those produced by istretinoin (Accutane®).

For a woman of normal weight, the recommended weight gain in pregnancy is 30 pounds. Of this, about 20–25 pounds is accounted for by the weight of the fetus, placenta, increased uterine and breast size, and increased bodily fluids. The remainder is due to fat.

Table 2.9 *Nutritional needs in pregnancy*

Nutrient	Requirements	
	Non-pregnant	Pregnant
Kilocalories (age 18 years)	2200	2500
Calcium (mg)	1200	1200
Cobalamin (vitamin B$_{12}$) (µg)	2.0	2.2
Folate (µg)	180	400
Iodine (µg)	150	175
Iron (mg ferrous iron)	15	30
Magnesium (mg)	280	320
Niacin (mg)	15	17
Phosphorus (mg)	1200	1200
Protein (g)	55	60
Pyridoxine (vitamin B$_6$) (mg)	1.6	2.2
Riboflavin (mg)	1.3	1.6
Thiamine (mg)	1.1	1.5
Vitamin A (µg)	800	800
Vitamin C (mg)	60	70
Vitamin E (mg)	8	10
Vitamin D (µg)	10	10
Vitamin K (µg)	55	65
Zinc (mg)	12	15

Adapted from Table 9.3 (National Research Council recommended daily dietary allowances) in Cunningham FG, MacDonald PC, Gant NF *et al*. *Williams' obstetrics*, 20th edn. Stamford, CT: Appleton & Lange, 1997: 256.

DISTINGUISHING BETWEEN PREGNANCY SYMPTOMS AND PSYCHIATRIC SYMPTOMS

A list of normal emotional symptoms in pregnancy overlaps with symptoms of depression, adjustment disorders, bulimia, anxiety disorders, and obsessive-compulsive disorder.

The hallmark symptoms of major depression are a sustained low mood or loss of pleasure (see Box 2.4).[13] An unwanted pregnancy can lead to a low mood, especially if the woman must continue the pregnancy without financial or emotional support, or if it means she must stay in an abusive relationship. Many women look forward to their pregnancy as a joyous time, and instead find that they are perplexed because they are often crying and physically uncomfortable, with frequent vomiting and frequent urination. In normal pregnancy, the low mood is not sustained and normal pleasure returns as the physical discomforts abate and an emotional acceptance of the pregnancy occurs (see Table 2.10, p.39).

Alterations in sleep and appetite are common, and pregnant women tire more easily. Awakening during the night, either to urinate or because of heartburn, is followed by a rapid return to sleep. Tiredness responds to a nap or rest period during the day. The changes are not of the same magnitude as the sleep, appetite and energy changes in major depression. Concentration remains normal during the pregnancy, and suicidal thoughts are not present. Ambivalent feelings are normal, such as wanting the baby but not the stretch marks or labor pains. Pregnant women often wonder if they will be good mothers, and guilty, ruminative and obsessive thoughts may occur in a normal pregnancy. The content of these thoughts usually includes keeping herself and the baby safe, trying to do everything for the baby's sake, and feeling guilt about taking a medication that might interfere with the pregnancy or harm the

---

Box 2.4 *Criteria for major depressive episode*

Five symptoms present for 2 or more weeks. The symptoms must be of marked severity and occur nearly every day. One of the five symptoms must be either depressed mood or loss of pleasure.

1 Depressed mood lasting nearly all day long on most days
2 Marked decrease in pleasure or interest in normal activities
3 Decreased or increased appetite, and decrease or increase in weight
4 Insomnia or hypersomnia
5 Psychomotor agitation or retardation
6 Fatigue or loss of energy
7 Feelings of worthlessness or guilt
8 Reduced ability to think or concentrate; indecisiveness
9 Recurrent thoughts of death; suicidal ideation

Symptoms must cause clinically significant distress or impairment, and must not be due to drugs of abuse, medication, medical illness or bereavement.

From American Psychiatric Association. *Diagnostic and statistical manual of mental disorders*, 4th edn. Washington, DC: American Psychiatric Association Press, 1994: 327.

---

baby. The thoughts are not all-consuming and they do not interfere with normal functioning, nor are they followed by compulsive rituals as in obsessive compulsive disorder, although the latter may be present in pregnancy.

Anxious thoughts are also common, and physical symptoms of increased heart rate, a sensation of needing to breathe, sweating and acid reflux may appear to be due to an anxiety disorder (see Table 2.11, p.40). However, in normal pregnancy the anxious thoughts are not generalized, and they pertain to the safety of the mother herself and the baby. Tachycardia (heart rate > 100 beats/min), hyperventilation, depersonalization and an overwhelming fear of death do not occur in normal pregnancy, and when present they indicate an anxiety or medical disorder.

Vomiting of pregnancy should be distinguished from bulimia nervosa. The latter is usually a pre-existing condition, although it may have gone undiagnosed. In bulimia there is a preoccupation with body image, and bingeing usually precedes vomiting. The normal vomiting of pregnancy may not be disturbing to a bulimic, and she may even seek foods that exacerbate the morning sickness.[73]

ROUTINE PRENATAL CARE

Prenatal visits should begin when the pregnancy is diagnosed. The objectives of prenatal care are to establish an approximate delivery date, to identify and treat preventable disorders, and to reassure and educate the mother. Obstetrical visits take place monthly until 28 weeks, bimonthly until 36 weeks, and then weekly.

Accurate assignment of gestational age is critical because fetal morbidity and mortality are higher in premature and postmature pregnancies. Gestational age is established by the last normal menstrual period, uterine size in the first trimester, auscultation of the fetal heartbeat at 20 weeks, and fetal measurements on sonograms before 20 weeks. A simple rule for calculating the approximate delivery date is to take the first day of the last menses, subtract 3 months, and then add 1 week (see Box 2.5). Accurate gestational dating is also important for scheduling genetic testing. Sonographic estimates of fetal age are most reliable in the first trimester. After 20

Table 2.10 *Distinguishing pregnancy symptoms from psychiatric symptoms of major depression*

Normal pregnancy changes	Major depression
Mood. Initially labile, tearful. May be appropriately upset if partner is unsupportive or if there are financial problems. Self-esteem is usually normal	Persistent gloomy and pervasive thoughts, with low self-esteem
Pleasure. Normal sexual enjoyment. Joy and anticipation once the shock of pregnancy diagnosis has worn off and morning sickness has subsided	Decreased libido. Failure to enjoy the normal events of pregnancy
Guilt. Limited to single issues (e.g. failing to use contraception). Pride in achieving a pregnancy	Guilty feelings and low self-esteem, pervasive in other areas as well as conception and pregnancy. Marked feelings of not being able to be a competent parent
Sleep. Often awakened for voiding, or by heartburn, movement of the fetus or physical discomfort. Falls asleep rapidly once comfortable	Early morning awakening. Difficulty in falling asleep once awakened
Energy. May tire easily, but extra rest and daytime naps restore energy	Extra rest does not restore energy. Tired upon awakening
Psychomotor. Normal activity and normal thought processes. Activity decreased by discomforts of pregnant and increased size, but able to accomplish normal chores. A spurt of 'nesting' energy is common several weeks before delivery	Agitated, pacing activity, often without a goal. Markedly decreased activity (e.g. prolonged periods of time in bed, or resting on the couch)
Suicidal ideation. None. Thoughts of death associated with unwelcome pregnancies should resolve if the woman is offered adequate social support (e.g. home for single mothers, partners agrees to marry her, opportunity to finish high school, etc.)	Active suicidal thoughts, intentions or plans. Thoughts of death, needing the emotional pain to end, hopelessness, thinking the world would be better off without one
Concentration. Normal. Anxiety about pregnancy may cause mild memory or concentration disturbances. Ambivalence is common, (e.g. wanting the baby but not stretch marks or morning sickness)	Concentration and memory may be mildly to markedly impaired. Indecisiveness
Appetite. Appetite increased and weight gain normal once morning sickness has passed. Food enjoyment is normal, cravings may be normal	Food not pleasurable, resulting in weight loss. Failure to gain normal amount of weight in pregnancy. Hyperemesis may be exaggerated. Overeating in order to derive some comfort from food results in excessive weight gain

---

Box 2.5 *Calculation of delivery date*

1 Take first day of last normal menses
2 Subtract 3 months
3 Add 1 week
For example, first day of last normal menses was 5 July 1998, so the due date is 12 April 1999.

Table 2.11 *Distinguishing pregnancy symptoms from psychiatric symptoms of anxiety disorder*

Normal pregnancy changes	Anxiety disorder (panic attacks)
Agoraphobia not present	May be very anxious or totally unable to leave house
Heart rate increased by 10–15 beats/min not symptomatic. Occasional palpitations are common	Heart rate above 100 beats/min, especially during panic attack
Sweating	Sweating
Not tremulous	Trembling, shaky
Increased awareness of breathing	Shortness of breath, suffocating sensation
Normal swallowing. Increased salivation in first trimester	Choking sensation
No chest pain apart from heartburn	Chest pain (may be severe during panic attack)
Nausea in first trimester and sometimes in second and third trimesters	Nausea, sensation of stomach 'churning'
Postural hypotension, may feel dizzy at times and have occasional brief fainting spells (fainting in pregnancy always requires evaluation)	Dizziness to the point of passing out; recurs frequently
No derealization	Derealization, depersonalization
Normal sense of control. Some loss of bladder control from frequency. Sense of being in control of life generally, except for the restrictions of pregnancy	Fear of losing control is marked and causes avoidant behavior
Marked concern about staying as healthy as possible to care for her child	Actual fear of dying
Paresthesias, numbness associated with musculoskeletal strain and edema	Numbness worst during panic attacks
Some hot and cold flashes	Marked complaints of chills and hot flashes

weeks, measurements are less reliable because fetal size is affected not only by fetal age but also by maternal size and nutrition and other maternal and pregnancy factors (see Box 2.6).

During prenatal visits, the obstetrician assesses whether or not the fetus is growing and if the amniotic fluid volume is normal. A rule of thumb is that at 20 weeks the fetus weighs less than 1 pound (320 g) but has strong enough movements for the mother to detect them. At 30 weeks the fetus weighs 3 pounds (1700 g). In low-risk populations there is no proven value in performing ultrasound examinations if the pregnancy is progressing normally.[74]

Abnormalities are screened for prenatally. Many anatomic anomalies are detectable by ultrasound at 16–20 weeks. Alpha-fetoprotein (AFP) determinations are performed at 16–18 weeks. Elevated AFP levels occur with neural-tube defects, and low levels correlate with chromosomal anomalies. Abnormal AFP levels are also found in misdated pregnancies and multiple gestations. In women at increased risk for chromosomal anomalies, a chorionic villus sample can be taken at 10–13 weeks. Amniocentesis is usually performed between 15 and 18 weeks, although it can be done as early as 11–14 weeks. The testing is timed so that there is maximum likelihood of detecting fetal anomalies, but still time to allow for termination should

Box 2.6 *Components of an obstetric history*

Age
Ethnic origin
Socio-economic status
Marital status
Education
Housing
Employment
Nutrition
Drug and alcohol abuse
Previous pregnancies full term, abortions (spontaneous and induced), premature deliveries, term
   deliveries, birth weights, length of labor, prenatal complications, labor and delivery
   complications, health of living children
Family history
Genetic illnesses
Hypertension
Diabetes
Twinning
Past medical history
Endocrine history
Thyroid history
Menstrual history, last menstrual period
Illnesses
Surgery
Blood clotting abnormalities
Emotional or nervous illness
Complete physical examination with attention to size of uterus and size of pelvic bones

a serious anomaly be discovered. Chorionic villus sampling produces earlier results and may be more psychologically acceptable to many patients.

Prenatal blood tests reveal treatable conditions such as anemia, gestational diabetes, isoimmunization and infectious disease (e.g. beta-streptococcus, HIV, hepatitis B, herpes, and other sexually transmitted diseases). Immune status to rubella is checked so that those who are not immune can be vaccinated immediately after delivery. Urine tests detect asymptomatic infection, glycosuria and albumin. Routine testing for other conditions (e.g. cytomegalovirus, toxoplasmosis or tuberculosis) is of no proven value and is only undertaken if clinically indicated.

Education and reassurance are important for the mother, as is maintaining a good rapport so that she will continue in prenatal care. During visits, the discomforts of pregnancy are managed and questions about the fetus can be answered. The mother is informed about the signs and symptoms of pregnancy complications, and instructed to call her obstetrician if they occur (see Box 2.7). She is also educated about the labor and delivery process and advised when to go to the hospital.

NORMAL LABOR AND DELIVERY

Labor is defined as regular contractions that result in cervical dilation. On average, in nulliparous women it lasts 9 h and in multiparous women, it lasts 5.5h. Patients often report longer durations

Box 2.7 *Warning signs during pregnancy that require evaluation*

Bleeding
- First trimester – any bleeding that is as much or more than a normal menses
- Second and third trimesters – any bleeding

Labor signs
- Painful contractions before 37 weeks
- Loss of amniotic fluid
- Unexplained vaginal discharge
- Signs of normal labor:
  'bloody show' – a bloody mucous plug may precede the onset of labor and is considered normal
  regular contractions 5 min apart for 2 h (nulliparous) or 1 h (multiparous)

Fainting

Urinary tract
- Dysuria
- Fever

Pre-eclampsia
- Elevated blood pressure (> 140/90 mmHg)
- Facial edema
- Headache, blurred vision and epigastric symptoms are signs of incipient seizures
- Weight gain > 2 pounds/week after mid-pregnancy

Decrease in fetal movement

of labor because they time labor onset from the first painful contraction, not from the time when the obstetrician thinks the cervix has started to dilate. Labor is divided into three stages, namely dilation, pushing, and expulsion of the placenta. The first stage is the longest (on average 8 h in nulliparous women and 5 h in multiparous women) and is divided into three phases - the latent phase, active phase and deceleration phase (see Figure 2.1). The latent phase is a phase of very slow dilation, and may last as long as 20 h in a nulliparous woman. The active phase begins once 3–4 cm of cervical dilation is reached, and dilation then progresses at a rate of 1 cm/h. The third phase is a deceleration or transitional phase between 8–10 cm dilation. The transition stage can be quite painful, and it is normal for the patient to be quite irritable during this stage.

The second stage of labor consists of pushing the baby down the birth canal. It lasts on average 20 min for a multiparous woman and 50 min for a nulliparous woman. The second stage ends with delivery of the baby. The third stage involves expulsion of the placenta and lasts an average of 10–15 min.

Most parous women agree that labor is painful. It is a state of stress with elevations in the stress hormones cortisol, epinephrine and norepinephrine. Endorphins are also elevated. The underlying emotional state of the patient contributes significantly to the pain of labor, with anxiety intensifying the pain. Interventions to relieve anxiety are associated with a 33% reduction in pain, a more functional labor, less need for analgesia, and fewer Cesarean sections. About 25% of nulliparous women describe the pain of labor as excruciating, and a further 25% describe it as relatively minor.[75]

Abuse victims may find that labor triggers traumatic memories and the pain may seem unbearable. Some abuse survivors cope by demanding to be in charge of the labor and delivery process, sometimes presenting a written list of demands, refusing to deliver in a traditional delivery room, and refusing to authorize an episiotomy or a Cesarean section. If a list of demands is presented this does not necessarily mean that the woman has been abused, but it should lead to a discussion of why she feels that she needs to protect herself with such a list. Other abuse victims have been so traumatized that they dissociate from painful stimuli

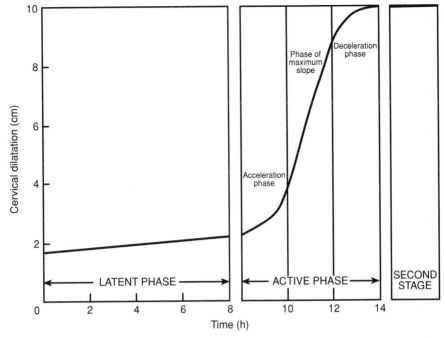

Figure 2.1 *The stages of labor in parturition. (Adapted from Cunningham et al. 1997, with permission)*

and do not complain. These women are usually considered 'good' patients. Lederman found that women who were generally assertive in most aspects of their daily lives entered labor with more confidence and more reasonable expectations about the labor process. Less assertive women experienced more anxiety during labor, and they described fears of being rendered helpless, being victimized or even dying.[76] The nature of labor also determines a woman's tolerance. Six hours of contractions lasting only 30–45 s each can be tolerated by many women, whereas 20 h of labor with contractions lasting 60–90 s each result in most women asking for analgesia. Regardless of the emotional state, labor is extremely painful and there are case reports of post-traumatic stress disorder resulting from childbirth.[77]

Labor causes increases in the adrenergic agents epinephrine and norepinephrine. Their vasoconstrictive effect can decrease uterine blood flow and labor slows down as a result. In fact, this mechanism is used to arrest premature labor. Beta-adrenergic agents inhibit uterine contractions, and two beta-adrenergic agents (ritodrine and terbutaline) are used to stop labor in women with premature labor. Relieving stress improves labor (e.g. an injection of meperidine (Demerol) may actually increase uterine activity). In addition, during labors with epidural anesthesia the fetus appears to be less stressed. Fetal blood samplings indicate that the fetus shows fewer acid–base alterations if the mother has epidural anesthesia as opposed to no anesthesia. Emotional preparation, such as the childbirth psychoprophylaxis popularized by Lamaze, relieves stress through focused breathing and the presence of a supportive person throughout the entire labor.[78]

EMOTIONAL AND ETHICAL PROBLEMS DURING LABOR

Some women may refuse to be examined during labor, which may be puzzling to the obstetrician, or may even provoke an annoyed or angry reaction. Usually such patients are young or non-English-speaking. It is rarely necessary to restrain a woman for examination and an examination, under anesthesia is a better option. Refusal to be examined may be associated with a pregnancy that is the result of rape or incest, a woman feeling very unsafe, or a previous traumatic experience involving a physician or authority figure.

Women sometimes make homicidal or suicidal threats, especially between 8 cm and complete cervical dilation, when contractions are often more intense and the normal emotional state is highly irritable. Comments in the throes of labor such as 'I want to die' or 'I'll kill him [for getting me pregnant]' should be evaluated if the thoughts persist after delivery. Invasive medical treatment (e.g. fetal monitoring, Cesarean section) may be refused. The commonest reasons for refusal are fear, lack of education, a need to remain in control, and rational choice. The delivery team may disagree with a woman's choice, but that does not make her choice irrational. However, a psychiatric consultation may be obtained, as it is important to establish that the woman's judgement is not impaired by depression or delirium. In severe depressions, Coverdale and colleagues recommend directive counseling to assist a woman in making a choice, especially if the fetus is viable.[79]

DELIVERY

Deliveries in the USA follow trends. Compared to 30 years ago, the incidence of Cesarean sections is higher, the incidence of forceps deliveries is lower, and the preferred anesthesia is either local or epidural. Compared to European countries, the incidence of Cesarean sections is almost twice as high.[80] Birthing suites have become more desirable, and staff routinely

Table 2.12 *Types of delivery*

Type	Explanation
Spontaneous vaginal delivery	Normal delivery, mother expels infant with or without episiotomy
Low forceps delivery	Head at perineum, forceps reduce delivery time and maternal pushing effort. Used in cases of fetal distress or maternal exhaustion. Low fetal morbidity
Mid forceps delivery	Head at level of ischial spines. Head must sometimes be rotated by forceps. Difficult procedure with higher fetal morbidity
High forceps delivery	Head not engaged in pelvis. High maternal and fetal morbidity. Older procedure used before Cesarean section became available. Now only performed for severe fetal distress if Cesarean section cannot be performed
Cesarean section	Performed when vaginal delivery is not safe or possible
Low transverse Cesarean section	Uterine incision in lower segment. Less blood loss and most common method
Vertical Cesarean section	Used for breech, transverse lie, large fetus or difficult Cesarean extraction. Risk of uterine rupture in future pregnancies
Cesarean hysterectomy	Preplanned in cases of carcinoma or carcinoma *in situ*. Emergency for severe hemorrhage postpartum (e.g. uterine artery laceration or placenta accreta). Transfusion is often needed

include the supportive partner or labor coach during the entire labor and delivery process. However, alternatives such as freestanding birthing centers, birthing chairs and ambulation during labor have no proven advantage.

Fetal monitoring is frequently used despite the debate as to whether continuous monitoring is any more effective than intermittent careful auscultation for producing a healthy baby at delivery. Forceps deliveries are more common if a woman has epidural anesthesia, because the relaxation of the pelvic musculature and the reduced maternal pushing force both tend to prolong the second stage of labor. Episiotomy (i.e. cutting the perineum to facilitate delivery) was once thought to reduce the incidence of anal sphincter lacerations, vaginal prolapse in later years, and postpartum pain. None of these benefits has been proven, and episiotomy is no longer routinely indicated.

Cesarean section is the method of delivery for 22% of births.[80] The common indications for Cesarean section are breech presentation, dystocia, fetal distress and previous Cesarean section (see Box 2.8). Vaginal birth after Cesarean section is an option for some women, and carries a 1 in 1000 risk of uterine rupture and fetal demise.

Box 2.8 *Indications for Cesarean section*

Previous Cesarean section
- Trial of labor not indicated
- Patient declines risk

Hemorrhage
- Placenta previa
- Abruptio placenta
- Severe cervicitis
- Uterine rupture

Failure to progress in labor
- Dystocia
- Failed induction of labor

Malpresentation
- Breech
- Transverse lie
- Twins with breech/cephalic presentation

Fetal distress

Fetal anomaly
- Enlarged thyroid
- Known congenital defect (e.g. spina bifida, diaphragmatic hernia)

Maternal anomaly
- Obstruction of vaginal outlet (e.g. tumor, condylomata)

POSTPARTUM

Marked changes in hormonal and fluid levels occur during the first 72 h postpartum. Immediately after delivery of the placenta, hormone levels fall. Edematous fluid immediately re-enters the vascular system, followed by a diuresis of excess fluid over the first 2–3 days. Fluid shifts are critical for patients with cardiac disease and for those taking medications that are distributed mainly in the vascular space (e.g. lithium). Pulmonary edema and congestive failure can occur immediately postpartum in patients with mitral stenosis.[81] Lithium toxicity may occur on the second or third day postpartum as diuresis occurs and the fluid compartment contracts.

The length of stay postpartum should be longer than 24 h, to ensure that the mother is sufficiently physically and mentally rested to cope with the physical and mental challenges of a new baby.

Cognitive and memory deficits have been noted on the first postpartum day. It does not seem prudent to send a new mother home with an important set of instructions on the very day when her mind is least able to remember those instructions. During labor and delivery, a woman may have gone without food and sleep for more than 24 h, endured 24 h of pain, had more than 2 h of exhausting physical exertion during pushing, sustained lacerations at delivery, and sustained a blood loss of up to 500 mL. Common sense would suggest that she will need more than a few hours to recuperate before assuming the new duties of motherhood.

COMPLICATED PREGNANCIES

Pregnancy is assumed to be a healthy time. Therefore complications are upsetting and mothers often look for something or someone to blame – often themselves or the obstetrician. Complications may be acute (e.g. Cesarean section or hemorrhage) or chronic (e.g. hypertension or threatened premature labor) (see Box 2.9).

Chronic complications often require bed rest and abstinence from intercourse. It may be necessary for the mother to stop work earlier than anticipated, resulting in an unexpected loss of income. In addition, there may be anxiety as to whether the baby will be normal, or guilt about having caused the complication. Disappointment at not having a normal pregnancy may be an additional source of anxiety. It may be necessary for an in-law or other relative to move into the home to help care for the younger children, marital and family stress may result, and supportive counseling may be needed for the couple. Maternal and fetal testing can add to the couple's anxiety.

Common antenatal tests include the following:

1. biophysical profile – a sonographic assessment of fetal movements, tone, breathing, heart rate, umbilical blood flow, amniotic fluid volume and evoked fetal responses;
2. stress test – in which the fetal heart is monitored while several mild contractions are induced; and,
3. non-stress test – in which the relationship between the fetal heartbeat and fetal movement is monitored.

ADVANCED MATERNAL AGE

Advanced maternal age is considered to be 35 years or older. The incidence of fertility and pregnancy complications gradually increases with age, but the incidence of infertility complications rises markedly by the age of 35 years. The proportion of women who delay childbirth has increased, with approximately 20% of women over 30 years old having no children.[82]

The incidence of most pregnancy complications increases significantly after 35 years of age. Both maternal and fetal mortality increase, and infertility, spontaneous abortions, chromosomal abnormalities and non-chromosomal birth defects are more frequent. There is also an increased frequency of macrosomic infants, abnormal labors, inductions of labor, Cesarean sections, premature rupture of membranes, vaginal bleeding, placenta previa, low Apgar scores, and neonatal complications requiring ICU admission. The majority of complications

---

Box 2.9 *Pregnancy complications*

Advanced maternal age
- Maternal age over 35 years by itself is not a risk, but it increases the risk of hypertension, diabetes, hemorrhage and fetal anomalies. Prenatal testing genetic testing, and counseling are often needed

Abnormal fetal growth
- Fetal growth retardation
- Macrosomia
- Complications at delivery, associated with gestational diabetes

Early/late delivery
- Prematurity – higher perinatal mortality
- Post-term – higher perinatal morbidity and mortality

Multifetal
- Twins:
     Fraternal
     Identical
- Triplets and higher order

Fetal problems
- Anomalies
- Rh isoimmunization
- Infections

Gestational diabetes

Hemorrhage
- Abruption
- Placenta previa
- Retained placenta
- Uterine atony
- Shock and disseminated intravascular coagulation

Hyperemesis gravidarum

Hypertension
- Pregnancy induced
     Eclampsia
     Pre-eclampsia
- Pregnancy associated
     Chronic hypertension

Labor complications
- Failure to progress
- Fetal distress
- Dysfunctional labor

Pregnancy losses

---

are due to underlying illnesses that tend to manifest with increasing maternal age. These include hypertension, diabetes, cardiovascular disease and collagen vascular disease.[83]

MACROSOMIA

A macrosomic infant weighs more than 4000 g. This occurs more commonly with gestational diabetes, prolonged gestation, advanced maternal age, and in infants of large parents. Labor may be prolonged and there is a higher incidence of Cesarean delivery and shoulder dystocia in such cases.

PREMATURE DELIVERY AND FETAL GROWTH RETARDATION

A birth weight of less than 2500 g is considered to be a low birth weight, and this may be due to prematurity or fetal growth restriction. Fetal growth restriction – or growth retardation, is defined as an infant weighing less than 2500 g at 40 weeks. It occurs in 3–10% of births.[84] Common causes of growth restriction are congenital anomalies, hypertension and intrauterine infections.

Prematurity, is the leading cause of infant mortality and is defined as a birth occurring before 37 weeks' gestational age. In the USA, approximately 16% of births are premature.

Extremely low-birth-weight infants (less than 1000 g) have a 50% rate of either death or major morbidity. Major morbidity is defined as oxygen dependence, necrotizing enterocolitis or grades III/IV periventricular bleeds. Between weights of 1000 g and 1250 g the risk of mortality and major morbidity drops to 30%. Above 1500 g the risk is about 10%.

Fetal growth retardation and premature delivery are associated with the same risk factors (see Box 2.10). Both occur more commonly in pregnancies complicated by poor weight gain, alcohol and/or drug abuse, and tobacco use. In addition, fetal growth retardation may be associated with chromosomal aberrations, teratogen exposure, infection (e.g. cytomegalovirus, tuberculosis, listeriosis, hepatitis) and chronic medical illness (e.g. collagen vascular disease, renal disease, hypoxia, anemia).[84]

Treatment of prematurity consists of bed rest, beta-adrenergic agonist therapy and steroids. Ritodrine and terbutaline (tocolytics) are used to suppress or delay premature labor, but are associated with only limited success, and may cause pulmonary edema and hyperglycemia. The tocolytics are useful for forestalling labor until betamethasone has had time to act.

Betamethasone (a corticosteroid) helps the fetal lungs to mature. Tocolytics and steroids may reduce the incidence and severity of respiratory distress syndrome. Ampicillin, used to treat a potential beta-streptococcus infection, is sometimes given antenatally in an attempt to prevent preterm labor. A variety of other drugs have a partial effect in inhibiting labor. These

---

Box 2.10 *Causes of small infant*

Maternal factors
- Small mother
- Poor nutrition
- Chronic illnesses
- Renal disease
- Vascular disease
- Anemia
- Hypoxia
- Hypertension
- Chronic hypertension
- Pre-eclampsia

Fetal causes
- Infections
- CMV (cytomegalovirus)
- Toxoplasmosis
- Listeria

- Tuberculosis
- Syphilis
- Others (hepatitis, etc.)
- Congenital anomalies
- Chromosomal anomalies
- Trisomies 18, 21

Drug and chemical exposure
- Smoking
- Alcohol
- Antineoplastic agents
- Cocaine
- Heroin
- Amphetamines
- Beta-blockers

Prematurity

include magnesium sulfate, prostaglandin inhibitors and calcium-channel blockers. Intravenous alcohol is no longer used.

The best route of delivery for the premature infant is controversial. Cesarean section has not been demonstrated to protect premature infants from intraventricular hemorrhage or cerebral palsy.

POST-DATES PREGNANCY

A post-dates pregnancy is one that is more than 42 weeks from the first day of the last menses. The most common cause of 'post-dates' is an incorrectly calculated due date. Some post-dates infants may have the 'postmaturity syndrome' of wrinkled skin, body wasting, long fingernails and thick meconium. Other post-term infants grow to large sizes, some greater than 4000 g, and are at risk of failure to progress in labor, or of shoulder dystocia. Amniotic fluid volume decreases after 40 weeks, and the incidence of cord accidents and intrauterine deaths is higher than for term pregnancies.

At 42 weeks an attempt may be made to induce labor. If the induction is unsuccessful, the obstetrician may wait several days to attempt another induction, or perform a Cesarean section. Going beyond the due date can be distressing for some women, whose concerns shift from the fear of labor to a desire to end the pregnancy, and questions of why the baby has not been delivered.

MULTIFETAL PREGNANCIES

Twinning occurs in about 1% of pregnancies in the USA, and its incidence is higher in blacks (about 2%). Monozygotic twinning occurs at a stable rate of 1 in 250 worldwide. Dizygotic twinning varies according to race, family history and maternal age.[85] Fertility treatments with follicle-stimulating hormone (FSH) increase the likelihood of there being two or more fetuses by 30%. Mothers are advised to bed rest for much of the pregnancy. Despite bed rest, multiple fetuses are usually delivered prematurely, and the higher morbidity and mortality are primarily a result of the complications of prematurity. Twin pregnancies have an increased frequency of congenital anomalies and a threefold increased risk of spontaneous abortion. Monochorionic, monoamnionic twins have an increased risk of being conjoined (i.e. 'Siamese twins') or of having twin–twin transfusions.

With triplet or higher-order pregnancies, maternal complications are greatly increased in frequency, and the risk of very low birth weight due to prematurity is also greatly increased. Greater overall viability can be achieved by reducing the number of fetuses to twins or triplets. This is termed selective reduction. The usual method of fetal reduction involves injecting potassium chloride either into the umbilical vein or directly into the fetal heart.

The decision to terminate one or more fetuses is difficult for couples. Most grieve for a period of time, but eventually reach an emotional acceptance without developing a major depression.[86] Couples should be aware that one potential complication of selective reduction may include death of one or more of the remaining fetuses.

FETAL ANOMALIES

Many parents wish merely that their child will be healthy. About 6–7% of newborns are born with a congenital anomaly (see Box 2.11), and about 3% of these are identifiable at birth (see Table 2.13).

Box 2.11 *Etiologies of fetal anomalies*

Genetic	Chromosomal and single-gene defects	10–25%
Fetal infections	Cytomegalovirus, syphilis, rubella, toxoplasmosis, other	3–5%
Maternal disease	Diabetes, alcohol abuse, seizure disorders, others	4%
Drugs and medications	Isotretinoin, alcohol, methotresate, etc.	< 1%
Unknown or multifactorial		65–75%

Adapted from Table 39–1 (Etiology of human malformations during the first year of life). In: Cunningham FG, MacDonald PC, Gant NF *et al.* (eds) *Williams' obstetrics*, 20th edn. Stamford, CT: Appleton & Lange, 1997: 896.

Table 2.13 *Fetal anomalies*

Type	Incidence	Description	Prognosis
Trisomy 21	1 in 660	Down's syndrome	Cardiac defects
Trisomy 18	3 in 1000	Edward syndrome	Multiple anomalies, death
Diaphragmatic hernia	1–5 in 10 000	Hole in diaphragm	Survival depends on degree of defect
Cardiac	8 in 1000	–	Survival rate is high
Spina bifida	5 in 10 000	Open spinal cord	Survival depends on severity of defect
Multiple congenital anomalies	1–10 in 10 000	–	Survival depends on degree of defect
Potter's	3 in 10 000	Renal insufficiency, pulmonary hypoplasia	Death
Anencephaly	3.4 in 10 000	Absence of brain	Death
Clubfoot	1 in 1000	Malformed talipes	Surgically correctable
Renal agenesis	1.5 in 10 000	Absent kidneys	Death
Abdominal wall defect	6.1 in 10 000	Exstrophy of abdominal organs	Survival depends on degree of defect

About 25% of these anomalies are chromosomal, and approximately 10% are due to drug exposure, intrauterine infection or maternal disease (e.g. alcoholism, diabetes, epilepsy). The majority of anomalies are unexplained.

Chromosomal anomalies occur in 10–25% of infants with birth defects. Pregnancies in which the fetuses have chromosomal anomalies are more likely to end in stillbirth or spontaneous abortion. Chromosomal anomalies include trisomy (especially trisomy 21 or Down's syndrome), deletions, translocations and inversions. Abnormalities may also occur in sex chromosomes (e.g. Turner's syndrome and Klinefelter's syndrome). Single-gene mutations also occur. Inherited abnormalities, which are less likely to be detected at birth, include dominant and X-linked disorders. In addition, trinucleotide-repeat disorders and fragile X-syndrome are chromosomal anomalies associated with birth defects.

Multifactorial defects are thought to be due to the interaction between genes and the environment. They include neural-tube defects, anencephaly, congenital heart disease, clubfeet, congenital hip dislocation, cleft palate and pyloric stenosis (see Box 2.12). Defects of unknown etiology include hydrocephaly, renal agenesis, abdominal wall defects and diaphragmatic hernia.

Box 2.12 *Birth defects*

Head and spine
- Cystic hygroma, lymphangiectasia
- Facial deformities (including Pierre Robin's syndrome)
- Holoprosencephaly
- Hydrencephalocele
- Hydrocephaly (including Dandy-Walker syndrome)
- Hypertelorism
- Meningomyelocele
- Microcephaly (including Meckel's syndrome)
- Neural-tube defects
- Anencephaly
- Spina bifida (including Arnold-Chiara syndrome)

Internal anatomy
- Diaphragmatic hernia
- Jejunal atresia
- Situs inversus viscerum
- Omphalocele, gastroschisis (history or elevated alpha-fetoprotein)
- Infantile polycystic kidney disease
- Renal agenesis (including Potter's syndrome)
- Renal anomalies (miscellaneous)

Skeleton and limbs
- Achondrogenesis
- Achondroplasia
- Acrocephalosyndactyly (Apert's syndrome)
- Adactyly
- Asphyxiating thoracic dysplasia
- Camptomelic dysplasia
- Cartilage hair hypoplasia (McKusick)
- Chondroectodermal dysplasia (Ellis van Creveld syndrome)
- Diastrophic dysplasia
- Ectrodactyly
- Fanconi's anemia
- Osteogenesis imperfecta
- Osteopetrosis
- Polydactyly
- Robert's syndrome
- Meckel's syndrome (microcephaly, dwarfism)
- Skeletal dysplasia (miscellaneous)
- Spondyloepiphyseal dysplasia
- Spondylothoracic dysplasia
- Thanatophoric dysplasia
- Thrombocytopenia with absent radii syndrome

If a defect incompatible with life (e.g. anencephaly) is discovered prior to delivery, a couple may be faced with the option of a late abortion (see Box 2.13). Experimental fetal surgery may be an option in other cases (e.g. hydronephrosis). Timed Cesarean section with a pediatric surgery team prepared to operate immediately after delivery is an option in still other cases (e.g. diaphragmatic hernia, certain cardiac defects).

Box 2.13 *Abnormalities found in third trimester*

Anencephaly
Microcephaly
Hydrocephaly
Cystic teratoma
Cystic hygroma
Intrathoracic cyst
Pleural effusion
Diaphragmatic hernia
Situs inversus viscerum
Duodenal atresia
Ileal volvulus

Abdominal cyst
Omental cyst
Gastroschisis
Omphalocele
Ovarian cyst
Potter's syndrome
Displastic kidneys
Urethral obstruction
Sacrococcygeal teratoma
Thanatophoric dysplasia
Multiple anomalies

RH ISOIMMUNIZATION

Rh isoimmunization is now uncommon, since Rh immune globulin is given regularly to Rh-negative women to prevent the formation of antibodies to Rh-positive blood. Antibody formation occurs in response to Rh-positive blood, usually fetal cells from an Rh-positive pregnancy that enter the maternal bloodstream. This can occur during a term pregnancy, or it may take place at the time of a miscarriage, amniocentesis or previous pregnancy. Once an Rh-negative mother has developed antibodies, her future pregnancies are at risk. Her antibodies enter the fetal circulation, causing hemolysis, jaundice and cardiac failure. This may require early delivery of the infant, who can then be treated with light therapy and transfusions.

PERINATAL INFECTIONS

Maternal infections may be transmitted to the fetus by transmission through the placenta, or through contact with the birth canal at delivery. Infections are associated with congenital anomalies, fetal growth retardation, chorioamnionitis, premature delivery and stillbirth. Infections that cross the placenta include the TORCH viruses (toxoplasmosis, other rubella, cytomegalovirus and herpes). Infections that are transmitted during passage through the birth canal include gonorrhea, chlamydia, condylomata and candidiasis. The influenza virus crosses transplacentally, but does not appear to cause anomalies or fetal infection. Group B streptococcus is associated with chorioamnionitis and neonatal infections. Some infections can be prevented in the infant by treatment with immune globulin immediately postpartum (e.g. hepatitis B, varicella zoster). Others can be prevented by treatment *in utero* (e.g. herpes, HIV, syphilis). Unfortunately, many intrauterine infections are not diagnosed until the neonatal period.

GESTATIONAL DIABETES

Gestational diabetes, defined as a fasting plasma glucose level of more than 105 mg/dl during pregnancy, is associated with large infants and with stillbirths. Most cases can be managed by diet. About 50% of women with gestational diabetes will develop diabetes during their lifetime.[87]

HEMORRHAGE

Hemorrhage is one of the three main causes of maternal mortality. About 4% of parturients hemorrhage in pregnancy. In the first trimester, bleeding may be due to an incomplete abortion. A ruptured tubal pregnancy causes internal bleeding. In the second and third trimesters, placenta previa and placental abruption are the most common causes of hemorrhage. Blood loss at delivery may be from perineal or vaginal lacerations. Postpartum blood loss is usually caused by uterine atony or a retained placenta.

Placenta previa is a placenta located low on the uterine wall, covering part or all of the cervix. The incidence is 1 in 400 deliveries, and advanced maternal age is a risk factor. The first episode of bleeding is usually not severe, but the second bleed may be profuse. The bleeding is painless, and diagnosis is by made sonogram. Vaginal examination is contraindicated, as sticking a finger through the placenta may cause exsanguinating hemorrhage.

Placental abruption is the separation of the placenta from the uterine wall before delivery. It occurs in approximately 1 in 150 deliveries and is fatal to the fetus in 1 in 850 deliveries. Hemorrhage may be visible, or concealed between the placenta and the uterine wall. In contrast to the painless bleeding of placenta previa, the patient with an abruption has severe abdominal pain. Risk factors include hypertension, premature rupture of the membranes, cigarette smoking, alcohol, heroin and cocaine.

HYPEREMESIS GRAVIDARUM

More than 50% of women experience nausea and vomiting during the first trimester. The vomiting is related to levels of HCG, with severe nausea and vomiting correlating with high levels of HCG. After 14 weeks, when HCG levels decline naturally, vomiting usually subsides. Reassurance and conservative measures such as small frequent meals and the consumption of crackers or ginger ale are helpful for most women. Anti-emetics are needed if dehydration and weight loss are problematic.

Hyperemesis gravidarum, or prolonged vomiting with dehydration, occurs in less than 1% of pregnant women. It requires hospitalization and intravenous hydration. A variety of anti-emetics and psychological treatments have been used to control vomiting. Interpersonal psychotherapy, family therapy and hypnosis have been found to be successful. Hospitalization is helpful because it removes the woman from a stressful home situation.[88]

HYPERTENSION

Hypertension is common in pregnancy, especially in teenagers and mothers over 40 years of age. It is categorized as follows:

1. transient hypertension – a mild condition diagnosed only in retrospect;
2. pregnancy – induced hypertension, hypertension, pre-eclampsia, eclampsia; or
3. chronic underlying hypertension that is exacerbated by pregnancy.

Pre-eclampsia is diagnosed with the triad of hypertension, proteinuria and edema. The placenta is underperfused and the maternal blood volume is constricted. If left untreated, pre-eclampsia may progress to eclampsia with convulsions and extreme hypertension. Severe pre-eclampsia and eclampsia always require immediate delivery because of the increased risk of seizures, blindness, cerebrovascular accident and maternal and fetal death. A diastolic blood pressure of 105 mmHg with 4+ proteinuria is associated with a 10% risk of fetal death.[89]

Although edema occurs normally in pregnancy, the edema of pre-eclampsia is marked in the hands and feet, and facial edema is also present. Edema of the face and a diastolic blood pressure of 90 mmHg should prompt intervention. Mild cases may be managed with bed rest. Symptoms of headache, epigastric pain and visual disturbances are more ominous signs that may warrant intervention before convulsions occur. Magnesium sulfate, administered intravenously or intramuscularly, usually prevents convulsions. However, the treatment is delivery of the fetus. The HELLP syndrome (HELLP is an acronym for the associated complications of Hemolysis, Elevated Liver enzymes and Low Platelet counts) is a variant of severe pre-eclampsia.

Chronic hypertension is a relative contraindication to pregnancy because of the 10–50% risk of superimposed pre-eclampsia. Antihypertensives are sometimes continued during the pregnancies of hypertensive women. Methyldopa is the first-line antihypertensive during pregnancy. Beta-blockers are effective but are associated with low birth weight. Angiotensin-converting enzyme inhibitors should be avoided because of the risk of fetal death.

LABOR AND DELIVERY COMPLICATIONS

The onset of labor may be premature or delayed.

Labor duration may be precipitous, with delivery of the baby prior to arriving at the delivery room. More problematically, the labor may be prolonged. If hydration and analgesia are not effective, the labor and delivery process can be speeded up by oxytocin administration (to strengthen contractions), a forceps delivery, or a Cesarean section. Other indications for Cesarean section are slowing of the fetal heart (indicating distress), and the onset of bleeding.

The emotional state of the mother needs attention. A supportive person should be present throughout the process. Comfort measures should be addressed, including the patient's choice of anesthesia and comfortable positioning of her baby during pushing and delivery. Critical comments should be avoided. A single mother needs emotional support, not criticism, during labor and delivery. A frightened woman who is screaming needs the cause of her pain and anxiety to be addressed, and should not be told to shut up. It should be noted that, in postpartum psychoses, women are sometimes delusional about being injured by the delivery nurse or doctor.

PREGNANCY LOSSES

Pregnancy loss may occur before implantation, with the only evidence of pregnancy being the presence of low levels of HCG or a slight change in the menstrual cycle. Losses in the first trimester occur more commonly in women who are older or who have illnesses (e.g. poorly controlled diabetes). Chromosomal anomalies account for more than 25% of these cases. Risk factors for first-trimester abortion include smoking, alcohol, and a family history of chromosomal abnormalities. Other risk factors for first-trimester abortion are exposure to toxins (e.g. lead, arsenic or benzene), the presence of antiphospholipid antibodies (e.g. lupus anticoagulant) and high doses of radiation. However, the risk of fatal birth defects is associated with doses of more than 10 rads to the fetus. The average chest X-ray involves a dose of less than 1 rad to the mother and less than 0.01 rad to the fetus. Chronic infections, with the exception of *Mycoplasma* and *Ureaplasma*, are not associated with first-trimester abortions. Nausea and vomiting of pregnancy do not cause abortions. Ectopic pregnancies (usually tubal pregnancies) become symptomatic in the first trimester.

In the second trimester, pregnancy loss may be due to an incompetent cervix. Second- and third-trimester losses are usually associated with congenital anomalies, underlying medical illness (e.g. renal failure or hypertension), premature labor or uterine anomalies. Recurrent pregnancy loss (two or more) may be an indication for karyotyping the couple, as they may carry a chromosomal abnormality that results in a non-viable fetus. A small number of losses are accidental, such as stabbing or gunshot wounds. Recuperating from pregnancy loss involves emotional as well as physical recovery.

Medically, an early first-trimester pregnancy loss involves little more than a heavy menstrual period (see Box 2.14). If a dilation and curettage (D&C) is necessary, a general or

> **Box 2.14** *Causes of pregnancy loss*
>
> Miscarriage
> - Spontaneous abortion – entire pregnancy is expelled
> - Incomplete abortion – entire placenta and embryo are not expelled. A D&C is necessary to remove retained products and stop bleeding
> - Missed abortion – embryo has stopped growing. If spontaneous abortion does not occur shortly, a D&C is necessary
>
> Fetal demise (death prior to delivery)
> - Unexplained
> - Immunological (e.g. antiphospholipid antibodies)
> - Cord accident – umbilical cord becomes tangled round a fetal limb or wrapped around the neck and shuts off the blood supply
> - Infection
> - Placental insufficiency – placenta may be small or infarcted. Associated with hypertension, collagen vascular disease and hypoxia
> - Genetic

local anesthetic is used. The patient is given medication (oxytocin or methergine), to help the uterus contract as well as a non-steroidal anti-inflammatory or a codeine-containing analgesic, and is then discharged several hours later. Apart from abstaining from coitus for 2 weeks, the patient is allowed to resume her normal activities on the next day. However, emotional changes do occur, including normal reactions of depressed mood, regrets, guilt and wondering. The painful contractions and blood loss of a miscarriage are distressing to most women. However, first-trimester pregnancy losses (either miscarriages or elective terminations of pregnancy) do not predispose to psychiatric disorders. Depression and psychosis are less common after such losses than after a delivery in the last trimester of pregnancy.

Pregnancy losses that occur at the end of the first trimester (at 12–14 weeks) are associated with heavier and more painful bleeding. If bleeding is profuse, a transfusion may be necessary. A loss at this stage can be more devastating, because by this time the couple will probably have announced the pregnancy. Physical recovery may take 2–6 weeks.

ACCIDENTAL DEATHS IN PREGNANCY

Deaths are infrequent during pregnancy (see Table 2.14). Maternal mortality in the USA is 8.5 per 100 000 live births. The commonest causes of death are embolism, hypertension and hemorrhage. Death rates are highest for women over 35 years of age. Accidental deaths account for 39% of maternal deaths. These include deaths due to homicide (63%), suicide (13%), motor-vehicle accidents (12%) and drug overdoses (7%). About 50% of these deaths are associated with illegal drug use.[90]

DRUG OVERDOSE

The substances most commonly ingested in overdose during pregnancy are acetaminophen, aspirin and iron (see Table 2.15).[91] Fortunately, as in non-pregnant women, the majority of suicide attempts are not fatal. All overdoses require an examination of the motivating factors. Was the mother depressed and attempting suicide? Was she upset, without social support, and

Table 2.14 *Causes of maternal death (overall maternal death rate is 8.5 per 100 000 deliveries*

Causes	Incidence (%)
Medical causes	61
Embolism	17
Hypertension	12
Ectopic pregnancy	10
Hemorrhage	9
Stroke	8
Anesthesia	7
Abortion related	5
Cardiomyopathy	4
Infection	3.5
Other	16
Accidental causes	39
Homicide	63
Suicide	13
Motor vehicle accident	12
Overdose	7
Other	5

Table 2.15 *Effects of drug overdoses during pregnancy*

Drug	Embryofetal effects
Acetaminophen	Not associated with fetal anomalies Cases of spontaneous abortions, fetal death, fetal hepatotoxicity, maternal hepatotoxicity and maternal death Treat with *N*-acetylcysteine
Aspirin	Not associated with fetal anomalies Tinnitus in mother Hyperventilation in mother and fetus Fetal and maternal death Treat with activated charcoal and supportive therapy
Iron	Fetus often survives. Cases of spontaneous abortion Maternal effects include metabolic acidosis, death, hepatic necrosis, gastrointestinal hemorrhage, cardiac collapse Treat with deferoxamine
Tricyclic antidepressants	Anticholinergic toxicity (tachycardia, agitation, hyperpyrexia, cardiac arrhythmias from prolonged QT interval) Maternal coma and death Treatment is supportive
Quinine	Fetal deafness and ototoxicity. Other congenital anomalies Maternal death Treatment is supportive
Ergotamine	Premature contractions, tetanic contractions. Fetal death from hypoxia, poor placental perfusion Treat with prazosin (nitroprusside causes cyanide to accumulate in fetal liver, and is therefore contraindicated)
Benzodiazepines	Respiratory depression in mother and fetus Floppy infant Treat with flumazenil if seizure risk is low
Prozac	No case reports
Diphenhydramine	Oxytocin-like effect

not knowing what to do? Was the overdose an attempt to abort the pregnancy? The drugs most commonly used to attempt abortion are quinine and ergotamine.

The maternal effects of an overdose and management of the acute overdose are similar in pregnant and non-pregnant females. *N*-acetylcysteine should be administered promptly for acetaminophen overdose. Deferoxamine may be given for iron overdose. Physostigmine reverses the anticholinergic effects of tricyclic antidepressants.

Among psychotropic drugs, benzodiazepines are most commonly ingested in suicide attempts. Flumazenil may be given for benzodiazepine overdose, unless there is a high risk of seizures.

Fetal effects vary according to the gestational age at the time of ingestion and the particular substance ingested. Most compounds cross the placenta and may be toxic to the fetus. The fetal liver and kidneys are immature. Hepatic metabolism and renal clearance are reduced. For example, the fetus cannot metabolize a large dose of acetaminophen, which is in fact protective, since it is the metabolite of acetaminophen – and not the drug itself – which is toxic. Teratogenic drugs are most toxic to the conceptus when ingested during the first trimester. The fetal effect in the second and third trimesters varies according to the drug.

Excessive amounts of drugs are sometimes taken in the hope of inducing labor. Castor oil and prostaglandins have been used in this way, and Brost and colleagues reported a case of diphenhydramine overdose causing contractions.[92]

SPECIAL CIRCUMSTANCES

Teenage pregnancy

Teenage pregnancy accounts for 20% of births, although teenage birth rates have dropped since 1990. Poor nutrition is common among teenagers, and they have higher rates of pre-eclampsia, low-birth-weight and very-low-birth-weight infants than women do in their twenties and thirties (see Box 2.15). Girls under 16 years of age are especially prone to prema-

---

Box 2.15 *Problems of teenage pregnancy*

Medical
- Nutrition
- Need for prenatal care
- Risk of prematurity
- Contraception postpartum

Social support
- Housing
- Education
- Single parenthood
  Choice of aborting, being a single parent, marrying, or placing the child for adoption may have been forced on the teenager against her will
  Preventing injury or death of infant
  Addressing special needs of premature infant

Psychiatric
- Higher-risk factors for postpartum depression:
  Pre-existing depression
  Lack of a supportive partner
  Pre-existing anxiety
  Pre-existing substance abuse

---

ture delivery.[93] In addition, their babies have increased rates of accidents, infections and infant mortality. However, there is no increase in chromosomal anomalies.[94]

Teenagers who become pregnant have higher rates of psychiatric disorders (depression, anxiety or substance abuse) than non-pregnant teenagers. However, fewer than 10% of teenagers place their babies for adoption.[95] Most of the increased morbidity in teenage pregnancies correlate not with the young age of the mother, but with the presence of social factors such as inadequate prenatal care, poor nutrition, poverty, sexually transmitted infections, drug use, alcohol consumption and cigarette smoking.

Giving infants up for adoption

Open adoptions – both private and through agencies – are now common. Formerly, most adoptions were closed, the birth records being sealed and kept secret. However, adopted children have taught us that they have a psychological need to learn about their biologic parents. For this reason, open adoptions have become more common.

The obstetrician may be placed in a middle position between the pregnant patient and the prospective parents who are paying the obstetrical fee. When making decisions about prenatal care or delivery procedures (e.g. the type of anesthesia or who will be present in the delivery room), the obstetrician must consider the emotional and financial support that the prospective parents might provide, but should at the same time be careful not to be coerced into doing something that is not in the patient's best interest. Many women are motivated to do their very best to deliver a healthy infant even though they will not be raising the child. Occasionally, however, mothers are reluctant to undergo certain procedures (e.g. an amniocentesis if over the age of 35 years, or being confined to bed rest if hypertension occurs).

Surrogate mothers and gestational carriers also release their babies for adoption. A surrogate mother ovulates naturally and is inseminated with the sperm provided by the adopting couple (usually the father's own sperm). A gestational carrier provides neither egg nor sperm, but merely a hormonally primed uterus in which the embryo can grow. Surrogate mothers and gestational carriers are both altruistically motivated and in financial need.[96] Some of them are married. However, just as with other mothers who give infants up for adoption, the gestational carrier or surrogate mother bonds with the fetus and wishes the very best for it, although she knows that the child will not be hers after its birth. She may find it difficult to release the infant after birth. In contrast to adoption, where a woman is not obliged to release her infant until after delivery, these women have agreed in advance to release the infants. In Texas, the law requires a delay of at least 2 days until the adoption papers can be signed. The most famous case is that of Baby M, in which the surrogate mother did not want to release her infant. Most courts have ruled that biological mothers have parental rights, making the offspring the illegitimate child of the surrogate mother and the father who donated the sperm.[97,98]

PSYCHOLOGICAL NEEDS OF THE MALE PARTNER

The psychological needs of the male partner are often ignored or considered to be insignificant. However, the love and support of the husband are extremely important to a woman during pregnancy, and even more important postpartum. At the same time that a man is expected to provide increased emotional support, he is facing challenges of his own in dealing with his new role as a father and provider. Fathers have an increased incidence of depressive symptoms postpartum, especially if the mother is depressed.[99] The male partner can benefit from empathic listening and from education about the mother's emotional and physical reactions, which very probably differs from his own reactions.

For instance, during fertility treatments, men and women display different emotional reactions. Women are likely to discuss the procedure at length whereas men do not feel such a need. Men are reported to experience distress later rather than earlier in the fertility treatment. After a miscarriage, attention often focuses on the woman, even though the male partner's dreams of a son or daughter and family have also been dashed. The strains of dealing with a fetal death, a premature infant or a malformed child are often more than many couples can cope with, and the divorce rate is twice the national average among couples who lose a child.[100]

Some men may develop physical symptoms in pregnancy. Toothache, abdominal cramps and nausea have been reported. The Couvade syndrome is defined as labor-like abdominal pains in a male. Pseudocyesis can occur in men, but is rare.

REFERENCES

1. Herrenkohl LR. The impact of prenatal stress on the developing fetus and child. In: Cohen RL (ed). *Psychiatric consultations in childbirth settings: parent and child oriented approaches.* New York: Plenum Publishing, 1988: 21–35.
2. Horton JA (ed.) Reproductive health. In: *The women's health data book: a profile of women's health in the United States.* Washington, DC: Elsevier; 1995: 5–15.
3. US Census Bureau. Vital statistic. In: *Statistical abstract of the United States, 1995: the national data book,* 115th edn. Washington, DC: Department of Commerce, 1995: 71–85.
4. Cunningham FG, MacDonald PC, Gant NF et al. (eds). *Williams obstetrics* 20th edn. Stamford, CT: Appleton & Lange, 1997: 464.
5. Kulin NA, Pastuszak A, Sage SR et al. Pregnancy outcome following maternal use of the new selective serotonin reuptake inhibitors: a prospective controlled multicenter study. *Journal of the American Medical Association* 1998; **279**: 609–10.
6. Chambers CD, Johnson KA, Dick LM, Felix RJ, Jones KL. Birth outcomes in pregnant women taking fluoxetine. *New England Journal of Medicine* 1996; **335**: 1010–15.
7. Brinch M, Isager T, Tolstrup K. Anorexia nervosa and motherhood: reproduction pattern and mothering behavior in 50 women [corrected and republished article originally printed in *Acta Psychiatrica Scandinavica* 1988; **77**: 98–104] *Acta Psychiatrica Scandinavica* 1988; **77**: 611–17.
8. Stewart DE. Reproductive functions in eating disorders. *Annals of Medicine* 1992; **24**: 287–91.
9. Willis DC, Rand CS. Pregnancy in bulimic women. *Obstetrics and Gynecology* 1988; **71**: 708–10.
10. Lingam R, McCluskey S. Eating disorders associated with hyperemesis gravidarum. *Journal of Psychosomatic Research* 1996; **40**: 231–4.
11. McGrath ME, Hogan JW, Peipert JF. A prevalence survey of abuse and screening for abuse in urgent care patients. *Obstetrics and Gynecology* 1998; **91**: 511–14.
12. Poole GV, Martin JN, Perry KG, Griswold JA, Lambert CG, Rhodes RS. Trauma in pregnancy: the role of interpersonal violence. *American Journal of Obstetrics and Gynecology* 1996; **174**: 1873–8.
13. American Psychiatric Association. *Diagnostic and statistical manual of mental disorders.* 4th edn. Washington, DC: American Psychiatric Association Press, 1994: 327.
14. Blacker CM, Ginsburg KA, Leach RE, Randolph J, Moshissi KS. Unexplained infertility. Evaluation of the luteal phase: results of the National Center for Infertility Research at Michigan. *Fertility and Sterility* 1997; **67**: 437–2.
15. Demyttenaere K, Nijs P, Evers-Kiebooms G, Koninckx P. The effect of a specific emotional stressor on prolactin, cortisol, and testosterone concentrations in women varies with their trait anxiety. *Fertility and Sterililty* 1989; **52**: 942–8.

16. Demyttenaere K, Nijs P, Steeno O, Konincks P, Evers Kiebooms G. Anxiety and conception rates in donor insemination. *Journal of Psychosomatic Obstetrics and Gynaecology* 1988; **8**: 175.

17. Wasser SK, Isenberg DY. Reproductive failure among women: pathology or adaptation? *Journal of Psychosomatic Obstetrics and Gynaecology* 1986; **5**: 153–75.

18. Boivin J, Taefman JE. Stress level across stages of *in vitro* fertilization in subsequently pregnant and nonpregnant women. *Fertility and Sterililty* 1995; **64**: 802–10.

19. Stoleru S, Cornet D, Vaugeois P *et al*. The influence of psychological factors on the outcome of the fertilization step of *in vitro* fertilization. *Journal of Psychosomatic Obstetrics and Gynecology* 1997; **18**: 189–202.

20. Sarrel PM, DeCherney AH. Psychotherapeutic intervention for treatment of couples with secondary infertility. *Fertility and Sterility* 1985; **43**: 897–900.

21. Rubenstein BB. An emotional factor in infertility: a psychosomatic approach. *Fertility and Sterility* 1951; **2**: 80–6.

22. Domar AD, Seibel MM, Benson J. The mind/body program for infertility: a new behavioral treatment approach for women with infertility. *Fertility and Sterility* 1990; **53**: 246–9.

23. Lamb EJ, Leurgans S. Does adoption affect subsequent fertility? *American Journal of Obstetrics and Gynecology* 1979; **134**: 138–44.

24. Murray JL, Abraham GE. Pseudocyesis: a review. *Obstetrics and Gynaecology* 1978; **51**: 627–31.

25. Whelan CI, Stewart DE. Pseudocyesis - a review and report of six cases. *International Journal of Psychiatry in Medicine* 1990; **20**: 97–108.

26. Culpepper L, Jack BW. Preconception care. In: Cherry SH, Merkatz IR (eds) *Complications of pregnancy: medical, surgical, gynecologic, psychosocial and perinatal*. 4th edn. New York: Williams & Wilkins, 1991:306–15.

27. Oates M. Management of major mental illness in pregnancy and the puerperium. *Baillieres Clinical Obstetrics and Gynaecology* 1989; **4**: 905–20.

28. Elam-Evans L, Adams M, Gaggiullo P, Kiely JL, Marks JS. Trends in the percentage of women who received no prenatal care in the United States, 1980–1992: contributions of the demographic and risk effects. *Obstetrics and Gynaecology* 1996; **87**: 575–80.

29. Herzberg BN, Johnson AL, Brown S. Depressive symptoms and oral contraceptives. *British Medical Journal* 1970; **4**: 142–5.

30. Wagner KD. Major depression and anxiety disorders associated with Norplant. *Journal of Clinical Psychiatry* 1996; **57**: 152–7.

31. Buekens P. Variations in provision and uptake of antenatal care. *Baillieres Clinical Obstetrics and Gynaecology* 1990; **4**: 187–205.

32. Cohen RL. Models of consultation and liaison: general principles. In: Cohen RL (ed.) *Psychiatric consultations in childbirth settings. Parent and child oriented approaches*. New York: Plenum Publishing,1988: 107–13.

33. Hartman KE, Thorp JM, Pahel-Short L, Koch M. A randomized controlled trial of smoking cessation intervention in pregnancy in an academic clinic. *Obstetrics and Gynaecology* 1996; **87**: 621–6.

34. Gabbe SG. Neibyl JR, Simpsom JL (eds). *Obstetrics: normal and problem pregnancies*. New York: Churchill Livingstone, 1996: 1142.

35. Jacobson JL. Intellectual impairment in children exposed to polychlorinated biphenyls *in utero*. *New England Journal of Medicine* 1996; **335**: 783–9.

36. Little BB, Van Beveren TT, Glilstrap LC. Cannabinoid use during pregnancy. In: Gilstrap LC, Little BB (eds) *Drugs and pregnancy*, 2nd edn. New York: Chapman & Hall, 1998: 416.

37. Little BB, Gilstrap LC. Tobacco use in pregnancy. In: Gilstrap LC, Little BB (eds) *Drugs and pregnancy*, 2nd edn. New York: Chapman & Hall, 1998: 463–71.

38. Little BB, Van Beveren TT, Gilstrap LC. Alcohol use during pregnancy and maternal alcoholism. In: Gilstrap LC, Little BB (eds) *Drugs and pregnancy*, 2nd edn. New York: Chapman & Hall, 1998: 395–404.

39. Little BB, Van Beveren TT, Gilstrap LC. Cocaine abuse during pregnancy. In: Gilstrap LC, Little BB (eds) *Drugs and pregnancy*, 2nd edn. New York: Chapman & Hall, 1998: 426–31.

40. Little BB. Immunosuppressant therapy during gestation. *Seminars in perinatology* 1997; **21**: 143–8.

41. Nicholson HS, Byrne J. Fertility and pregnancy after treatment for cancer during childhood or adolescence. *Cancer* 1993; **71** (Supplement 10): 3392–9.

42. Crosby E, St-Jean B, Reid D, Elliott RD. Obstetrical anesthesia and analgesia in chronic spinal cord-injured women. *Canadian Journal of Anaesthesia* 1992; **39**: 487–94.

43. Little BB, Snell LM, Wendel GD, Gilstrap LC, Johnston WL, Gluck KL. Prevalence of HIV in pregnant intravenous drug users in Dallas, Texas. *Texas Medicine* 1991; **87**: 81–3.

44. American College of Obstetricians and Gynecologists *Educational bulletin. Human immunodeficiency virus infections in pregnancy*. Washington, DC: American College of Obstetrics and Gynecologists, 1997.

45. Cantrell DT, Gilstrap LC, Little BB. Anticonvulsant drugs during pregnancy. In: Gilstrap LC, Little BB (eds) *Drugs and pregnancy*, 2nd edn. New York: Chapman & Hall, 1998: 137–47.

46. Stephens EH. Projections of impaired fecundity among women in the United States: 1995 to 2020. *Fertility and Sterility* 1996; **66**: 205–9.

47. Potashnik G, Lerner-Geva L, Genkin L, Chetrit A, Lunenfeld E, Porath A. Fertility drugs and the risk of breast and ovarian cancers: results of a long-term follow-up study. *Fertility and Sterility* 1999; **71**: 853–9.

48. Williams KE. Psychopathology and psychopharmacology in the infertile patient. In: Burns LH, Covington SN (eds) *Infertility counseling a comprehensive handbook for clinicians*. New York: Parthenon, 1999: 78.

49. American Society for Reproductive Medicine. *Practice Committee Report. Induction of ovarian follicle development and ovulation with exogenous gonadotropins*. Washington, DC: American Society for Reproductive Medicine, 1998.

50. McMahon CA, Ungerer JA, Tennant C, Saunder D. Psychosocial adjustment and the quality of the mother–child relationship at 4 months postpartum after conception by *in vitro* fertilization. *Fertility and Sterility* 1997; **68**: 492–500.

51. Society for Assisted Reproductive Technology and American Society for Reproductive Medicine. Assisted reproductive technology in the United States and Canada: 1995 results generated from the American Society for Reproductive Medicine/Society for Assisted Reproductive Technology Registry. *Fertility and Sterility* 1997; **60**: 389–98.

52. Thorpe EM, Ling FW. Sex and sexuality in pregnancy. In: Sciarra JJ (ed.) *Obstetrics and Gynecology. Vol. 2*. Philadelphia, PA: Lippincott, 1995: 1–7.

53. Bogein LY. Changes in sexuality in women and men during pregnancy. *Archives of Sexual Behavior* 1991; **20**: 35–45.

54. Alder EM. Sexual behaviour in pregnancy, after childbirth and during breast-feeding. *Baillieres Clinical Obsterics and Gynaecology* 1989; **3**: 805–21.

55. Solberg DA, Butler J, Wagner N. Sexual behavior in pregnancy. *New England Journal of Medicine* 1973; **24**: 1098–103.

56. Alder EM, Cook A, Davidson D, West C, Bancroft J. Hormones, mood and sexuality in lactating women. *British Journal of Psychiatry* 1986; **148**: 74–79.

57. Robson KM, Brant HA and Kumar *British Journal of Obstetrics and Gynaecology* 1981; **88**: 882–9.

58. Munjack DJ. The recognition and management of desire phase sexual dysfunction. In: Sciarra (ed.) *Gynecology and Obstetrics. Vol. 6*. Philadelphia, PA: JP Lippincott, 1995: 1–15.

59. Kayner CE, Zagar JA. Breast-feeding and sexual response. *Journal of Family Practice* 1983; **17**: 69–73.

60. Glazner CM. Sexual function after childbirth: women's experiences, persistent morbidity and lack of professional recognition. *British Journal of Obstetrics and Gynaecology* 1997; **104**: 330–5.

61. Cunningham FG, MacDonald PC, Gant NF *et al*. Maternal adaptations to pregnancy. In: *Williams obstetrics*, 20th edn. Stamford, CT: Appleton & Lange, 1997: 215–17.

62. Cherry SH, Merkatz JR (eds) *Complications of pregnancy: medical, surgical, gynecologic, psychological and perinatal*, 4th edn. New York: Williams & Wilkins, 1991: 1227–62

63. Cunningham FG, MacDonald PC, Gant NF *et al*. Maternal adaptations to pregnancy. In: *Williams obstetrics*, 20th edn. Stamford, CT: Appleton & Lange, 1997: 210.

64. Gleicher N, Myers SA. Physiologic changes in normal pregnancy. In: Gleicher N (ed.) *Principles and practice of medical therapy in pregnancy* 2nd edn. Norwalk, CT: Appleton & Lange, 1992: 41.

65. Lawson W, Biller HF. Ear, nose and throat disorders in pregnancy. In: Cherry SH, Merkatz IR (eds) *Complications of pregnancy: medical, surgical, gynecologic, psychosocial and perinatal*, 4th edn. New York: Williams & Wilkins, 1991: 618.

66. Pruzansky ME, Siffert RS, Levy RN. Orthopaedic complications. In: Cherry SH, Merkatz IR (eds) *Complications of pregnancy: medical, surgical, gynecologic, psychosocial and perinatal*, 4th edn. New York: Williams & Wilkins, 1991: 1001–2.

67. Gabbe SG, Neibyl JR, Simpsom JL (eds). *Obstetrics: normal and problem pregnancies*. New York: Churchill Livingstone, 1996: 142.

68. Brunner DP, Munch M, Biedermann K, Huch R, Huch A, Borbely AA. Changes in sleep and sleep electroencephalogram during pregnancy. *Sleep* 1994; **17**: 576–82.

69. Driver HS, Shapiro CM. A longitudinal study of sleep stages in young women during pregnancy and postpartum. *Sleep* 1992; **15**: 499–53.

70. Swain AM, O'Hara MW, Starr KR, Gorman LL. A prospective study of sleep, mood and cognitive function in postpartum and non-postpartum women. *Obstetrics and Gynecology* 1997; **90**: 381–6.

71. American College of Obstetricians and Gynecologists. *Nutrition during pregnancy*. Technical Bulletin No. 179. Washington, DC: American College of Obstetricians and Gynecologists, 1993.

72. American College of Obstetricians and Gynecologists. *Vitamin A supplementation during pregnancy*. Committee Opinion No 196. Washington, DC: American College of Obstetricians and Gynecologists, 1998.

73. Lingam R, McCluskey S. Eating disorders associated with hyperemesis gravidarum. *Journal of Psychosomatic Research* 1996; **40**: 231–4.

74. American College of Obstetricians and Gynecologists. *Practice patterns. Routine ultrasound in low-risk pregnancy*. Washington, DC: American College of Obstetrics and Gynecology, 1997.

75. Cunningham FG, MacDonald PC, Gant NF *et al*. (eds) Multifocal pregnancy. In: *Williams obstetrics* 20th edn. Stamford, CT: Appleton & Lange, 1997: 896.

76. Lederman RP. *Psychosocial adaptation in pregnancy. Assessment of seven dimensions of maternal development*, 2nd edn. New York: Springer, 1996.

77. Rhodes N, Hutchinson S. Labor experiences of childhood sexual abuse survivors. *Birth* 1994; **21**: 213–19.

78. Gibbs CP. Obstetrical anesthesia. In: Gabbe SG, Neibyl JR, Simpson JL (eds) *Obstetrics: normal and problem pregnancies*. New York: Churchill Livingstone, 1986: 427–9.

79. Coverdale JM, Chervenak FA, McCullough LB, Bayer T. Ethically justified clinically comprehensive guidelines for the management of the depressed pregnant patient. *American Journal of Obstetrics and Gynecology* 1996; **474**: 169–73.

80. Cunningham FG, MacDonald PC, Gant NF *et al*. (eds) Dystocia due to abnormalities in presentations, position or development of the fetus. In: *Williams obstetrics*, 20th edn. Stamford, CT: Appleton & Lange, 1997: 510–11.

81. Shea MJ, Bleske BE, Santinga JT, Das SK. Heart disease in pregnancy. In: Sciarra JJ (ed.) *Obstetrics and Gynecology. Vol. 2.*. Philadelphia, PA: JP Lippincott, 1995: 10.

82. Cunningham FG, MacDonald PC, Gant NF *et al*. (eds) Forceps delivery and related techniques. In: *Williams obstetrics*, 20th edn. Stamford, CT: Appleton & Lange, 1997: 572.

83. Bianco A, Stone J, Lynch L, Lapinski R, Berkowitz G, Berkowtiz R. Pregnancy outcome at age 40 and older. *Obstetrics and Gynecology* 1996; **6**: 917–22.

84. Cunningham FG, MacDonald PC, Gant NF *et al.* (eds) Obsterical hemorrhage. In: *Williams obstetrics*, 20th edn. Stamford, CT: Appleton & Lange, 1997: 839–43.

85. Cunningham FG, MacDonald PC, Gant NF *et al.* (eds) Preterm and post-term pregnancy and fetal growth retardation. In: *Williams obstetrics*, 20th edn. Stamford, CT: Appleton & Lange, 1997:860–5.

86. Covington SN and Burns LH. Pregnancy after infertility. In: Burns LH, Covington SN (eds) *Infertility counseling: a comprehensive handbook for clinicians*. New York: Parthenon, 1999: 436.

87. Cunningham FG, MacDonald PC, Gant NF *et al.* (eds) Ectopic pregnancy. In: *Williams obstetrics*, 20th edn. Stamford, CT: Appleton & Lange, 1997: 1206.

88. Gise LH. Psychiatric implications of pregnancy. In: Cherry SH, Merkatz IR (eds) *Complications of pregnancy: Medical, surgical, gynecologic, psychosocial and perinatal*, 4th edn. New York: Williams & Wilkins, 1991: 216–20.

89. Cunningham FG, MacDonald PC, Gant NF *et al.* (eds) Ectopic pregnancy. In: *Williams obstetrics*, 20th edn. Stamford, CT: Appleton & Lange, 1997: 695.

90. Dannenberg AL, Lawson HW, Dorfman SF, Ashton DM, Carter DM, Grahan EH. Homicide and other injuries as causes of maternal death in New York City, 1987 through 1991. *American Journal of Obstetrics and Gynecology* 1995; **172**: 1557–64.

91. Little BB, Gilstrap LC, Van Beveren TT. Drug overdoses during pregnancy. In: Gilstrap LC, Little BB (eds) *Drugs and pregnancy*, 2nd edn. New York: Chapman & Hall, 1998: 377–94.

92. Brost BD, Scardo JA, Newman RB. Diphenhydramine overdose during pregnancy: lessons from the past. *American Journal of Obstetrics and Gynecology* 1996; **175**: 1376–7.

93. Cunningham FG, MacDonald PC, Gant NF *et al.* (eds) Forceps delivery and related techniques. In: *Williams obstetrics*, 20th edn. Stamford, CT: Appleton & Lange, 1997: 571.

94. Little BB, Ramin SM, Cambridge BS *et al.* Risk of chromosomal abnormalities with emphasis on live-born offspring of young mothers. *American Journal of Human Genetics* 1995; **57**: 1178–85.

95. Kessler RC, Berglund PA, Foster CL, Saunders WB, Stang PE, Walters EE. Social consequences of psychiatric disorders. II. Teenage parenthood. *American Journal of Psychiatry* 1997; **154**: 1405–11.

96. Braverman AM, Corson SL. Characteristics of participants in a gestational carrier program. *Journal of Assisted Reproduction and Genetics* 1992; **9**: 353–7.

97. Kermani EJ. Issues of child custody and our moral values in the era of new medical technology. *Journal of the American Academy of Child and Adolescent Psychiatry* 1992; **31**: 533–8.

98. Healy JM. The Baby M case: findings and implications. *Connecticut Medicine* 1987; **51**: 407.

99. Deater-Deckard K, Pickering K, Dunn JF, Golding J. Avon longitudinal study of pregnancy and childhood study team. Family structure and depressive symptoms in men preceding and following the birth of a child. *American Journal of Psychiatry* 1998; **155**: 818–235.

100. Dameron GW. Sexuality. In: Gleicher N, Buttino L (eds) *Principles and practice of medical therapy in pregnancy*, 2nd edn. Norwalk, CT: Appleton & Lange, 1994: 206.

3

Clinical assessment and counseling of the pregnant psychiatric patient and those contemplating pregnancy

BERTIS B. LITTLE AND KIMBERLY A. YONKERS

INTRODUCTION

A few disease categories have been viewed quite differently from most others by both ancient and modern societies. Birth defects, cancer, mental retardation, psychiatric illness and hereditary diseases are regarded as stigmatizing diseases, in that their occurrence is consciously or unconsciously perceived by the affected individual or their family as an affliction or punishment. In ancient Babylonia, mothers who delivered a child with some type of birth defect were punished, because it was believed that the malformed child represented retribution for acts of misbehavior. Historically, fathers or mothers of malformed infants were ridiculed, criticized, persecuted or even prosecuted.[1,2] Folklore and superstition dominated the field, and such maladies were attributed to evil spirits, fornication with animals, lewd thoughts or other immoral acts. In the 1600s, the idea of seeking compensation for the birth of a malformed child would probably never have arisen. In fact, the opposite was the case for a farm worker in New Haven, Connecticut, named George Spencer, who was sentenced to death in 1642 because he owned a swine that gave birth to malformed pigs.

More than a 1000 trials involving malformed infants have been recorded since the execution of George Spencer. Injustices may not be as extreme as in his case,[2,3] but they still occur. Since the 1960s injustices have tended to favor the affected plaintiff.[4] Drug or chemical-related causes of maternal complications, congenital anomalies and fetal toxicity are unique because they are presumed to be preventable. However, there is a narrow window of opportunity within which it is possible to act with preventative measures (see Figure 3.1). Thus, as potentially preventable causes of 'damage,' they are often the focus of malpractice litigation. Attorneys recognize that in some instances such adverse outcomes could have been avoided, and litigation ensues despite the fact that the window of opportunity for intervening prudently may not have existed for the physician. More importantly, the drug exposure may not be teratogenic. Patients and attorneys often have the perception that a large number of infants are born with congenital anomalies or other deficits because they were affected by intrauterine exposure to drugs or medications. In fact, fewer than 1% of congenital malformations (birth defects) are due to drugs prescribed by physicians or chemicals in the environment (see Figure 3.2).[5]

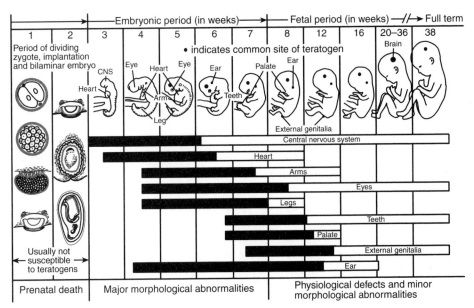

Figure 3.1 *Timing of prenatal developmental events (reproduced from Airens and Simonis[6], with permission).*

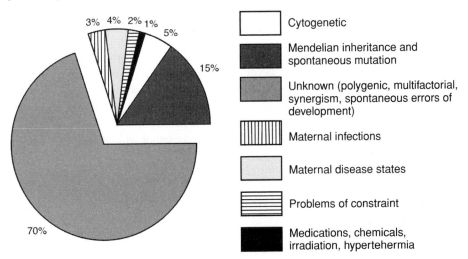

Figure 3.2 *Etiology of congenital anomalies by cause (compiled from Beckman and Brent[23]).*

More importantly, serious congenital malformations occur in approximately 3% of live offspring. Since exposure to drugs, chemicals and physical agents occurs quite commonly (50–90% of cases), it can readily be understood why the occurrence of a congenital malformation and exposure to such agents could be mistakenly concluded to have a causal basis. However, physicians or employers may be blamed even if the drugs or medications are not known to cause congenital anomalies when used during pregnancy. It is well documented scientifically that among known causes of birth defects, drug or medication exposure during pregnancy ranks last, although such exposure ranks high on the list of litigation. Perhaps the area of greatest concern for pregnant patients who must chronically use a medication to maintain their health is concern for the safety of their unborn child. Birth defects are among the greatest fears of these patients, as is abnormal mental development.

Knowledge of the effects of prenatal exposure and the opportunity for intervention are the key factors in the evaluation and prevention of morbidity and mortality due to drug and chemical exposure during pregnancy. It is difficult to intervene and encourage drug discontinuation, as most pregnant women do not present for prenatal care until embryogenesis is complete (i.e. after 58 days postconception). Intervention is further complicated by the fact that many women are unaware of the potential adverse affects of drugs and chemicals during pregnancy. For example, in a study of 1600 recently delivered women, more than 60% had never heard of fetal alcohol syndrome and were reportedly unaware of the adverse effects of alcohol on pregnancy.[7]

Clearly, patient education prior to conception is the most effective form of intervention, but there are many social and cultural barriers to overcome in this process. For example, many obstetrical patients have culturally based 'folk etiologies' for the occurrence of birth defects and other adverse pregnancy outcomes that are not usually correlated with medically accepted causes. Folk explanations must therefore be taken into account when informing the obstetrical patient of the risks to pregnancy of medications, drugs and chemicals. Folk etiologies for congenital anomalies are founded on culturally influenced notions and rationale, and are usually culture-specific. Examples include the 'evil eye' or 'working roots' explanations for abnormalities. The idea that birth defects are caused by maternal sins is also common in certain cultures. Inbreeding is almost universally accepted as a cause of adverse pregnancy outcomes, but this is based on religious rather than biological reasoning.

MAGNITUDE OF THE PROBLEM

Women use a wide variety of medications during pregnancy, but the prevalence varies from one country to another.[8,9] In an older community survey, 97% of the pregnant women surveyed took prescribed drugs and two-thirds took self-administered drugs.[15] In an Australian study, 66% of women took prescribed drugs during their pregnancy.[11] According to two community surveys, 70% of pregnant women in the USA took prescribed drugs[11,12] and according to another study 85% of pregnant Egyptian women took medications during pregnancy.[13]

In England, only 35% of pregnant women took drugs or medications during pregnancy, and only 6% used medications other than vitamin or iron supplements during the first trimester.[14] In Michigan, women received an average of 3.1 prescriptions for medications other than vitamins or iron during their pregnancies.[15] Medications commonly taken during pregnancy included anti-emetics, antacids, antihistamines, analgesics, antibiotics, tranquilizers, hypnotics, nutritional supplements and diuretics. Clearly, medication use during pregnancy is a frequent event, although its safety may be questionable in many instances.

Frequently, pregnant women take prescription drugs that are not intended for use during pregnancy. Some of these medications are taken before the pregnant state is recognized, and some are taken without or against the physician's advice once the pregnancy is recognized.[8,9] In practice, physicians frequently have to determine whether a medication or drug may be harmful to a pregnant woman or her unborn child after the exposure has occurred. Substance abuse during pregnancy is also prevalent, and is discussed in detail in Chapters 12 and 13. Briefly, an estimated 10–20% of pregnant women use illicit substances and/or alcohol during their pregnancies. In 1999, cocaine appeared to be the most frequently used illegal substance (Chasnoff, personal communication).

CLINICAL EVALUATION

Information that will assist physicians in elucidating the effects of psychotropic exposure on human pregnancy is discussed under the specific psychopathology. Clinical evaluation of potentially teratogenic and/or toxic exposures must consider maternal, embryonic and fetal aspects of pregnancy.

TERATOGENS

A teratogen is defined as any agent, physical force or other factor that can induce a congenital anomaly through alteration of normal development during any stage of embryogenesis.[16] Such agents include drugs and other chemicals, and physical forces such as ionizing radiation. Teratogenic maternal diseases include disorders such as diabetes mellitus and phenylketonuria. Any of the agents that cause defects during the postembryonic (fetal) period have the potential to give rise to adverse fetal effects. However, not all agents or factors that are teratogens have adverse fetal effects, and vice versa.

The period of the embryo is described as the growth of undifferentiated cells into specialized cells that are arranged in specific ways (i.e. organs and specialized tissues). These specialized cell lines or lineages increase in number and change in structure and arrangement, giving rise to organs and tissues. Some organs and tissues are formed earlier than others. For example, the brain and spine form earlier than the face and endocrine system. After embryogenesis (58–60 days postconception) is complete, the conceptus is a fetus (see Figure 3.1). With few exceptions, the morphological architecture for a normal (or abnormal) human is laid down during the embryonic period, and these structures simply grow in size and develop normal physiologic function during the fetal period. Birth defects may be induced during the fetal period through a fetal effect, although congenital anomalies are usually induced during the critical embryonic period. For example, a structure that was formed normally during embryogenesis can be damaged during the fetal period, and the resulting malformation may appear to have arisen during morphogenesis. A classic example of a fetal effect is hemorrhaging due to coumadin exposure, which may induce brain or eye defects despite the fact that these structures were formed normally during the embryonic period.

Animal studies

Animal models are poor predictors of whether a drug or chemical is a human teratogen. The sensitivity and specificity of animal models for human teratogenicity are related directly to the particular species used. Non-human primates are better predictors of human teratogenicity and fetotoxicity than are non-primate models, because the former are phylogenetically close to humans. Interpretation of animal teratology experiments is further complicated by the use of dosages that are many times higher than those given to humans, so that maternal toxic effects may confound the interpretation of fetal outcome. In addition, the metabolism and absorption of drugs and chemicals often vary greatly between different species. Inter-species differences in placentation, pharmacodynamics, embryonic development and innate predisposition to various congenital anomalies are well recognized. Of approximately 2000 drugs and chemicals tested in animal models, 55% were found to have teratogenic effects.[7]

Animal teratology studies are traditionally used to evaluate the safety of medications for use during human pregnancy, and are an accepted part of the Food and Drug Administration (FDA) drug approval process. Consequently, human teratogens are discovered only after numerous children have already been born with malformations. The main problem with animal teratology studies is that the most frequently used models are rodents, which are phylogenetically distant from humans. Rodent physiology, metabolism and ontogenetic development are quite different from those of humans. It is important to note that the sensitivity and specificity of rodent studies are both less than 60%.[17] Teratology studies using non-human primates are considerably better predictors of which medications may be harmful when given during human pregnancy, with a sensitivity and specificity of more than 90%. However, non-human primate studies are whole orders of magnitude more expensive than rodent teratology studies, and for this reason few drugs are evaluated in primates. Unfortunately, the ultimate assessment of the safety of medication use in pregnancy must come from human studies.[16,17]

Human studies

Human teratogens are identified by careful interpretation of data obtained from several different kinds of reports, including case reports, clinical series and epidemiologic studies.[16,18–20] Case reports and clinical series often provide the first evidence that an agent is teratogenic in humans. A recurrent pattern of birth defects in babies who experienced similar well-defined exposures at common points during embryogenesis suggests that the agent in question may be teratogenic. Although they are important for generating hypotheses, case reports cannot provide reliable quantitative estimates of the risk of anomalies in an exposed pregnancy. Quantitative estimates of the strength and statistical significance of associations between exposure of pregnant women to agents and the development of abnormalities in their offspring may only be obtained via epidemiological studies. It is important to note that most hypotheses are subsequently shown to be incorrect. For example, a high incidence of environmental exposure to spermicides by pregnant women who have children with congenital anomalies in their offspring is a coincidental occurrence.

CRITICAL TIME PERIODS

Three specific periods of development *in utero* are critical, namely preimplantation, the period of the embryo and the time of the fetus. Any evaluation of drugs and medications for use during pregnancy must consider these time periods differentially, because the effects on the unborn child are dependent on the time of exposure (Figure 3.1).

Preimplantation

On conception (penetration of the ovum by the spermatid to form a single diploid cell) no physiologic interface between the mother and the conceptus exists. Theoretically, the first week postconception is the 'protected period.' This is the time that elapses until the blastocyst attaches to the wall of the uterus and begins to form chorionic villi and build the maternoplacental and embroplacental vascular interfaces necessary for the mother's circulation to deliver oxygen and other nutrients to the conceptus. Based on current understanding of pre-embryonic biology, before implantation the conceptus is protected from drugs or medications that may be transported in the maternal circulation because there is no formal biological interface between the blastocyst and the mother. However, there are some exceptions in which passive diffusion of small amounts of medication may occur (e.g. mitomycin C).

Embryonic development

The period of the embryo is a critical stage of development for the genesis or inception of birth defects. This stage occurs from the time of implantation until 58–60 days postconception. The structures that comprise organs and tissues of the unborn baby are being formed during this period, which is also termed organogenesis. Errors that occur in the formation of these structures are manifested as malformations (congenital anomalies) at birth, and are deemed to be birth defects. Teratogens are agents that cause abnormal physical or physiological embryonic development by acting during the period of the embryo, or organogenesis.[21] Malformations that are lethal to the embryo present as spontaneous abortion which often occurs before the pregnancy is recognized. Similarly, some substances are directly toxic to the embryo (e.g. methotrexate). The critical times for the development of various organs and structures of the human embryo are shown in Figure 3.1.

Fetal development

Changes in certain cellular structures (e.g. the brain's neuronal arrangement) occur during the fetal period. The predominant fetal event is hyperplastic growth (i.e. increase in cell number). Organs and other tissues become larger via cellular proliferation. The thyroid appears early in the fetal period, and the genesis of other fetal endocrine functions takes place soon after embryogenesis is complete. The majority of potential adverse effects during fetal development consist of growth retardation and maldevelopment due to interrupted cell migration.[21] However, malformations in organ structures that were formed normally during embryogenesis may occur (e.g. with fetal cocaine or warfarin exposure). If blood flow to an organ or structure is interrupted or obstructed, an organ or structure could undergo necrosis and be resolved. This may even produce a defect that mimics a teratogenic effect when the true origin of the defect would be in fact fetotoxicity.

Drugs reach the embryo and fetus through the placenta. The placenta can metabolize certain drugs before they reach the embryofetal compartment, but the extent to which there is a protective effect is unknown. An estimated 99% of drugs can cross the placenta, in most cases by simple diffusion. However, drugs that are composed of large molecules (i.e. molecular weight > 1000) generally do not cross the placenta unless there is an active transport system (e.g. antibodies). In addition, some characteristics of molecules other than size interfere with placental transport. Drugs that are highly polar have little potential for placental passage, and the same is true for drugs that are tightly bound to maternal serum proteins.[22] Some drugs may accumulate in the embryofetal compartment because of the poor potential for transfer back to the maternal circulation. Lipid-soluble drugs are easily transported from the mother to the fetus, and vice versa. However, although water-soluble drugs are readily transferred to the fetus, transfer back to the mother's circulation is not easily achieved. In general, water-soluble drugs tend to accumulate in the amniotic fluid (i.e. the fetal compartment).

POTENTIAL ADVERSE EFFECTS AND SPONTANEOUS ABORTION

It is estimated that 50% of early pregnancies (0–58 days) end in spontaneous abortion, and recent findings from *in-vitro* fertilization studies suggest that the majority of these cases may be caused by abnormal chromosomal constitution. Of fetuses surviving 59–126 days of gestation, 15–20% may abort, and the risk decreases to 1–2% by 18–20 weeks (127–140 days). After this early fetal period, up until 28 weeks (196 days), surviving conceptuses have a similar risk of approximately 2% for spontaneous abortion.[23]

Congenital anomalies

Approximately 3.5–5% of congenital anomalies are detected at birth.[24] This figure is thought to underestimate the true frequency of anomalies by as much as twofold. Only 50% of birth defects are detected at birth, and 100% detection of anomalies is not usually achieved until about 5 years of age. The frequency of congenital anomalies is higher among stillbirths and miscarriages, and is especially high among early (i.e. first-trimester) miscarriages.[25]

Fetal effects

Fetal effects are of four primary types, namely damage to structures or organs that are formed normally during embryogenesis, damage to systems undergoing histogenesis during the fetal period, growth retardation, or fetal death or stillbirth. Any or all of these fetal effects can occur concomitantly. Fetal effects may be caused by a teratogen, but may also be generated by agents that have no apparent potential to produce abnormal embryonic development. Organs, structures or functions that have developed normally during embryogenesis can be damaged by some environmental exposures during the fetal period. The most frequently observed effect of agents given during pregnancy and outside the period of embryogenesis is fetal growth retardation. However, it is often difficult to distinguish the effects of the agents from those of the disease entity being treated. For example, propranolol is associated with fetal growth retardation, but the maternal disease for which the drug is given (hypertension) is also associated with fetal growth retardation in the absence of antihypertensive therapy. Some agents that are teratogenic may be associated with fetal growth retardation, and the latter may occur in the absence of embryonic damage. An increased risk of fetal death and stillbirth is associated with exposure to some agents during pregnancy.

Neonatal and postnatal effects

Developmental delay is frequently associated with the action of teratogens, but is also observed in association with the fetal effects of drugs that are apparently not teratogenic. For example, after exposure *in utero* to glucocorticoids and immunosuppressants, the immune systems of infants may be suppressed and thus rendered susceptible to infection. Certain drugs are associated with adverse neonatal effects, such as difficulty in adapting to life outside the womb. These same drugs are not necessarily associated with teratogenic effects. Transient metabolic abnormalities, withdrawal and hypoglycemia are well-documented neonatal effects of certain medications and non-medical drugs. Infants that are exposed prenatally to heroin, which is not a teratogen, frequently experience mild to moderate postnatal growth and developmental delays.[8,9] Examples of other adverse neonatal effects include floppy infant syndrome following the use of benzodiazepines near term, patent ductus arteriosus with the use of prostaglandin synthetase inhibitors (NSAIDs) such as aspirin or indomethacin, and gray baby syndrome with high-dose chloramphenicol near the time of delivery.

MATERNAL PHYSIOLOGY DURING PREGNANCY

Profound physiological changes occur during pregnancy (see Chapter 2). Maternal enzymes, particularly cholinesterases, show lowered activity. The maternal blood volume increases dramatically during pregnancy, perhaps by 40–50%, to support the requirements of the developing fetus. The distribution of drugs in this increased blood volume may lower serum concentrations. Absorption of drugs occurs with about the same kinetics as in the non-pregnant adult. However, renal clearance is increased and some enzyme activity is down-regulated. Decreased levels of enzyme activity are exacerbated somewhat by the increased blood volume, thereby decreasing the overall effective serum concentration of a given dose. Concomitantly, increased renal output may result in an increased clearance index for most drugs.[26] Drugs that are tightly bound to the serum proteins have little opportunity to cross the placenta or enter breast-milk. Consequently, increased demands are placed on cardiovascular, hepatic and renal systems. In addition, the gravid uterus is vulnerable to a variety of effects that are not present in the non-pregnant state (e.g. hemorrhage, rupture or preterm contraction).

PRENATAL DIAGNOSIS

Medication exposure or substance use during pregnancy, including that which is chronic, is not necessarily an indication for pregnancy termination. However, it is an indication for prenatal diagnosis. Although prenatal diagnosis cannot rule out defects that are not related to structural abnormalities, major congenital anomalies (e.g. spina bifida, structured heart defects and limb reduction) can usually be determined prenatally. Three types of prenatal diagnosis can be used to screen for congenital anomalies and other fetal complications following the use of medications or drugs during pregnancy, namely high-resolution ultrasound, maternal serum alpha-fetoprotein (MSAFP) and fetal echocardiography. Ultrasound studies are useful in assessment of fetal growth and in the possible detection of specific structural anomalies of major organs. MSAFP is important for screening pregnancies for open neural-tube or other open defects (e.g. gastroschisis). Although amniocentesis may be performed to assess an abnormal alpha-fetoprotein level, with the exception of colchicine, a karyotype study is not indicated in the setting of drug or alcohol exposure. Fetal echocardiography is used to screen for cardiovascular defects such as valvular defects and vascular stenosis (which cannot be detected with the basic ultrasound four-chamber view of the heart).

During counseling, the patient should be advised of the limitations of prenatal diagnosis not only with regard to the limitations on what can be detected (i.e. gross structural abnormalities), but also in terms of its reliability in detecting defects prenatally (ranging from 40%

to 90%).[27] Counseling of patients who have been exposed to drugs or other environmental agents during pregnancy is difficult for several reasons. Many patients experience anxiety about such exposure because they fear that their child will be born with birth defects. This anxiety is heightened because the mother frequently feels guilt, believing that she may have damaged her baby through some action of her own. Cultural beliefs about the causes of congenital anomalies differ from scientific explanations, and generally place blame on the mother. Other factors, such as the patient's educational background, socio-economic status and ethnic-specific culture, may also present an obstacle to communication during counseling. These influences come into play when counseling patients who have been or are exposed to potential teratogens. It is important to establish a good rapport with the patient, ensure confidentiality and establish a basis for the patient's trust. The counselor must convey to the patient his or her understanding of their concerns, and explain that the purpose of the consultation is to deal directly with those concerns by ascertaining the magnitude of the risk of an adverse pregnancy outcome due to the drug exposure.

GENERAL PRINCIPLES OF COUNSELING

Patients are frequently dissatisfied with the counseling they receive for exposure to potential teratogens during pregnancy, due to two major issues that cause them anxiety. First, the physician is frequently unable to obtain adequate information to enable him or her to make meaningful statements about the medical risks and whether the pregnancy was adversely affected by the drug exposure. Secondly, most patients do not understand the difference between an embryo and a fetus. Consequently, they may be unable to grasp the importance of the concept of 'critical periods' unless they have been given a proper briefing during the consultation. The first phase is embryonic development, during which period the structure, or architecture, of the baby is established. Embryonic age must be differentiated from menstrual age, which is 2 weeks longer than embryonic age. It should be briefly explained to the patient that organs take shape and the body assumes the form it will have thereafter by the day 58 postconception (see Figure 3.1). All of the major structures, including the heart, brain, liver, kidneys and limbs, have formed by this time. Fetal development during the remainder of pregnancy (the second phase of development) is primarily devoted to the growth of these organs and structures and to augmentation of their function. This heuristic approach to counseling the patient helps her to understand that most congenital anomalies are due to early exposures, often before the pregnancy is recognized. This ameliorates any anxiety and guilt. This information should be conveyed early in the consultation and the patient will then understand why certain questions are so important. Possession of such knowledge also increases patient co-operation and rapport.

PRECONCEPTIONAL COUNSELING

Ideally, all counseling with regard to drug or medication use during pregnancy should take place before conception, because the opportunity to prevent possible adverse effects is then optimal. Preconceptional counseling should include all the components of a consultation during the pregnancy, with one exception. Recommendations regarding medication use during pregnancy will be for a preventive purpose, and only medically indicated drugs and medications that are known to be safe would be recommended for continued use during attempts to conceive and during gestation.

COUNSELING THE EXPOSED GRAVIDA

Counseling for drug or medication exposure during pregnancy should follow the protocol outlined in the flow diagram in Figure 3.3. The concept of background risk for major congenital anomalies should be explained in a manner that is tailored to the patient's level of understanding. This concept is particularly important because it conveys to the patient that, even if the drug to which she has been exposed is harmless, no guarantee can be given that the fetus she is carrying will not have a congenital anomaly. Notwithstanding other risk factors, the risk for major congenital anomalies is approximately 3.5–5%. Other identified risks (e.g. family history, maternal disease status, etc.) are generally considered to be additive to background risk.

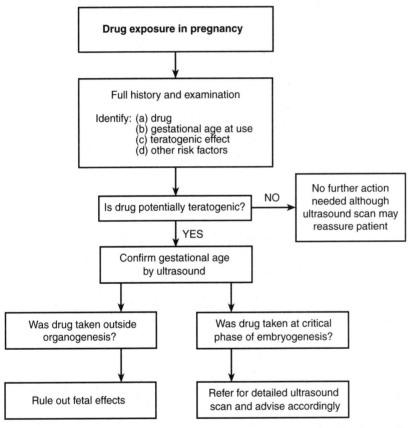

Figure 3.3 *Protocol for evaluation of prenatal exposure to drugs (modified from Rubin[15]).*

An important component of counseling is the determination of exactly what drugs were taken, the dosage, timing and duration of exposure, the patient's health history and her present state of health. A thorough physical examination should be used to determine the present state of health. In addition, a medical genetic pedigree that includes the patient's parents, as well as the baby's father's parents, brothers and sisters, and nieces and nephews, should be constructed (see Figure 3.4). The current state of health of all individuals in the pedigree should also be elicited. For those individuals in the pedigree who are no longer living, the cause of death (e.g. whether it was due to a birth defect or a heritable disorder)

UNIVERSITY OF TEXAS HEALTH SCIENCE CENTER AT DALLAS
DEPARTMENT OF OBSTETRICS AND GYNECOLOGY
DIVISION OF CLINICAL GENETICS

FAMILY HISTORY

PATIENT NAME Jane Doe   AGE 36

Constructed by VRK
DATE 1/1/88

REASON FOR REFERRAL Advanced Maternal Age

Husband/FOB

                              Patient   John Doe - Age 38

Health history History of Urinary tract Infections,
                Family History of Neurfibromatosis

Medications Prenatal Vitamins   Same

X-rays None

Alcohol None   Smoking 1/2 PPD

High risk ethnic group Non Jewish; Non Mediterranean; White

Bleeding/Cramping No

Treatment No

Other pregnancy complications None

COMMENTS: No FH Birth Defects or Genetic Diseases   CONSANGUINITY: (NO)   YES

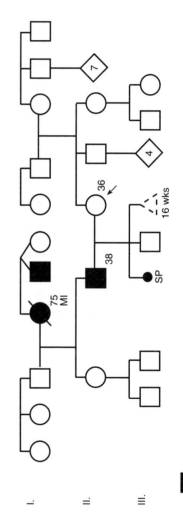

■ Neurofibromatosis

Figure 3.4 (a) Medical genetic pedigree.

PEDIGREE SYMBOLS

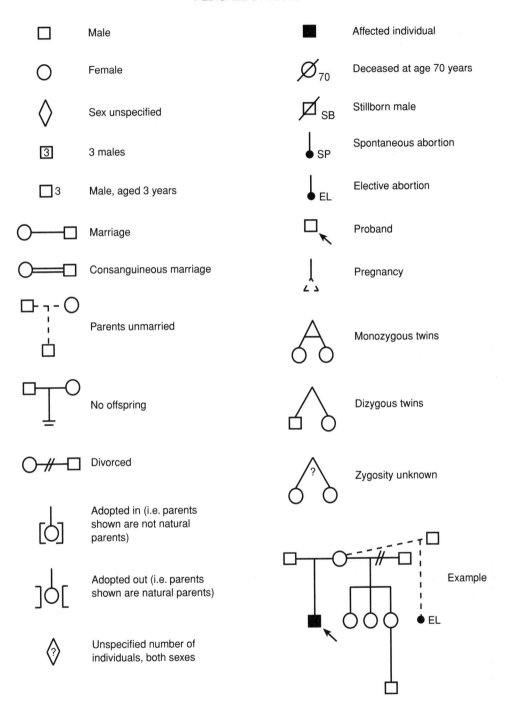

□	Male	■	Affected individual
○	Female	Ø₇₀	Deceased at age 70 years
◇	Sex unspecified		Stillborn male (SB)
3	3 males		Spontaneous abortion (SP)
□3	Male, aged 3 years		Elective abortion (EL)
○—□	Marriage		Proband
○=□	Consanguineous marriage		Pregnancy
	Parents unmarried		Monozygous twins
	No offspring		Dizygous twins
○—//—□	Divorced		Zygosity unknown
	Adopted in (i.e. parents shown are not natural parents)		
	Adopted out (i.e. parents shown are natural parents)		Example
◇?	Unspecified number of individuals, both sexes		

Figure 3.4 *(b) Pedigree symbols.*

Sample Prenatal Genetic Screen*

Name _____ Patient# _____ Date _____

1. Will you be 35 years or older when the baby is due?	Yes_____	No _____
2. Have you, the baby's father, or anyone in either of your families ever had any of the following disorders?	Yes_____	No_____
• Down's syndrome (mongolism)	Yes_____	No_____
• Other chromosomal abnormality	Yes_____	No_____
• Neural tube defect, i.e. spina bifida (meningomyelocele or open spine), anencephaly	Yes_____	No_____
• Hemophilia	Yes_____	No_____
• Muscular dystrophy	Yes_____	No_____
• Cystic fibrosis	Yes_____	No_____

If yes, indicate the relationship of the affected person to you or to the baby's father: _____

3. Do you or the baby's father have a birth defect?   Yes_____ No_____
If yes, who has the defect and what is it? _____

4. In any previous marriages, have you or the baby's father had a
child, born dead or alive, with a birth defect not listed in
question 2 above?   Yes_____ No_____
If yes, what was the defect and who had it? _____

5. Do you or the baby's father have any close relatives with mental retardation?   Yes_____ No_____
If yes, indicate the relationship of the affected person to you or the baby's father: _____
Indicate the cause, if known: _____

6. Do you, the baby's father, or a close relative in either of your families have a birth
defect, any familial disorder, or a chromosomal abnormality not listed above?   Yes_____ No_____
If yes, indicate the condition and the relationship of the affected person to you or to the
baby's father: _____
_____

7. In any previous marriages, have you or the baby's father had a still born child or three
or more first-trimester spontaneous pregnancy losses?   Yes_____ No_____
Have either of you had a chromosomal study?   Yes_____ No_____
If yes, indicate who and the results: _____
_____

8. If you or the baby's father are of Jewish ancestry, have either of you been screened for
Tay-Sachs disease?   Yes_____ No_____
If yes, indicate who and the results: _____
_____

9. If you or the baby's father are black, have either of you been screened for sickle-cell
trait?   Yes_____ No_____
If yes, indicate who and the results: _____

10. If you or the baby's father are of Italian, Greek, or Mediterranean background, have
either of you been tested for β-thalassemia?   Yes_____ No_____
If yes indicate who and the results: _____
_____

11. If you or the baby's father are of Philippine or Southeast Asian ancestry, have either of
you been tested for α-thalassemia?   Yes_____ No_____
If yes, indicate who and the results: _____
_____

12. Excluding iron and vitamins, have you taken any medications or recreational drugs
since being pregnant or since your last menstrual period? (include non-prescription
drugs)   Yes_____ No_____
If yes, give name of medication and time taken during pregnancy: _____
_____

*Any patient replying 'YES' to questions should be offered appropriate counseling. If the patient declines further counseling or testing, this should be noted in the chart. Given that genetics is a field in a state of flux, alterations or updates to this form will be required periodically.

Figure 3.4 *(c) Questionnaire.*

should be determined. It is also important to ask whether the patient's family or the baby's father's family have any members who are mentally retarded, or who have a chromosomal abnormality, Down's syndrome or mongolism, congenital heart disease, spina bifida or some other neural-tube defect, or any other inherited disease. If such risk factors are discovered, it is important to explore these avenues further, and it may be desirable to refer the patient for a medical genetic consultation and evaluation.

The next step in the consultation is to determine whether or not the agent(s) have known teratogenic potential. This is the most difficult part of the evaluation because there is insufficient information to make such a determination for more than 60% of medications. The most up-to-date and reliable source of information on drug or medication use during pregnancy is TERIS, a computerized database available for use either on IBM-compatible personal computers or on-line by subscription (see Table 3.1). If it can be ascertained that the agent has no teratogenic risks or adverse fetal effects associated with its use during pregnancy, then no further action is required except to document this in the medical record and counsel the patient accordingly. However, one should never assume that the absence of data indicates an absence of risk. Some patients may benefit from reassurance offered by high-resolution ultrasound to confirm fetal well-being, and this procedure should be offered if the patient's anxiety is not relieved by counseling. However, the limitations of diagnostic ultrasound must be mentioned in the consultation.

If the drug is known to be unsafe for use during pregnancy, or if there are reasons to suspect that a drug with unknown risks is associated with congenital anomalies, then the gestational age should be confirmed by ultrasound. It is essential to base the risk assessment and counseling on embryonic age, not menstrual age. If the exposure occurred during embryogenesis, then it is necessary to perform high-resolution ultrasound in an attempt to detect damage to specific organ systems or structures that were being formed at the time of exposure. If the ultrasound scan is normal, then it is reasonable to reassure the patient of the apparently normal fetal structure (within the limits of the sensitivity and specificity of ultrasound, which range from 40% to 90% for gross structural abnormalities when the procedure is performed by an experienced sonographer). If the exposure occurred during the fetal period, it is again important to evaluate the possible fetal effects of the medication.

Table 3.1 *Sources of information on potential teratogens for counseling*

Computerized database

ReproTox, Columbia Women's Hospital, Washington, DC (202) 293–5138
TERIS – Department of Pediatrics, University of Washington, Seattle (206) 543–4365
TOXLINE, National Library of Medicine, Bethesda, MD (800) 638–8480

Published volumes

Schardein JL. *Chemically induced birth defects* New York: Marcel Dekker, 1993.
Shephard TH. *Catalog of teratogenic agents*, 8th edn. Baltimore, MD: Johns Hopkins University Press, 1995.
Gilstrap LC, Little BB (eds) *Drugs and pregnancy*, 2nd edn. New York: Chapman and Hall, 1998.
Briggs GG, Freeman RK, Yaffe SJ. *Drugs in pregnancy and lactation*, 4th edn. Baltimore, MD: Williams & Wilkins, 1994.
Niebyl JR. *Drug use in pregnancy*. Philadelphia, PA: Lea & Febiger, 1998.
Berkowits RL, Coustan DR, Mochizuki TK. *Handbook for prescribing during pregnancy*. Boston, MA: Little, Brown & Co., 1986.
Rubin PC. *Prescribing in Pregnancy*. London: BMJ publications, 1986.
Friedman JM, Polifka, JE. *Teratogenic effects of drugs: a resource for clinicians (TERIS)* Baltimore, MD: Johns Hopkins University Press, 2000.

If defects are detected, it is necessary to describe them in detail to the patient and to give a prognosis (as accurately as available medical knowledge will allow) regarding the outcome of pregnancy and postnatal development. Prognostication should include medically documented risk figures to aid the patient in making a decision about the disposition of the pregnancy. Ethically, pregnancy termination should not be recommended to the patient, her family and significant others. This option should be discussed, but the ultimate decision of whether to continue the pregnancy should be left to the patient, her family and significant others. The role of teratogen counseling is ultimately to provide the patient with as much information as possible, and to encourage her to make her own decision as to whether or not to continue the pregnancy. The counselor must be aware that some patients are seeking justification for pregnancy termination, and may attempt to manipulate the situation to this end.

In 1979, the Food and Drug Administration (FDA) attempted to improve labeling policies for the use of medications during pregnancy. Five risk categories that addressed potential adverse fetal effects, including congenital anomalies, were developed. Although it is an improvement over the previous labeling disclaimers, this classification is still less than perfect.[5]

According to the *Physicians' Desk Reference*,[28] the categories devised by the FDA are 'based on the degree to which available information has ruled out risk to the fetus, balanced against the drug's potential benefits to the patient.' Although these were intended to provide management guidelines about teratogenic risks, one study has found that FDA categories show little if any correlation with teratogenic risk. Friedman and colleagues[29] compared the teratogenic risk of the 157 most frequently prescribed drugs according to TERIS (Teratogen Information System), a computerized database of clinical teratology data, with the FDA pregnancy categories (where available). These authors pointed out that 'any classification of agents according to teratogenic risk is incomplete because the risk to a given patient is determined by all of the conditions of exposure.' Paramount importance must also be ascribed to drug dose, route of administration and timing of exposure, as well as exposure to multiple agents during the pregnancy.[29] The information on the package insert, which is jointly prepared by the FDA and the pharmaceutical company, fails to provide details about known risks, does not discuss the option of pregnancy interruption, and provides anxiety-provoking details that are irrelevant (e.g. this drug crosses the placental barrier).[5]

INFORMED CONSENT AND POST-EXPOSURE COUNSELING

Before obtaining informed consent regarding medication exposure during pregnancy, the dose, route of administration and timing of exposure must be ascertained as accurately as possible. Even if an agent is a potential teratogen that poses a significant risk, or a proven teratogen such as thalidomide, the actual risk to the fetus may be minimal or non-existent if the timing of exposure occurred during late pregnancy or after the period of organogenesis. In contrast, some teratogens (e.g. radioactive iodine or the angiotensin-converting-enzyme inhibitors) may only be harmful after early organogenesis.[30]

After a detailed history has been obtained, the patient should be given 'full disclosure' of the known or suspected risk of the agent, as well as the various therapeutic and diagnostic options that are available. This information should be accurate, but also presented in a form that is easily understood. All such information and counseling should be fully documented in the patient's chart.

All counseling on drug or medication exposure should be conducted by a clinician who is knowledgeable in both teratology and counseling. Taking the whole clinical picture into account, one should utilize a resource such as TERIS as well as other teratogen information resources to obtain the most up-to-date and accurate information possible on the potential teratogenic effects of a specific agent. Experienced counselors may also have their own personal reprint collection on the subject of teratogens. We include all such information in the patient's chart, and it is used as an adjunct in the counseling of each drug- or chemical-exposed pregnant patient.

Needless to say, litigation may result from inexperience in the field of teratology, lack of information or misinformation, especially if the latter leads to an otherwise unwanted pregnancy termination. Brent has suggested that the following labeling might prove useful for many agents, and when providing patients with details prior to requesting their informed consent: 'The risk of spontaneous malformations is much greater than any risk of the drug that could be hypothesized from available information. . . .'[5] Thus the patient could be advised that the risk of a specific drug is less (or at least no greater) than the 3–5% risk of congenital anomalies in the general population, and that termination of pregnancy is not warranted on the basis of such a risk.[5] For agents such as methotrexate that carry a significant risk, Brent has suggested the following statement: 'The embryotoxic risks of methotrexate have been evaluated by human and animal teratologic studies. An inadvertent or therapeutic exposure during pregnancy imposes an increased risk substantially greater than the spontaneous risk.'[5]

In counseling, one could also make the following statement: 'Although this agent may be associated with an increased risk of malformation when utilized in the first 8 to 10 (menstrual) weeks of pregnancy, it would not be expected to be associated with significant risk when given in the latter half of pregnancy.' In the case of an agent such as tetracycline, one might state: 'It is logical to conclude that tetracycline would not be expected to cause yellow-brown discoloration of the teeth when given during the first 16 to 20 weeks of pregnancy.'

Another suggested statement would be as follows: 'Although the actual teratogenic risk of this agent is unknown, given the dose and route of administration, the fetal risk of this preparation is negligible to non-existent, since little to none of it reaches the fetus.'

Other sources of information on the teratogenic risk of specific agents that may be useful in counseling patients include *Drugs and Pregnancy*,[31] TERIS,[32] *Shepard's Catalog of Teratogenic Agents*,[16] *A Reference Guide to Fetal and Neonatal Risk*[33] and *Chemically Induced Birth Defects*.[17]

SUMMARY

In summary, the clinician must be cognizant of the fact that many patients as well as attorneys believe that most congenital malformations must be secondary to a drug or medication that was taken during gestation. Counseling of such patients requires a significant degree of both knowledge and skill, and should include information regarding the risks and benefits of both drug administration and drug discontinuation. It is hoped that the building of a relationship of trust between the patient and her physicians before conception will facilitate the best possible outcome for both mother and baby.

REFERENCES

1. Warkany J, Kalter H. Maternal impressions and congenital malformations. *Plastic and Reconstructive Surgery* 1962; **30**: 628.
2. Landauer W. Hybridization between animals and man as a cause of congenital malformations. *Extra Archives of Anatomy, Histology and Embryology: normales et experimental* (Supplement): 1961; 44–155.
3. Hoadley CJ. *Records of the colony and plantation of New Haven from 1638 to 1649*. Hartford, CT: Case, Tiffany & Co., 1857.
4. Brent RL. Medicolegal aspects of teratology. *Journal of Pediatrics* 1967; **71**: 288–98.
5. Brent RL: Drugs and pregnancy: are the insert warnings too dire? *Contemporary Obstetrics and Gynecology* 1982; **20**: 42.
6. Airens ES, Simonis AM. De invlsed can Chemischestoffen op het angebaren kind. *Natuuren Technieke* 1974; **43**: 4.
7. Madry KG, Fredlund EV, Wallisch LS, Spence RT. *1990 Texas Survey of Postpartum and Drug-Exposed Infants*. Austin, TX: Texas Commission on Alcohol and Drug Abuse, 1991.
8. Little BB, Gilstrap LC, Cunningham FG *et al*. Medication use during pregnancy part 1. Concepts of human teratology. In: Pritchard J, MacDonald P, Gant N (eds) *Williams' obstetrics*, 18th edn. *Supplement 10*. Norwalk, CT: Appleton & Lange, 1991: 1–15.
9. Nelson MM, Forfar JO. Association between drugs administered during pregnancy and congenital abnormalities of the fetus. *British Medical Journal* 1971; **1**: 523–7.
10. Abdul-Hadi B, Torok J, Mezey G. Drug utilization study during pregnancy. *Acta Pharmaceutica Hungarica* 1995; **65**: 69–75.
11. Fitzgerald M. Prescription and over-the-counter drug use during pregnancy. *Journal of the American Academy of Nurse Practitioners* 1995; **7**: 87–9.
12. Rubin JD, Ferencz C, Loffredo C. Use of prescription and non-prescription drugs in pregnancy. The Baltimore-Washington Infant Study Group. *Journal of Clinical Epidemiology* 1993; **46**: 581–9.
13. Rizk MA, Abdel-Aziz F, Ashmawy AA, Mahmoud AA, Abuzeid TM. Knowledge and practices of pregnant women in relation to the intake of drugs during pregnancy. *Journal of the Egyptian Public Health Association* 1993; **68**: 567–91.
14. Rubin PC. *Prescribing in pregnancy*. London. BMJ publications, 1986.
15. Piper JM, Baum C, Kennedy DL. Prescription drug use before and during pregnancy in a Medicaid population. *American Journal of Obstetrics and Gynecology* 1987; **157**: 148–56.
16. Shepard TH. *Catalog of teratogenic agents*, 8th edn. Baltimore, MD: Johns Hopkins University Press, 1995.
17. Schardein JL. *Chemically induced birth defects* 2nd edn. New York: Marcel Dekker, 1993.
18. Brent RL. Drugs and pregnancy: are the insert warnings too dire? *Contemporary Obstetrics and Gynecology* 1982; **20**: 42.
19. Brent RL. Evaluating the alleged teratogenicity of environmental exposure. *Clinical Perinatology* 1986; **13**: 609–13.
20. Cordero JF, Oakley GP Jr. Drug exposure during pregnancy: some epidemiological considerations. *Clinical Obstetrics and Gynecology* 1983; **26**: 418–28.
21. Jones KL. *Smith's recognizable patterns of human malformation*, 4th edn. Philadelphia, PA: WB Saunders, 1988.
22. Beck FB, Lloyd JB. Comparative placental transfer. In: Wilson JG, Fraser FC (eds) *Handbook of teratology. Vol. 3*. New York: Plenum, 1977: 155–83.
23. Kallen B. Miscarriage or spontaneous abortion? *Epidemiology of Human Reproduction* 1988; **3**: 11–18.

24. Brent RL, Beckman DA. Environmental teratogens. *Bulletin of the New York Academy of Medicine* 1990; **66**: 123–63.
25. Thompson MW, Innes RR, Willard HF. *Genetics in medicine*, 5th edn. Philadelphia, PA: WB Saunders, 1991.
26. Little BB. Pharmacokinetics during pregnancy: evidence-based maternal dose formulation. *Obstetrics and Gynecology*, 1999; **93**: 858–68.
27. Davis GK, Farquhar CM, Allan LD, Crawford DC, Chapman MG. Structural cardiac abnormalities in the fetus: reliability of prenatal diagnosis and outcome. *British Journal of Obstetrics and Gynaecology* 1990; **97**: 27–31.
28. *Physicians' desk reference*, 45th edn. Oradell, NJ: Medical Economics, 1991.
29. Friedman JM, Little BB, Brent RL, Cordero JF, Hanson JW, Shepard TH. Potential human teratogenicity of frequently prescribed drugs. *Obstetrics and Gynecology* 1990; **75**: 594–7.
30. Brent RL, Beckman DA. Angiotensin-converting enzyme inhibitors, an embryopathic class of drugs with unique properties: information for clinical teratology counselors. *Teratology* 1991; **43**: 543–6.
31. Gilstrap LC, Little BB (eds) *Drugs and pregnancy*, 2nd edn. New York: Chapman and Hall, 1998.
32. Friedman JM, Polifka JE. *Teratogenic effects of drugs. A resource for clinicians (TERIS)*, 2nd edn. Baltimore, MD: Johns Hopkins University Press, 2000.
33. Briggs GG, Freeman RK, Yaffe SJ. *A reference guide to fetal and neonatal risk*, 5th edn. Baltimore, MD: Williams & Wilkins, 1998.

4

Somatic treatments in depression: concerns during pregnancy and breastfeeding

A. CHRIS HEATH AND KIMBERLY A. YONKERS

INTRODUCTION

Despite popular opinion in the medical field that pregnancy is protective against exacerbations of psychiatric illness, there is a significant incidence of both recurrent and new-onset illness in the prenatal period.[1-3] However, decisions concerning the use of medications during pregnancy are complicated. The physician must be able to discuss with his or her patient the known and potential risks and benefits of various treatment options.

The hazards of not treating depression during pregnancy are multiple. The potential consequences to the mother of untreated depression include malnutrition, functional impairment and suicide. The increased incidence of depression and impaired cognitive development in children of mothers with postpartum depression is well documented.[4-8] There is some evidence that neonates born to mothers who are depressed during pregnancy are more irritable than their counterparts born to well mothers when measured as early as 8–72 hours after birth, suggesting a direct negative effect of depression on the fetus even before birth.[9]

Decisions regarding the initiation of pharmacotherapy require consideration of the effects on the fetus. Data on immediate risks are limited, and little is known about potential long-term risks, but some clinical and theoretical evidence informs these discussions. The purpose of this chapter is to provide a resource for clinicians who may treat pregnant depressed patients. We shall examine human data as well as potentially important animal data on antidepressant medications, and throughout the chapter we shall evaluate each class of antidepressant medication for indications of morphologic as well as functional teratogenicity. Clinical and preclinical empirical studies will be reviewed, as well as theoretical evidence where appropriate. Finally, the evidence regarding the safety of breastfeeding while taking these medications will be examined.

SELECTIVE SEROTONIN REUPTAKE INHIBITORS (SSRIs)

Animal data

Studies of fluoxetine and paroxetine in rats and rabbits[10–12] have shown that these compounds are unlikely to cause physical malformations at doses up to 43 mg/kg/day (40 times the maximum human dose (MHD*)) in daily doses through the period of organogenesis. Fetal toxicity (death or resorption) does occur at high doses, but a direct causal relationship with the medication is not clearly established, since maternal toxicity also occurs at these doses. Specifically, impairment of maternal weight gain, which begins to occur at doses higher than 12 mg/kg in rats and rabbits, may cause the increased rate of fetal death and resorption seen at doses higher than 20 mg/kg.[10–12] Although craniofacial malformations have been seen in mouse embryos in whole embryo culture in-vitro at 10M concentrations of fluoxetine and sertraline (4 mg/kg),[13] this has not been seen in any in-vivo studies.

The increased rate of hematomas observed in rats at birth is concerning. In one study,[14] 29% of rat pups exposed to fluoxetine at 5.6 mg/kg/day from day 7 of gestation until the day of birth had hematomas on examination, whereas control rats had a 2% incidence. Stanford and Pattan[14] postulated a 5-HT-associated platelet function impairment with fluoxetine exposure, citing a case study of eight patients with bleeding disorders while taking fluoxetine. A case report describes a neonate born with petechiae and a subdural hematoma who was exposed to fluoxetine in utero.[15] Some caution is therefore indicated, especially with pregnancies that may involve coagulation disorders.

No gross behavioral teratogenicity has been seen in animals exposed to fluoxetine. In rats exposed to 12 mg/kg fluoxetine during the period of organogenesis, there was no subsequent impairment of performance in maze learning, startle habituation, the amount of motor activity, or passive-avoidance tests.[10] Although tests of gross anatomic and behavioral teratogenicity have been negative, there is evidence that 5-HT affects the growth of serotonergic neurons prenatally.[16,17] This opens up the possibility of lasting effects of SSRIs on these neurons, for which our measures of behavioral teratogenicity in animals may not be sensitive enough. There are increases in 5-HT synthesis in rat brain between gestational days 12 and 15,[16,18] which may correlate with a particularly sensitive period for serotonergic neurons. This is a cause for concern, since gestational days 12–15 in the rat are outside the generally accepted period of organogenesis, namely days 1–8.[19] A complex developmental scheme[16,17] has been postulated in which growth of serotonergic neurons is inhibited by feedback collaterals until the correct stage is reached, at which time 5-HT axons are signaled by changes in the neurotransmitter milieu to grow and connect with more distant nuclei.[16,17] Changes in this milieu caused by SSRIs could affect this growth. A similar process may occur in humans. A sharp increase in 5-HT$_{1A}$ receptor density which is observed in human fetal brains between gestational weeks 16 and 22 is analogous to the rat developmental situation. This binding activity is three to four times as dense during this period as in the adult human brain. The brains of

* MHD for fluoxetine and paroxetine is 1 mg/kg/day.

Down's syndrome-affected fetuses have inappropriately low levels of these receptors,[20] which suggest a neurodevelopmental role for 5-HT in humans.

Indeed, there are changes in 5-HT function in rats that have been exposed during gestation to antidepressants affecting this neurotransmitter. In rats exposed to 10 mg/kg/day of fluoxetine from gestational days 13 to 20, the density of hypothalamic 5-HT$_{2A/2C}$ receptors was significantly (35%) decreased at day 70 of life (early adulthood) compared to controls.[21] Decreased 5-HT reuptake activity has been found as late as 25 days postpartum in rats exposed in the last 15 days of gestation to clomipramine and fluoxetine, but was not found with desipramine.[22] This is a site-specific effect – 5-HT transporter densities show both negative and positive changes (relative to controls), depending on anatomic location, in pre-adolescent rats exposed to fluoxetine between gestational days 13 and 20.[18] These changes in reuptake transporters may not be permanent in the offspring, since there were no differences compared to controls in exposed adult animals.[18,22]

Serotonin levels are also affected by gestational exposure to SSRIs. In rats exposed to 10 mg/kg/day fluoxetine during gestational days 13–20, a 28% decrease in 5-HT concentration was seen in the frontal cortex of prepubescent animals. By adulthood, this change was no longer present, but a 28% decrease in 5-HT concentration was seen in the midbrain, compared to untreated controls.[23] These changes were very localized, and no change in total brain 5-HIAA, the major metabolite of 5-HT, was detected. The levels of dopamine and norepinephrine remained unchanged from those of controls.

There are few data on the possible implications of these changes in 5-HT function in adult humans. Given the possibility of changes in serotonergic neuron growth with SSRI-induced neurotransmitter changes, a theoretical effect on the incidence of psychiatric illnesses related to 5-HT in offspring exposed to SSRIs may exist. However, when considering the more definite risks to the pregnant woman and her fetus from untreated depression, the scales seem to weigh in favor of treatment, especially when psychiatric symptoms lead to impaired function.

Human data

There have been several studies on the use of SSRIs during pregnancy. The bulk of these are naturalistic studies which include women who contact or are referred to a Teratology Information Service (TIS).[24,25] Although these databases are important sources of information, they are subject to reporting bias, and reports emanating from them have not included a comparison group of women who are depressed but untreated. These databases have therefore not controlled for risks to the fetus which may arise from the depressive illness itself. Four such studies have been published on the risks of SSRIs.[26–29]

Pastuszak and colleagues prospectively studied 128 women taking fluoxetine in the first trimester of pregnancy.[26] They used a matched control group of 128 non-depressed women exposed to non-teratogens* and a depressed control group consisting of 74 matched probands taking TCAs. They found no differences in the incidence of major malformations, and no change in birth weight between the three populations. They did observe a non-significant increase in miscarriage rates in treated groups (see Table 4.1). However, they did not address an apparent increase in neonatal complications – 12%, 8.6% and 1.6% in the TCA-treated, fluoxetine-treated and control groups, respectively. Neonatal complications[26] included minor malformations such as clubfoot (considered to be major malformations in some other studies), as well as non-structural events such as apnea.

* Pastuszak and colleagues,[26] as well as other groups,[27–29] used an untreated control group consulting a TIS for exposure to drugs and procedures not considered teratogenic, such as dental radiography and acetaminophen use. Goldstein and colleagues[30,31] used historic control groups from the literature.

Table 4.1 *Rates of miscarriage and elective abortion in antidepressant trials*[*]

Trial	Miscarriage			Elective abortion		
	SSRI	TCA	Controls	SSRI	TCA	Controls
Pastuszac et al.[26]	13.5	12.2	6.8	8.1	6.8	2.7
Chambers et al.[27]	10.0	N/A	8.5	9.6	N/A	2.7
Nulman et al.[28]	13.6	9.3	N/A	8.0	1.6	N/A
Kulin et al.[29]	13.8	N/A	8.9	6.8	N/A	3.8
Goldstein et al.[†30,31]	13.3	N/A	N/A	N/A	N/A	N/A

[*] Numbers are expressed as a percentage of the total number of patients.
[†] Elective abortions were 'excluded from tabulations' in the study by Goldstein *et al.*
N/A, not available.

Chambers and colleagues[27] compared 228 women taking fluoxetine, most of whom took this medication during the first trimester, with 254 women who were exposed to non-teratogens. Although there was no increase in major malformations in the treated group, there was an increase in the number of neonates with three minor malformations (15.5% vs. 3.7%; $P = 0.03$) as rated by an examiner blinded to the treatment conditions. Notably, the rate of a single occurrence of minor malformation was higher in the untreated group (77.8% vs. 57.7%; $P = 0.002$). These researchers saw a significantly increased number of infants who were of low birth weight (less than the tenth percentile), required admission to special-care nurseries and experienced poor neonatal adaptation born to women who received fluoxetine in the third trimester, compared to women who stopped fluoxetine early on, or untreated controls. Birth weight was not affected by antidepressant treatment in the study by Pastuszak and colleagues,[26] or in studies by Nulman and colleagues,[28] and Kulin and colleagues.[29] Here again, in the study by Chambers and colleagues[27] the rate of spontaneous abortions was slightly but non-significantly higher in fluoxetine-treated mothers. The rate of therapeutic abortion was significantly higher in the treated group (9.6% vs. 2.7%; $P = 0.002$).

Nulman and colleagues[28] compared women taking TCAs ($n = 80$) or fluoxetine ($n = 55$), beginning in their first trimester, with untreated women ($n = 84$). They found no increase in major malformations or perinatal complications with drug treatment, but they did not report on the occurrence of minor malformations. There was a 9.3% incidence of spontaneous abortion in the TCA-treated group, and a 13.6% incidence of spontaneous abortion in the fluoxetine-treated. However, the rate in the control group was not reported. An important component of this paper was the evaluation of childhood development after the neonatal period. After examining children between 16 months and 7 years of age, they found no differences in IQ or language development between treated and untreated groups.

The most recent of the TIS publications[29] reported outcomes for women exposed to paroxetine, sertraline and fluvoxamine. Among 267 women exposed to these drugs, there was no increase in the rate of major malformations over matched controls ($n = 267$), and birth weights were also equivalent. Importantly, major malformation was defined conservatively, including such conditions as clubfoot. These researchers made no mention of the incidence of neonatal complications, but they did find a non-significant increase in the rate of spontaneous abortions (13.5% vs. 8.9%) in patients who were treated with the target SSRIs compared to controls.

Two reports from the Eli Lilly fluoxetine database have been published.[30,31] Both were prospective (exposure was reported to Lilly before the outcome was known). One included data on 796 women who took fluoxetine during the first trimester.[31] These patients were compared with historical standards from the literature. The rates of major malformation were 3.5% and 4%, and the rates of minor malformations were 0.2% and 2.3% fluoxetine-exposed and historical controls, respectively. In this report, the rate of spontaneous abortion was 13.3%, for which there was no comparable control group. Rates of therapeutic abortion were not reported.

Another report from the Eli Lilly database[30] evaluated women taking fluoxetine during the third trimester, in order to obtain information on the side-effects or withdrawal effects in the neonate. In a sample of 115 neonates, they found six with irritability and four with somnolence – common side-effects of fluoxetine. The authors note that these are common events in neonates in general, but they do not cite the rate of such neonatal difficulties in control groups. Withdrawal effects of fluoxetine in neonates are in fact rare, only three reports of such events being found in the literature, namely opisthotonos and restlessness with fluoxetine,[32] increased respiratory rate and jitteriness with paroxetine,[33] and petechiae and a subdural hematoma with fluoxetine.[14] If these problems were a common occurrence, there would probably be more case reports of such withdrawal effects.

Overall, these studies argue strongly that there is no increased risk of major malformations with fluoxetine,[26–28,30,31] and the same is probably true for sertraline, paroxetine and fluvoxamine.[29] Although Chambers and colleagues[27] found an increased incidence of infants with at least three minor malformations in the fluoxetine-treated group, the rate of single minor malformations was higher in the untreated group, consistent with the findings of Goldstein and colleagues (Table 4.2).[31] Moreover, Chambers and colleagues[27] have been criticized for drawing conclusions regarding the incidence of combinations of deformities when they had no depressed, untreated control group.[24,34,35] In reply to these criticisms, they point out that they controlled for smoking, alcohol intake and maternal weight gain through regression model analysis – variables that probably covary with ongoing maternal depression.[36]

A major concern is the trend towards higher rates of miscarriage noted by all of the research groups that have addressed this problem.[26–29,31] Although this could be an effect of the medications, it may also be an effect of the underlying depression. More speculative but not impossible is the conclusion drawn by Pastuszak and colleagues that some women may be reporting miscarriages when they in fact had therapeutic abortions.[26]

There is a higher risk of elective abortions among women taking these medications (see Table 4.1). This is consistent with the fear that many women have of the effect of medications on the fetus. In one study, women presenting for TIS consultation were asked to guess the rate of malformation with the questioned medication before consultation. In this study, the mean estimate by the women was 24% (a very high rate), even when considering medications known to be non-teratogenic.[37] This perception may result in pressure on a woman to obtain an elective abortion. Rates of elective abortion in women who became pregnant while enrolled in therapeutic trials of fluoxetine have been as high as 30%.[30] Such data argue for the importance of educational programs such as TIS, as well as physician–patient communication about the risks of any medication exposure to the developing fetus.

Table 4.2 *Rates of malformations and complications in antidepressant trails*[*]

Trial	Major anomalies			Minor anomilies		
	SSRI	TCA	Controls	SSRI	TCA	Controls
Pastuszac et al.[†26]	3.4	0	3.0	8.6	12.0	1.6
Chambers et al.[27]	5.5	N/A	4.0	57.7	N/A	77.8
Nulman et al.[28]	3.6	3.8	2.4	N/A	N/A	N/A
Kulin et al.[29]	3.8	N/A	3.8	N/A	N/A	N/A
Goldstein et al.[30,31]	3.5	N/A	4.0	0.2	N/A	2.3

[*] Numbers are expressed as a percentage of the total number of patients.
[†] Minor malformations in the trial by Pastuszac et al. are included in 'neonatal complications'; data for the latter are shown here.
N/A, not available.

There appear to be sufficient data to support the use of fluoxetine[26–28,30,31] during pregnancy when some degree of impairment from psychiatric symptoms is present. A similar argument can be made for paroxetine, sertraline and fluvoxamine, although there are fewer data available on these medications.[29] Consideration should be given to the trends seen in the human literature towards increased rates of miscarriage associated with the use of these medications. However, these trends did not reach the level of significance, and numerous potential confounding conditions exist. The animal data reflecting changes in neurotransmitters in the short- to intermediate-term postpartum period have not been supported by short-term infant behavioral difficulties in humans, but more long-term studies are needed.

TRICYCLIC ANTIDEPRESSANTS (TCAs)

Animal data

A review of the effects of TCAs on malformations in animals finds little support for physical teratogenicity in rodents at levels comparable to therapeutic doses in humans (2–4 mg/kg/day). During rabbit and mouse testing, there was no increase in malformations among exposed compared to control animals when doses up to 15 mg/kg of imipramine[38,39] or amitriptyline[40] were used daily during the period of organogenesis. Presumably this could be extrapolated to a similar conclusion for the metabolites of these medications, namely desipramine and nortriptyline. Three of 39 neonate rabbits exposed to amitriptyline at a dose of 15 mg/kg/day showed stunted growth (1 in 76 control neonates showed stunted growth), but none were malformed, and neither stunting nor malformations were seen in mice at this dose.[40] At higher doses of these medications, there was a dose-dependent increase in malformations resulting in 50% of neonates having malformations at 60–100 mg/kg/day in hamsters,[41–43] mice,[40,44] and rabbits.[40] These malformations tended to manifest in the brain, with increasing severity as well as frequency at higher doses.[41–44] However, these higher doses were also associated with maternal toxicity (maternal LD_{50} = 70–140 mg/kg/day),[44] suggesting, as seems to be the case with the SSRIs, that the effects on the fetus may be at least partially related to maternal toxicity. A pilot study of the effects of gestational exposure in monkeys was initially negative at 1 to 10 times the human dose. It was terminated prematurely when the authors felt that the collective data on humans indicated that TCAs were safe during pregnancy.[45]

Maprotiline has been evaluated in two animal studies, and has not shown the central nervous system (CNS) defects related to high-dose amitriptyline and imipramine, despite similar maternal toxicity. In fact, no external or visceral abnormalities were seen at daily dosing of up to 40 mg/kg (10 times the maximum human dose) during organogenesis*, although ossification patterns were less mature in fetuses exposed to 30–40 mg/kg in mice and rats[46] and rabbits.[47] Doxepin appeared to be particularly devoid of deleterious effects, with no external, visceral or skeletal abnormalities at doses as high as 270 mg/kg (70 times the maximum human dose) during the organogenic period in rats.† However, it is unclear whether a consistent examination for CNS defects was performed. Apart from the group that received the highest dose (270 mg/kg/day), 90% of neonates in both control and treated groups survived to weaning, which also supports the minimal teratogenicity of doxepin at these doses in rodents.[48]

---

* The therapeutic human dose range for of maprotiline is 1–3 mg/kg/day.
† The therapeutic human dose range for doxepin is 1–4 mg/kg/day.

Two other observations of note can be gleaned from the animal data on TCAs. First, inbred strains of mice are more sensitive to teratogenic compounds than outbred strains,[44] suggesting the existence of inter-individual and possibly inter-racial differences in sensitivities to these effects. Second, the combination of TCAs and benzodiazepines may potentiate the teratogenicity of TCAs,[41,43] arguing for the need to use increased caution when combining therapies, especially during organogenesis.

The findings of studies of behavioral teratogenicity raise some concern about TCAs. Mild decreases in some tests of motility have been seen in offspring exposed *in utero* to TCAs, even at doses close to human therapeutic doses. Chronic doses of imipramine at 5 mg/kg/day during the period of organogenesis led to mild decreases in exploratory behavior in young rat offspring, although learning was not impaired.[49] Another group used similar dosing of 0, 5 and 10 mg/kg/day imipramine, and found a consistently decreased startle response in the adult offspring of treated pregnant rats.[50] Amitriptyline, desipramine and clomipramine at 10 mg/kg/day, administered on day 10 of gestation through delivery, caused a decrease in avoidance behavior in adult rats (but no decrease in ambulation).[51] Finally, administration of clomipramine at a daily dose of 10 mg/kg during organogenesis was related to increased social interaction[19] and decreased movement[52] at postnatal day (PND) 25 (the equivalent of late childhood). Taken together, these studies suggest the possibility of mild but lasting effects of TCAs on behavior when used during the period of organogenesis. Although these changes do not interfere with learning in rodents, the nature of these effects cannot be extrapolated to humans without more complete testing.

Human data

Although much of the data concerning TCAs and physical mutations is difficult to interpret because of methodologic problems with this research, there is a large amount of data in the literature which, as a whole, does not support deleterious effects of these medications. An early case study of 24 patients in which women were exposed to TCAs (mostly imipramine, $n = 20$) found no abnormalities in the offspring.[53] This was followed by a report of three infants exposed to imipramine *in utero* with limb abnormalities,[54] which caused alarm among both the medical and lay press.[55,56] Of note, this occurred only 10 years after the discovery of similar defects in infants exposed to thalidomide, a drug that does not show teratogenicity in many animal models.[57] A subsequent outpouring of data from registries of pregnancies[56,58] and malformations,[55,59,60] including a very large database kept by the World Health Organization,[55] showed no disproportionate association between malformations and TCA (mostly imipramine, with some data on amitriptyline) exposure *in utero*.[55,56,58–60] In a similar study of 50 282 mother–child pairs, none of the 59 infants exposed to TCAs *in utero* had malformations.[57] The most recent of these uncontrolled case series is a survey by McElhatton and colleagues of women presenting to a TIS clinic in Europe.[25] This study included 283 women taking various TCAs beginning in the first trimester, and 174 women who took other prescription medications in addition to the antidepressant. There was no increase in malformation rates compared to historical controls, and no clustering of specific anomalies. However, these authors did find what they considered to be a high incidence of neonatal disorders such as drowsiness and withdrawal symptoms (e.g. hypothermia, cyanosis). These occurred in 9.6% of neonates exposed to TCAs plus another medication, and in 4.6% of those exposed to TCAs alone. The rates of spontaneous abortion were 11% for those exposed to TCAs alone, and 13.2% for those exposed to TCAs plus other medication, which were within normal limits according to the authors, although several groups that have addressed this question have found lower rates of miscarriage in their untreated, non-depressed control groups.[26,27,29] The rates of elective abortion were 10.1% and 20.7% for the two groups, respectively.

As reviewed earlier, two studies have compared neonates exposed to TCAs or fluoxetine *in utero* with unexposed controls. Nulman and colleagues found no increased rate of malformations and no IQ or language development problems between 16 months and 7 years of age in children exposed to TCAs during the first trimester.[28] Pastuszak and colleagues, found a significant increase in neonatal complications and a non-significant increase in miscarriage in both fluoxetine- and TCA-treated groups compared to an untreated control group.[26]

The question of perinatal complications due to TCAs in the neonatal period addressed by McElhatton and colleagues[25] is an important one, for which few data are available. However, several case reports indicate that infants born to women taking any of various TCAs at the time of birth show a trend towards anticholinergic effects such as irritability/jitteriness,[61-64] hypoactivity,[61,62,65,66] colon blockage,[67] and urinary retention.[68] Importantly, these effects tended to occur within a time period consistent with the elimination of these medications, which is extended in neonates because of an initially poorly developed cytochrome oxidative degradation pathway compared to that in adults.[69] Side-effects lasted for a few days[63,65,67,68,70] to a week,[61,62,64] and in one case were successfully treated with physostigmine.[66]

More concerning are two cases of neonates with seizures who had been exposed to clomipramine shortly before delivery.[70] The time-course of the seizures in one baby was 53 h, and the seizures were refractory to phenobarbital. The second neonate in this report had seizures that were also refractory to phenobarbital, but which were well controlled immediately with an intravenous bolus of clomipramine at 24 h of life, suggesting that they represented withdrawal seizures rather than a direct side-effect of the clomipramine.

Prentice and Brown have reported a single case of tachycardia in a fetus, possibly related to dothiepin use by the mother.[71] The mother took dothiepin from weeks 16 to 37 and experienced no problems up to week 34, but there was an increase in the fetal heart rate (to 180 beats/min) in week 37. This rate decreased to normal within 4 days after dothiepin was discontinued. As a single case with a questionable relationship between medication administration and an adverse event, this should not necessarily change our management of these patients in and of itself, but it is important to be aware of the possibility of such direct effects of any medication on the fetus.

Overall, the TCAs seem to have little morphological teratogenic potential. As with the SSRIs, we know little about the long-term health and development of children who have been exposed to these medications. Also true for studies of both SSRIs and TCAs is the trend towards an increased rate of miscarriage. It seems prudent to employ close obstetric follow-up for these cases, especially shortly after changes in medications.

The literature shows many examples of neonates with complications consistent with side-effects or withdrawal symptoms of TCAs.[61-70] It is difficult to make specific recommendations, as the incidence of such complications is unknown, as are the effects on the fetus of stopping these medications before delivery. Moreover, stopping the medications just before childbirth may subject the new mother and her infant to the burden of a postpartum depression, which carries its own risks. It is certainly wise to minimize the dose of these medications during pregnancy, and to avoid polypharmacy.

Another possibility is to lower the dose of TCAs for a week immediately before the expected or planned delivery, and to increase it again immediately after delivery. Above all, one must be aware of potential side-effects in the neonate, and use logical treatment strategies for their management when necessary.

BUPROPION

Although no controlled studies of bupropion use during pregnancy are available, this drug has been given a Pregnancy Category B designation by the Federal Drug Administration.[72] Other currently marketed antidepressants in the USA have been placed in Category C, because of reports of decreased newborn weight in animal pups exposed to those medications *in utero*. No such data have emerged for bupropion (personal communication, Larry Lim, Drug Information Branch, US Food & Drug Administration, July 1998). Bupropion doses of 7 to 11 times the maximum human dose in rats and rabbits show no definitive evidence of impaired fertility or harm to the fetus.[73] A slight increase in fetal abnormalities was found in two studies of rabbits, but no clustering of any specific abnormality was present.[73]

A registry is in place for identification of mothers taking bupropion. In October 1998, 15 mothers had been identified who took bupropion during their first trimester. Although no data have been published, six mothers had given birth to babies who had no birth defects, and the remaining nine mothers were still pregnant without complications (personal communication, Barbara Haight, Glaxo Wellcome Inc. October 1998).

MONOAMINE OXIDASE INHIBITORS (MAOIs)

The safety of MAOIs during pregnancy has been questioned, and these medications should be regarded as last-line treatments. However, there has been no documentation of consistent teratogenicity (as has been seen with thalidomide and ethanol, for instance). Moreover, two case reports of MAOIs treatment throughout pregnancy with a good outcome have been published.[74,75] The practitioner is sometimes faced with such difficult situations as a clinical depression that is only responsive to MAOIs, and then has to weigh the risks and benefits of such treatment for the pregnant patient. Although only two MAOIs, namely phenelzine and the non-hydrazine, tranylcypromine, are currently available in the USA (isocarboxazid is no longer available), the literature for all systemically administered MAOIs will be reviewed for trends in fetal toxicity that may be helpful in considering the ones currently available.

Animal data

The teratogenic potential of MAOIs has not been well studied in the literature.[75] No thorough studies of the teratogenicity of phenelzine have been published.[75] However, Poulson and Robson[76] reported lower weights of sexual organs after early gestational exposure of mice to a derivative of phenelzine. A study of tranylcypromine noted no negative effects on rat fetuses, although no systematic examination of the animals for malformations was reported.[78]

Few studies of behavioral teratogenicity have been conducted. A combination of clorgyline, a selective MAO type A inhibitor, and deprenyl, an MAO type B inhibitor (used in the treatment of Parkinson's disease) has been tested.[78] Pregnant rats were given doses throughout pregnancy that were comparable by weight to those used in humans. Some differences with untreated controls were noted. For example, the fetuses showed decreased weight gain throughout gestation, and the gestation times were longer. In addition, they showed decreased performance in tests of passive avoidance of noxious stimuli.[78] A study of exposure of pregnant rats to isocarboxazid or iproniazid* showed similar decreases in avoidance behavior in adult offspring when compared to controls – changes identical to those seen with TCA treatment.[51]

---

* Iproniazid is a relatively toxic MAOI that is used in the treatment of tuberculosis.

Increases in miscarriage rates have been found in animals exposed to MAOIs. Iproniazid causes an increased risk of fetal death and resorption in mice.[79,80] This was attributed to a direct toxic effect of serotonin on the placenta,[80–83] although other studies of iproniazid in rats have attributed the increased rate of miscarriage to a luteolytic effect,[77,84] which is reversible with progesterone treatment.[77,85] This postulated inhibitory effect on the corpus luteum may be mediated via prostaglandin synthesis. In rats, the increased miscarriage rate is reversible by aspirin administration.[84] Such an inhibitory effect on the corpus luteum is also consistent with the increased incidence of miscarriage during early gestation with iproniazid and isoniazid exposure, when viability is dependent on luteal production of progesterone. Viability during the late phases of pregnancy is less disrupted by iproniazid.[77,80] Isocarboxazid similarly causes an increased fetal mortality in rats during early pregnancy, but is associated with a much lower fetal mortality rate when administered later in pregnancy.[79] Phenelzine may also have deleterious effects on fetal viability during early pregnancy. Doses of 25 mg/kg/day (25 times the maximum human dose) on days 1 to 6 of gestation in mice caused a marked reduction in the rate of birth of live litters compared to untreated controls (36% vs. 67%);[76] no change in the rate of survival was observed when mice were treated later in gestation. Phenelzine showed increases in fetal mortality during early pregnancy (but post-implantation) in mouse fetuses,[85] consistent with the theory of luteolysis. For several derivatives of phenelzine, this effect was correlated with low progesterone levels, and was prevented by the administration of exogenous progesterone. Interestingly, tranylcypromine at doses comparable to those used in humans (1 mg/kg/day) and harmaline* (both non-hydrazine MAOIs) showed no effect on pregnancy viability in rats compared to untreated controls.[77] In this study, MO-911 (an experimental, non-hydrazine MAOI), iproniazid and three other experimental hydrazine MAOIs caused increases in fetal death rates when administered early in pregnancy. It may be that tranylcypromine (the only non-hydrazine MAOI marketed in the USA) is, for this reason, a wiser choice for use in pregnancy, especially early in gestation.

Some of the preclinical literature reporting increases in rates of fetal loss may be capturing a degree of induced infertility as well as direct fetal toxicity. These studies[76,77] used physical signs of copulation (rather than more definitive proof of pregnancy) as confirmation of conception. This method may overestimate the number of successful conceptions (and therefore mistake poor rates of fertility for higher rates of fetal death). Other groups confirmed pregnancy before MAOI treatment, and their rates of pregnancy loss therefore reflect actual fetal death.[80,84,85] Some experimental data directly implicate mechanisms of decreased fertility with MAOI treatment.[86] In rats, isocarboxazid has been seen to cause changes in the oviductal isthmus, including an unstable resting pressure and intermittent vigorous bursts of activity,[86] contributing to a lower rate of fertility in these animals. Although this effect on fertility could contribute to the decrease in birth rate observed when hydrazine MAOIs are given early in pregnancy,[76,77,80,84,85] it does not explain the losses of pregnancy during the later stages[76,77] or the beneficial effects of supplemental progesterone.[77,85] On the basis of the preclinical data currently available, there appear to be increases in the rates of both infertility and fetal death with the hydrazine MAOIs.[75–85] These effects are seen early in pregnancy, and progesterone augmentation may be partially protective against them. However, data are scarce and at times inconsistent.

Human data

The database on safety of MAOI use during pregnancy is very limited. It includes the two case reports noted above, as well as one cohort study.[57] In the large study by Heinonen and

---

* Harmaline, no longer used in the USA, was historically used in the treatment of Parkinson's disease.

colleagues[57] of human pregnancy and medication exposure, of the 21 mother–infant pairs exposed to MAOIs during pregnancy, three had malformations in the fetus, resulting in a relative risk of 2.21. However, there was no clustering of specific malformations.[57] If MAOI use is necessary during pregnancy, we must rely for the most part on the animal literature and clinical judgement as guidelines. On the basis of the data currently available, our initial statement of the need for caution remains true.

TRAZODONE

No controlled trials have investigated the incidence of malformations in babies exposed to trazodone *in utero*, although a population study of 229 101 Medicaid recipients in Michigan revealed only one major birth defect out of 100 babies exposed to trazodone (less than the four expected statistically).[87] Trazodone HCL causes increased fetal resorption and has other adverse effects on rat fetuses when given at 30–50 times the maximum human dose.[88] One of three rabbit studies revealed an increase in congenital abnormalities at doses of 15–50 times the maximum human dose.[88] These data do not reflect a high degree of teratogenic potential for trazodone.

MIRTAZAPINE

No human data have been published on the use of mirtazapine during pregnancy. According to the manufacturer (Organon Inc), studies using up to 20 times (in rats) and 17 times (in rabbits) the maximum human dose by weight have shown no increase in malformations. In rats, increased post-implantation losses, decreased birth weights, and an increase in deaths during the first 3 days of life were observed at 20 times the maximum human dose, but not at three times the maximum human dose (personal communication, Loree Levine, RPh, Organon Inc., July 1998). These data are reassuring, although human data are needed before any definitive statement can be made. A lack of malformations in animals exposed to a drug is not a guarantee against human teratogenicity, as shown by the lack of birth defects in many animal models exposed to thalidomide *in utero*.[57] However, a risk–benefit analysis must be performed for each case. The reader is encouraged to report to the manufacturer and/or pursue publication of any experience with new antidepressants and pregnancy, especially during the first trimester.

NEFAZODONE

As with mirtazapine, there are no human data available on the safety of nefazodone used during pregnancy. Doses in rabbits and rats of six and five times the maximum human dose, respectively, caused no increased rate of malformations, but decreased birth weights and decreased early pup survival rates were found in rats at five times the maximum human dose.[89]

VENLAFAXINE

No published data are available on venlafaxine use during pregnancy. Venlafaxine is reported by the manufacturer to cause no malformations in rats and rabbits exposed to 11 times (in rats) or 12 times (in rabbits) the maximum human dose (personal communication, Dominick Albano, RPh, MBA, Wyeth-Ayerst Pharmaceuticals, April 1999). The manufacturer describes 16 pregnancies during drug trials with venlafaxine. Five of these women delivered healthy, normal-weight babies at full term, five women had spontaneous abortions, one had an ectopic pregnancy, and six underwent elective abortions. One patient was lost to follow-up after conception. There have been many spontaneous reports of venlafaxine use during pregnancy. Some of these infants showed birth defects. There does not appear to be a clustering of abnormalities, but this is not yet clear from the available data (personal communication, Dominick Albano, RPh, MBA, Wyeth-Ayerst Pharmaceuticals, April 1999).

CITALOPRAM

No published data exist on citalopram exposure during pregnancy. Although a degree of teratogenicity occurred in rats exposed to 18 times the maximum human dose, none occurred at 9 times that dose. This teratogenicity is proposed to be secondary to poor maternal weight gain (personal communication, Kim Holliday, PharmD, Forest Pharmaceutical, Inc., May 1999). Over 100 reports of citalopram-exposed pregnancies have been presented to Forest Laboratories, the majority of which gave rise to normal births (personal communication, Kim Holliday, PharmD, Forest Pharmaceutical, Inc., May 1999). There was no mention of clustering of specific malformations or whether pregnancies were exposed during the first trimester. However, citalopram has been marketed in several countries, resulting in the treatment of 12 million patients over a 9-year period (personal communication, Kim Holliday, PharmD, Forest Pharmaceutical, Inc., May 1998). If specific major malformations occurred as a result of exposure to citalopram, they would probably have been reported, although the lack of such reports is no guarantee of safety in the absence of at least formal case study reports.

ELECTROCONVULSIVE THERAPY (ECT)

ECT is an effective treatment modality for melancholic depression, and should be considered for the severely depressed pregnant patient. Although ECT cannot rival the convenience and relatively low cost of antidepressant medications, a large body of literature shows the procedure to have few complications in the pregnant patient. As we have seen, this literature does not exist for many of the newer antidepressant medications. During ECT, medication exposure is minimal, and anesthetic agents can be selected to minimize transfer into the feto–placental system. Moreover, when depression is complicated by psychosis, ECT may be the treatment of choice during pregnancy, especially since little is known about the synergistic teratogenicity of combining antidepressant, antipsychotic and sedative medications.

As reviewed by Miller,[90] 300 cases of ECT during pregnancy have been reported in the literature. Of these, complications were noted in 9.3%, many of which had no apparent causal relationship with the ECT administration. Close temporal relationships occurred with transient fetal arrhythmias (five cases), vaginal bleeding (five cases) and uterine contractions or abdominal pain (four cases). However, no adverse effects on these infants were noted after delivery. Four cases in the literature report the occurrence of premature labor, but in these cases labor did not immediately follow the treatments, so could have been due to other causes. Adverse events in the infant are rarely seen in this literature, and the incidence of such effects may be no different to that in the untreated population, although no sham-ECT controlled trials have been reported on gravid patients. Adverse events noted include five miscarriages (1.6% of reported ECT treatments of pregnant patients), three stillbirths (each of which had other factors more likely to have been responsible for fetal death) and one case of respiratory distress at birth (few details given). Five cases of congenital abnormalities have been noted after ECT was given to the gravid mother. This was lower than the incidence of 2.2% seen in an historical control population,[91] and there was no clustering of specific abnormalities. Two of these mothers had also received insulin shock therapy, and one received ECT only after the period of organogenesis (week 20). None of the case reports of congenital abnormalities after ECT provided complete information about exposure to other potential teratogens.

Limited exposure of the fetus to medications is an argument for using ECT instead of chronic dosing of antidepressants. Medication exposure during modified ECT includes three classes of medications, namely hypnotics, paralytic agents and anticholinergics.[92] The hypnotics used are typically short-acting barbiturates which have not been shown to cause complications in pregnancy, except in rare cases with porphyria.[90] Succinylcholine, a paralytic agent commonly used for ECT, has minimal transfer across the placenta because of its quick degradation.[90,93] Use of anticholinergics is more complicated because of the potential side-effects. Although atropine crosses the placental barrier easily and may contribute to the transient fetal arrhythmias that are sometimes seen with ECT, glycopyrrolate, an alternatively used anticholinergic, has limited transfer across the placenta and does not affect the fetal heart rate.[90,93] If an anticholinergic is used, glycopyrrolate should be the medication of choice. However, use of an anticholinergic agent may increase the risk of regurgitation by lowering the esophageal sphincter tone. An informed decision has to be made in each case as to whether to use an anticholinergic agent, as is true of ECT in general.

Recommendations in the literature with regard to precautions during ECT on pregnant patients vary widely, ranging from little more than is typically done for treatments[94] to ensuring the presence of an obstetrician in the ECT suite during all treatments.[95] The practitioner must assess which precautions are required for safety of the fetus and which are more redundant, and issues of affordability and practicality must be considered. The literature supports the following additions to current ECT practices.

1 *Obstetric consultation.* There is agreement that an obstetrician should be a member of the consulting team, and there should be a pelvic examination on record for a patient prior to ECT.[90,95,96] The presence of an obstetrician during treatments is probably unnecessary in most cases,[90,94] although an assessment of uterine contractions and vaginal bleeding should be made at some point after each treatment.

2 *Fetal heart monitoring.* Most sources recommend fetal monitoring,[90,93,95,96] although transient fetal heart decelerations can be treated by procedural changes, and are not necessarily a contraindication to further treatment. Procedural changes include placing the patient in a slight left lateral position to decrease pressure on the arterial system,[90] and increasing oxygenation (although hyperventilation should be avoided*). Given the lack of reports of lasting fetal arrhythmias,[90] weekly non-stress tests of the fetus as recommended by Wise and colleagues[95] are probably unnecessary.

3 *Intubation.* Patients beyond the first trimester are at high risk for regurgitating stomach contents, and should therefore be treated as if they have a full stomach. Intubation should be considered on a case-by-case basis in these patients.

Given these additional precautions and the known efficacy of ECT, it represents a powerful tool for the treatment of severely depressed pregnant patients.

---

* Although pregnancy is accompanied by chronic mild hyperventilation, respiratory alkalosis caused by excessive hyperventilation (as is sometimes used to lower the seizure threshold during ECT) can hinder oxygen transfer from maternal to fetal hemoglobin and should be avoided.[93]

BREASTFEEDING

The American Academy of Pediatrics (AAP) recommends breastfeeding as the optimum form of nutrition for infants,[97] and the position of the AAP Committee on Drugs is weighted towards using timing and dosing strategies to minimize infant exposure, rather than discontinuation of breastfeeding, when medications are necessary.[98] Many mothers prefer to forego medication treatment rather than stop breastfeeding or expose their baby to medications through their breast-milk.[62] It is crucial that the practitioner is able to discuss competently with his or her patient the risks and benefits of taking these agents while breastfeeding.

A knowledge of some concepts of maternal and infant pharmacokinetics is necessary to enable one to select appropriate medication, design strategies to minimize levels in milk, and understand the metabolism of these drugs in infants. These concepts have been reviewed in depth by Anderson[69] and Atkinson and colleagues.[99] Above all, it should be remembered that, for most psychiatric medications, infants are exposed to much less medication through breast-milk than via the placental circulation.[69]

Most compounds with a molecular weight of < 200 Daltons pass into breast-milk by passive diffusion, consistent with a two-compartment model.[69,99] This diffusion occurs both into and out of the milk compartment, and is dependent on the following chemical characteristics of milk and plasma.

Protein binding Plasma contains much more protein (*c.* 75 g/L) than human breast-milk (8–9 g/L),[69] and medications that are tightly bound to protein tend to be retained in the plasma. Because of the high degree of protein-binding of SSRIs, this effect decreases the transfer of fluoxetine, sertraline and paroxetine (all of which show > 94% binding).[100]

Lipophilicity Milk contains 3–5% emulsified fat, and lipophilic drugs, (e.g. diazepam) can be concentrated in milk. One way to minimize exposure to these drugs is to feed the infant only foremilk (i.e. that expressed early in the feed), which is much lower in fat than hindmilk.[101] However, this is logistically difficult to achieve. Moreover, feeding only foremilk deprives the infant of important fat-derived calories, and the feeds must therefore be supplemented with formula.

Acid–base characteristics Milk is typically more acidic than plasma, and weak bases (such as most psychotropic medications) therefore tend to collect partition into milk, although this is probably not a major effect compared to other characteristics.

Time to maximal concentration (T_{max}) Antidepressants are distributed by passive diffusion, and their concentrations increase and decrease in relation to the T_{max} in plasma. Feeds can therefore be timed to avoid feeding at T_{max}.[69,101] However, such timing strategies are difficult for new mothers who are already overwhelmed by motherhood complicated by depression. A simple strategy is to take medications in the evening and use formula for night feedings, when maternal drug levels are higher. Because retrograde diffusion occurs, the first milk expression in the morning does not necessarily have a high drug concentration, and does not need to be pumped and wasted.[69]

There are significant differences between infant and adult pharmacodynamics, some of which are not clearly delineated for antidepressants.[69,99] Gastrointestinal absorption characteristics differ between infants and adults, and the protein-binding affinity for drugs is lower in infants. Lower activities of liver cytochrome oxidases and glucuronidation pathways in neonates cause slower metabolism and therefore higher serum levels of drugs metabolized via these pathways. These metabolic capacities are about 20% of the adult levels at birth, but between weeks 8 and 12 they increase to levels in excess of that of the adult. Glomerular filtration rates (GFR) for normal term infants are about one-third those of adults until they normalize at about 2 weeks of age (a post-conceptual age of 34 weeks for premature infants).

As reviewed by Chisholm and Kuller[102] and Wisner and colleagues,[103] numerous case studies report infrequent side-effects in infants who have been breastfed by mothers who are taking antidepressants. In cases where infant serum levels of the medication or its metabolites were measured, infant levels were mostly low or undetectable, with a few notable exceptions. One problem with this literature concerns the lower limits of quantification of antidepressant levels. This threshold has been about 1% of typical adult serum levels (2–4 ng/mL) for most antidepressants. The reader is encouraged to bear this in mind when levels are noted as being unmeasurably low.

SSRIs

One case of colic from maternal use of fluoxetine has been reported.[104] In this case, the infant's symptoms began between 1 and 10 weeks of age and were clearly related to periods of fluoxetine exposure. Colic symptoms were present for periods during which the baby nursed or was bottle-fed pumped breast milk, but they resolved when the baby was fed formula. Unfortunately, serum levels of fluoxetine were not measured in this baby. Another case reported transient mild irritability in an infant whose mother was started on fluoxetine 3 months after the birth.[105] This irritability was only noted by the father (a pediatrician), and not by the mother or the infant's pediatrician. Partly in response to these reports, the decision was made by the US Food and Drug Administration to include warnings against breastfeeding in the package insert for fluoxetine.[106] However, three case studies including a total of 16 infants (7–10 weeks of age) have reported no adverse reactions in infants exposed to fluoxetine through milk,[107–109] and serum fluoxetine and metabolite levels were unmeasurable (< 2 ng/mL) in the four infants in whom they were measured.[107,108] Yoshida and colleagues[107] reported normal developmental scores on the Bayley Scale of Infant Development at 12 months for four infants who were exposed to fluoxetine through breast-milk.

Four articles have reported on 24 infants (10–15 weeks of age) who were exposed to sertraline through breast-milk, none of whom showed adverse effects.[109–112] Levels of sertraline and its major metabolite desmethylsertraline were measured in all of these cases. Sertraline levels were undetectable (9 cases), unmeasurably low (< 2 ng/mL) (13 cases) or very low (3 ng/mL) (almost all cases). One case[111] had a high sertraline level close to therapeutic values (64 ng/mL, 55% of that of the mother). The authors did not consider that this was consistent with the mother's levels, and they suggested the possibilities of laboratory error or surreptitious administration of sertraline to the infant. The metabolite N-desmethylsertraline has widely varying levels in infants, ranging from undetectable to 8% of maternal levels.

Paroxetine has been documented to cause no adverse effects in one infant who was exposed to the drug 3 days after delivery.[113] This is consistent with reports of unmeasurably low levels of paroxetine in serum of 16 neonates being breastfed by mothers undergoing paroxetine treatment. Given the possibility of build-up of metabolites in neonates, who have an immature cytochrome oxidase system, paroxetine may be a better choice because of its lack of metabolites that are active on serotonin transporters.[114]

TCAs

No side-effects in breastfeeding infants have been seen in relation to exposure via breast-milk to imipramine, desipramine, amitriptyline or nortriptyline (n = 33 infants, 10–24 weeks of age).[62,115–122] Some of these studies reported infant serum levels. In a study of seven breastfeeding mother–infant pairs taking nortriptyline, unmeasurably low levels (< 4 ng/mL) of nortriptyline were found in the infants, although levels of a metabolite, hydroxynortriptyline, were present in low but detectable amounts in two infants.[122] The two infants with higher levels of metabolite were younger than 10 weeks. However, a later study by the same group found non-quantifiably low levels of nortriptyline and its metabolites in five infants younger than 10 weeks.[121] Desipramine and 2-hydroxydesipramine were not found in the serum of one infant (who was exposed to the medication through breast-milk).[116]

Detectable levels of doxepin have been found in two breastfed infants of women taking this medication. One (whose age was not noted) had a level of N-desmethyldoxepin that was 15% that of the mother, but an unmeasurably low doxepin level.[123] However, the other (8 weeks old) had N-desmethyldoxepin levels equal to the mother's, but almost undetectable doxepin levels.[124] This infant had symptoms of doxepin toxicity just after an increase in the mother's dose, including acute respiratory depression. However, the infant returned to normal within 24 h of discontinuation of breastfeeding.

Wisner and colleagues[125] examined four nursing mother–infant pairs taking clomipramine. None of these infants had side-effects, and all of the infants had undetectable or unmeasurably low levels of clomipramine and three of its metabolites, even though two of these infants were younger than 10 weeks.[125] An infant who displayed jitteriness and hypotonia after being born to a woman who took clomipramine throughout her pregnancy showed no symptoms when exposed to clomipramine through breast-milk at 7 days of age. The infant's serum level at 5 weeks of age was 2% of the mother's.[126]

Long-term follow-up has been investigated with one tricyclic antidepressant, namely dothiepin. Buist and Janson[127] studied 15 infants exposed to dothiepin through breast-milk. These infants showed no difference in cognitive development at the 3- to 5-year follow-up when compared to 15 control infants whose mothers were depressed but untreated during their infancy, or to 36 control infants whose mothers had no history of depression. Behavior scores were poorer in the group exposed to dothiepin, but this difference lost significance when other variables were factored in.

Bupropion

No studies of bupropion use during breastfeeding have been reported. Bupropion is relatively tightly bound (80%) to serum albumin,[73] and would probably partition into breast-milk to a minimal degree. However, several active metabolites attain high concentrations in patient serum,[73] making bupropion a potentially poor choice during breastfeeding of infants less than 2 months old.

MAOIs

No studies of the effects these medications have been performed in humans. Given the risk of side-effects in adults, consideration should be given to discontinuation of breastfeeding when these medications are to be used.

Trazodone

Trazodone is excreted in breast milk, and the infant's calculated dose is approximately 0.7% of that of the mother by weight.[128] The effects of trazodone on the newborn are unknown.

Mirtazapine

No studies of mirtazapine use during breastfeeding have been reported. Mirtazapine is 85% bound to serum albumin.[72] This drug does have metabolites, but those metabolites are present in low concentrations in human serum during steady-state pharmacokinetics.[72]

Nefazodone

No studies of nefazodone have been published with regard to use during breastfeeding. Nefazodone is 99% bound to serum protein. This and the short half-life of both the parent compound and the active metabolites[89] make it a potentially good choice for use during breastfeeding. However, some caution is advised in neonates, as there are multiple active metabolites. Moreover, both the parent compound and the metabolites may exhibit nonlinear pharmacokinetics, in that a given dose increase results in a greater than expected concentration increase.[89] If this medication is used during breastfeeding, close attention needs to be paid to potential side-effects in the infant.

Venlafaxine

One study has evaluated levels of venlafaxine and its metabolite, O-desmethylvenlafaxine (ODV), in breast-milk and exposed infants aged 2, 6 and 36 weeks. Venlafaxine and ODV appeared to concentrate in breast-milk, with milk/plasma ratios in the range 3.26–5.18. Although infant venlafaxine levels were undetectable (< 4% of maternal levels), ODV levels were 225, 100 and 23 µg/L for the 2-, 6- and 36-week-old infants (maternal ODV levels werein the range 375–800 µg/L). The infants showed no overt adverse effects.[129] Build-up of ODV in the younger infants is consistent with the poor oxidative metabolism seen in neonates. However, the lack of symptoms in these infants, and the relatively low levels of both the drug and its metabolite, are reassuring.

Citalopram

Two studies have examined infant levels of citalopram exposed through breast-milk. Jensen and colleagues[130] found significant levels of citalopram in a 2-month-old infant (15% of maternal levels). This is higher than that seen with other SSRIs (see above), consistent with the lower protein-binding (50%) observed with citalopram. No adverse effects were seen in that infant.[130] Another group found breast-milk concentrations in three cases consistent with weight-adjusted infant doses of 5%, 1.2% and 1.8% of that of the mother (infant levels were not measured).[131] The lowest relative dose was seen in breast-milk with an unusually high pH, consistent with a partitioning effect from the high pK_a of this drug. Effects on the infants were not noted.

ECT

There have been no studies of the effects of ECT on breastfeeding. Given the short duration of exposure to medications, there seems to be no contraindication to breastfeeding during courses of ECT.

SUMMARY OF BREASTFEEDING DATA

In general, infants exposed to most of the SSRIs and TCAs through breast-milk generally have low drug levels and few side-effects (with the exception of doxepin and possibly fluoxetine). Although this information does not rule out the risk of long-term side-effects, there is some evidence that cognitive problems are not present on intermediate-term follow-up after exposure to these agents. Risks of poor cognitive development and depression are certainly evident in children whose mothers are not treated for their postpartum depression,[6–8] arguing in favor of treatment. When using these agents, it is important to weigh the options with the mother, considering discontinuation of breastfeeding if side-effects occur in the infant, and minimizing medication doses where possible.

REFERENCES

1. Brockington I. *Motherhood and mental health*. New York: Oxford University Press, 1996.
2. Llewellyn AM, Stowe ZN, Nemeroff CB. Depression during pregnancy and the puerperium. *Journal of Clinical Psychiatry* 1997; **58**: 26–32.
3. Kumar R, Robson KM. A prospective study of emotional disorders in childbearing women. *British Journal of Psychiatry* 1984; **144**: 35–47.

4. Cogill SR, Caplan HL, Alexandra H, Robson KM, Kumar R. Impact of maternal postnatal depression on cognitive development of young children. *British Medical Journal* 1986; **292**: 1165–7.
5. Caplan HL, Cogill SR, Alexandra H, Robson KM, Katz R, Kumar R. Maternal depression and the emotional development of the child. *British Journal of Psychiatry* 1989; **154**: 818–22.
6. Downey G, Coyne JC. Children of depressed parents: an integrative review. *Psychological Bulletin* 1990; **108**: 50–76.
7. Murray L, Hipwell A, Hooper R, Stein A, Cooper P. The cognitive development of 5-year-old children of postnatally depressed mothers. *Journal of Child Psychology and Psychiatry* 1996; **37**: 927–35.
8. Cooper PJ, Murray L. The impact of psychological treatments of postpartum depression on maternal mood and infant development. In: *Postpartum depression and child development*. New York: Guilford Press, 1997: 206–18.
9. Zuckerman B, Bauchner H, Parker S, Cabral H. Maternal depressive symptoms during pregnancy, and newborn irritability. *Developmental and Behavioral Pediatrics* 1990; **11**: 190–4.
10. Vorhees CV, Acuff-Smith KD, Schilling MA, Fisher JE, Moran MS, Buelke-Sam J. A developmental neurotoxicity evaluation of the effects of prenatal exposure to fluoxetine in rats. *Fundamental and Applied Toxicology* 1994; **23**: 194–205.
11. Baldwin JA, Davidson EJ, Pritchard AL, Ridings JE. The reproductive toxicology of paroxetine. *Acta Psychiatrica Scandinavica* 1989; **80**: 37–9.
12. Byrd RA, Markham JK. Developmental toxicology studies of fluoxetine hydrochloride administered orally to rats and rabbits. *Fundamental and Applied Toxicology* 1994; **22**: 511–18.
13. Shuey DL, Sadler TW, Lauder JM. Serotonin as a regulator of craniofacial morphogenesis: site-specific malformations following exposure to serotonin uptake inhibitors. *Teratology* 1992; **46**: 367–78.
14. Stanford MS, Patton JH. *In utero* exposure to fluoxetine HCl increased hematoma frequency at birth. *Pharmacology, Biochemistry and Behavior* 1993; **45**: 959–62.
15. Mhanna MJ, Bennet JB, Izatt SD. Potential fluoxetine hydrochloride (Prozac) toxicity in a newborn. *Pediatrics* 1997; **100**: 158–9.
16. Mercado R, Hernandez RJ. A molecular recognizing system of serotonin in rat fetal axonal growth cones: uptake and high-affinity binding. *Developmental Brain Research* 1992; **69**: 133–7.
17. Whitaker-Azmitia PM, Azmitia EC. Autoregulation of fetal serotonergic neuronal development: role of high-affinity serotonin receptors. *Neuroscience Letters* 1986; **67**: 307–12.
18. Cabrera-Vera TM, Battaglia G. Prenatal exposure to fluoxetine (Prozac) produces site-specific and age-dependent alterations in brain serotonin transporters in rat progeny: evidence from autoradiographic studies. *Journal of Pharmacology and Experimental Therapeutics* 1998; **286**: 1474–81.
19. File SE, Tucker JC. Prenatal treatment with clomipramine: effects on the behaviour of male and female adolescent rats. *Psychopharmacology* 1984; **82**: 221–4.
20. Bar-Peled O, Gross-Isseroff R, Ben-Hur H, Hoskins I, Groner Y, Biegon A. Fetal human brain exhibits a prenatal peak in the density of serotonin 5-HT$_{1A}$ receptors. *Neuroscience Letters* 1991; **127**: 173–6.
21. Cabrera TM, Battaglia G. Delayed decreases in brain 5-hydroxytryptamine$_{2A/2C}$ receptor density and function in male rat progeny following prenatal fluoxetine. *Journal of Pharmacology and Experimental Therapeutics* 1994; **269**: 637–45.
22. Montero D, de Ceballos ML, Del Rio J. Down-regulation of 3H-imipramine binding sites in rat cerebral cortex after prenatal exposure to antidepressants. *Life Sciences* 1990; **46**: 1619–26.
23. Cabrera-Vera TM, Garcia F, Pinto W, Battaglia G. Effect of prenatal fluoxetine (Prozac) exposure on brain serotonin neurons in prepubescent and adult male rat offspring. *Journal of Pharmacology and Experimental Therapeutics* 1997; **280**: 138–45.

24. Loebstein R, Koren G. Pregnancy outcome and neurodevelopment of children exposed *in utero* to psychoactive drugs: the Motherisk experience. *Journal of Psychiatry and Neuroscience* 1997; **22**: 192–6.

25. McElhatton PR, Garbis HM, Elefant E *et al*. The outcome of pregnancy in 689 women exposed to therapeutic doses of antidepressants. A collaborative study of the European Network of Teratology Information Services (ENTIS). *Reproductive Toxicology* 1996; **10**: 285–94.

26. Pastuszak A, Schick-Boschetto B, Zuber C *et al*. Pregnancy outcome following first-trimester exposure to fluoxetine (Prozac). *Journal of the American Medical Association* 1993; **269**: 2246–8.

27. Chambers CD, Johnson KA, Dick LM, Felix RJ, Jones KL. Birth outcomes in pregnant women taking fluoxetine. *New England Journal of Medicine* 1996; **335**: 1010–15.

28. Nulman I, Rovet J, Stewart DE *et al*. Neurodevelopment of children exposed *in utero* to antidepressant drugs. *New England Journal of Medicine* 1997; **336**: 258–62.

29. Kulin NA, Pastuszak A, Sage SR *et al*. Pregnancy outcome following maternal use of the new selective serotonin reuptake inhibitors. *Journal of the American Medical Association* 1998; **279**: 609–10.

30. Goldstein DJ. Effects of third-trimester fluoxetine exposure on the newborn. *Journal of Clinical Psychopharmacology* 1995 **15**: 417–20.

31. Goldstein DJ, Corbin LA, Sundell KL. Effects of first-trimester fluoxetine exposure on the newborn. *Obstetrics and Gynecology* 1997; **89**: 713–18.

32. Spencer MJ. Fluoxetine hydrochloride (Prozac) toxicity in a neonate. *Pediatrics* 1993; **92**: 721–2.

33. Dahl ML, Olhager E, Ahlner J. Paroxetine withdrawal syndrome in a neonate. *British Journal of Psychiatry* 1997; **171**: 391–2.

34. Cohen LS, Rosenbaum JF. Birth outcomes in pregnant women taking fluoxetine. *New England Journal of Medicine* 1997; **336**: 872.

35. Goldstein DJ, Sundell KL, Corbin LA. Birth outcomes in pregnant women taking fluoxetine. *New England Journal of Medicine* 1997; **336**: 872–3.

36. Jones KL, Johnson KA, Chambers CD. Birth outcomes in pregnant women taking fluoxetine. *New England Journal of Medicine* 1997; **336**: 873.

37. Koren G, Bologa M, Long D, Feldman Y, Shear NH. Perception of teratogenic risk by pregnant women exposed to drugs and chemicals during the first trimester. *American Journal of Obstetrics and Gynecology* 1989; **160**: 190–94.

38. Harper KH, Palmer AK, Davies RE. Effect of imipramine upon the pregnancy of laboratory animals. *Arzneimittelforschung* 1965; **15**: 1218–21.

39. Larsen V. The teratogenic effects of thalidomide, imipramine HCL and imipramine-N-oxide HCL on white Danish rabbits. *Acta Pharmacologica Toxicologica* 1963; **20**: 186–200.

40. Khan I, Azam A. Study of teratogenic activity of trifluoperazine, amitriptyline, ethionamide and thalidomide in pregnant rabbits and mice. *Excerpta Medica International Congress Series* 1969; **181**: 235–42.

41. Beyer BK, Guram MS, Geber WF. Incidence and potentiation of external and internal fetal anomalies resulting from chlordiazepoxide and amitriptyline alone and in combination. *Teratology* 1984; **30**: 39–45.

42. Guram MS, Gill TS, Geber WF. Teratogenicity of imipramine and amitriptyline in fetal hamsters. *Research Communications in Psychology Psychiatry and Behavior* 1980; **5**: 275–82.

43. Guram MS, Gill TS, Geber WF. Comparative teratogenicity of chlordiazepoxide, amitriptyline, and a combination of the two compounds in the fetal hamster. *Neurotoxicology* 1982; **3**: 83–90.

44. Jurand A. Malformations of the central nervous system induced by neurotropic drugs in mouse embryos. *Development and Growth Differences* 1980; **22**: 61–78.

45. Hendricks AG. Teratologic evaluation of imipramine hydrochloride in Bonnet (*Macaca radiata*) and Rhesus (*Macaca mulatta*) monkeys. *Teratology* 1975; **1**: 219–22.

46. Esaki K, Tanioka Y, Tsukada M, Izumiyama K. Teratogenicity of maprotiline tested by oral administration in mice and rats. *Jitchuken Zenrinsho Kenkyuho* 1976; **2**: 69–77.

47. Hirooka T, Morimoto K, Tadokoro T *et al*. Teratogenicity test on maprotiline in rabbits. *Oyo Yakuri Pharmacometrics* 1978; **15**: 555–65.

48. Owaki Y, Momiyama H, Onodera N. Effects of doxepin hydrochloride administered to pregnant rats upon the fetuses and their postnatal development. *Oyo Yakuri Pharmacometrics* 1971; **5**: 913–24.

49. Coyle IR. Changes in developing behavior following prenatal administration of imipramine. *Pharmacology, Biochemistry and Behavior* 1975; **3**: 799–807.

50. Ali SF, Buelke-Sam J, Newport GD, Slikker W Jr. Early neurobehavioral and neurochemical alterations in rats prenatally exposed to imipramine. *Neurotoxicology* 1986; **7**: 365–80.

51. Drago F, Continella G, Alloro MC, Scapagnini U. Behavioral effects of perinatal administration of antidepressant drugs in the rat. *Neurobehavioral Toxicology and Teratology* 1985; **7**: 493–7.

52. DeCeballos ML, Benedi A, DeFelipe C, Del Rio J. Prenatal exposure of rats to antidepressants enhances agonist affinity of brain dopamine receptors and dopamine-mediated behavior. *European Journal of Pharmacology* 1985; **116**: 257–62.

53. Scanlon FJ. Use of antidepressant drugs during the first trimester. *Medical Journal of Australia* 1969; **2**: 1077.

54. McBride WG. Limb deformities associated with iminodibenzyl hydrochloride. *Medical Journal of Australia* 1972; **1**: 492.

55. Morrow AW. Limb deformities associated with iminodibenzyl hydrochloride. *Medical Journal of Australia* 1972; **1**: 658–9.

56. Crombie DL, Pinsent RJFH, Fleming D. Imipramine in pregnancy. *British Medical Journal* 1972; **1**: 292.

57. Heinonen OP, Slone D, Shapiro S. *Birth defects and drugs in pregnancy*. Littleton, MA: Publishing Sciences Group, 1977.

58. Kuenssberg EV, Knox JDE. Imipramine in pregnancy. *British Medical Journal* 1972; **2**: 292.

59. Idanpaan-Heikkila J, Saxen L. Possible teratogenicity of imipramine/chloropyramine. *Lancet* 1973; **2**: 282–3.

60. Rachelefsky GS, Flynt JW, Ebbin AJ, Wilson MG. Possible teratogenicity of tricyclic antidepressants. *Lancet* 1972; **1**: 838–9.

61. Eggermont E, Raveschot J, Deneve V, Casteels-Van Daele M. The adverse influence of imipramine on the adaptation of the newborn infant to extrauterine life. *Acta Paediatrica Belgica* 1972; **26**: 197–204.

62. Misri S, Sivertz K. Tricyclic drugs in pregnancy and lactation: a preliminary report. *International Journal of Psychiatry in Medicine* 1991; **21**: 157–71.

63. Musa AB, Smith CS. Neonatal effects of maternal clomipramine therapy. *Archives of Diseases in Childhood* 1979; **54**: 405.

64. Webster PAC. Withdrawal symptoms in neonates associated with maternal antidepressant therapy. *Lancet* 1973; **2**: 318–19.

65. Ostergaard GZ, Pederson SE. Neonatal effects of maternal clomipramine treatment. *Pediatrics* 1982; **69**: 233–4.

66. Vree PH, Zwart P. A neonate with amitriptyline intoxication. *Nederlands Tijdschrift Geneeskunde* 1985; **129**: 910–12.

67. Falterman CG, Richardson CJ. Small left colon syndrome associated with maternal ingestion of psychotropic drugs. *Journal of Pediatrics* 1980; **97**: 308–10.

68. Shearer WT, Schreiner RL, Marshall RE. Urinary retention in a neonate secondary to maternal ingestion of nortriptyline. *Journal of Pediatrics* 1972; **81**: 570–2.

69. Anderson PO. Drug use during breast-feeding. *Clinical Pharmacy* 1991; **10**: 595–624.

70. Cowe L, Lloyd DJ, Dawling S. Neonatal convulsions caused by withdrawal from maternal clomipramine. *British Medical Journal* 1982; **284**: 1837–8.

71. Prentice A, Brown R. Fetal tachyarrythmia and maternal antidepressant treatment. *British Medical Journal* 1989; **298**: 190.

72. Mosby-Year Book Inc. Mosby's GenRx, *The complete reference for generic and brand name drugs*, 8th edn. St Louis, MO: Mosby Year Book, 1998.

73. Glaxo Wellcome Inc. *Product information for Wellbutrin tablets*. Research Triangle Park, NC: Glaxo Wellcome Inc., 1998.

74. Pavy TJG, Kliffer AP. Anaesthetic management of labour and delivery in a woman taking long-term MAOI. *Canadian Journal of Anaesthesia* 1995; **42**: 618–20.

75. Gracious BL, Wisner KL. Phenelzine use throughout pregnancy and the puerperium: case report, review of the literature, and management recommendations. *Depression and Anxiety* 1997; **6**: 124–8.

76. Poulson E, Robson JM. Effect of phenelzine and some related compounds on pregnancy and on sexual development. *Journal of Endocrinology* 1964; **30**: 205–15.

77. Poulson E, Robson JM. The effect of amine oxidase inhibitors on pregnancy. *Journal of Endocrinology* 1963; **27**: 147–52.

78. Whitaker-Azmitia PM, Zhang X, Clarke C. Effects of gestational exposure to monoamine oxidase inhibitors in rats: preliminary behavioral and neurochemical studies. *Neuropsychopharmacology* 1994; **11**: 125–32.

79. Werboff J, Gottliev JS, Dembicki EL, Havlena J. Postnatal effect of antidepressant drugs administered during gestation. *Experimental Neurology* 1961; **3**: 542–55.

80. Poulson E, Botros M, Robson JM. Effect of 5-hydroxytryptamine and iproniazid on pregnancy. *Science* 1960; **131**: 1101–2.

81. Koren Z, Pfeifer Y, Sulman FG. Induction of legal abortion by intra-uterine instillation of pargyline hydrochloride (Eutonyl). *Journal of Reproduction and Fertility* 1966; **12**: 75–9.

82. Potts DM. Termination of pregnancy. *British Medical Bulletin* 1970; **26**: 65–71.

83. Lesinski J, Kurzepa ST, Samojlik E. Influence of phenelzine on 5-hydroxytryptamine level in rat placenta and fetuses. *American Journal of Obstetrics and Gynecology* 1967; **97**: 249–51.

84. Chatterjee A, Biswas L, Pal AK. Aspirin and the reversal of antifertility effect of iproniazid in rats. *Prostaglandins* 1974; **7**: 285–91.

85. Robson JM, Sullivan FM, Wilson C. The maintenance of pregnancy during the pre-implantation period in mice treated with phenelzine derivatives. *Journal of Endocrinology* 1971; **49**: 635–48.

86. Marsafi YM, Hafez ESE. Effect of adrenoceptor blockers and MAOI on postcoital utero-oviductal contractility, sperm transport, and sperm attachment to eggs in rabbits. *Archives of Andrology* 1981; **6**: 307–16.

87. Briggs GG. Trazodone. In: Briggs GG, Freeman RK, Yaffe SJ (eds) *Drugs in pregnancy and lactation*, 4th edn. Baltimore, MD: Williams and Wilkins, 1994, 835–6.

88. Bristol-Myers Squibb Company. *Product information for Desyrel tablets*. Princeton, NJ: Bristol-Myers Squibb Company, 1998.

89. Bristol-Myers Squibb Company. *Product information for Serzone tablets*, Princeton, NJ: Bristol-Myers Squibb Company, 1998.

90. Miller LJ. Use of electroconvulsive therapy during pregnancy. *Hospital and Community Psychiatry* 1994; **45**: 444–50.

91. Nelson K, Holmes LB. Malformations due to presumed spontaneous mutations in newborn infants. *New England Journal of Medicine* 1989; **320**: 19–23.

92. Abrams R: *Electroconvulsive therapy*, 2nd edn. New York: Oxford University Press, 1992.

93. Ferrill MJ, Kehoe WA, Jacisin JJ. ECT during pregnancy: physiologic and pharmacologic considerations. *Convulsive Therapy* 1992; **8**: 186–200.

94. Kalinowsky LB. ECT in pregnancy. *American Journal of Psychiatry* 1984; **141**: 1643.

95. Wise MG, Ward SC, Townsend-Parchman W, Gilstrap LC, Hauth JC. Case report of ECT during high-risk pregnancy. *American Journal of Psychiatry* 1984; **141**: 99–101.

96. Remick RA, Maurice WL. ECT in pregnancy. *American Journal of Psychiatry* 1978; **135**: 761–2.

97. American Academy of Pediatrics. The promotion of breast-feeding. *Pediatrics* 1982; **69**: 654–61.

98. American Academy of Pediatrics Committee on Drugs. The transfer of drugs and other chemicals into human milk. *Pediatrics* 1994; **93**: 137–50.

99. Atkinson HC, Begg EJ, Darlow BA. Drugs in human milk: clinical pharmacokinetic considerations. *Clinical Pharmacokinetics* 1988; **14**: 217–40.

100. Preskorn SH. Pharmacokinetics of antidepressants: why and how they are relevant to treatment. *Journal of Clinical Psychiatry* 1993; **54(S9)**:14–34.

101. Stowe ZN, Owens MJ, Landry JC et al. Sertraline and desmethylsertraline in human breast milk and nursing infants. *Amercian Journal of Psychiatry* 1997; **154**: 1255–60.

102. Chisholm CA, Kuller JA. A guide to the safety of CNS-active agents during breastfeeding. *Drug Safety* 1997; **17**: 127–42.

103. Wisne KL, Perel JM, Findling RL. Antidepressant treatment during breast-feeding. *American Journal of Psychiatry* 1996; **153**: 1132–7.

104. Lester BM, Cucca J, Andreozzi L, Flanagan P, Oh W. Possible association between fluoxetine hydrochloride and colic in an infant. *Journal of the American Academy of Child and Adolescent Psychiatry* 1993; **32**: 1253–5.

105. Isenberg KE. Excretion of fluoxetine in human breast milk. *Journal of Clinical Psychiatry* 1990; **51**: 169.

106. Nightingale SL. Fluoxetine labelling revised to identify phenytoin interaction and to recommend against use in nursing mothers. *Journal of the American Medical Association* 1994; **271**: 1067.

107. Yoshida K, Smith B, Craggs M, Kumar RC. Fluoxetine in breast-milk and developmental outcome of breast-fed infants. *British Journal of Psychiatry* 1998; **172**: 175–9.

108. Taddio A, Ito S, Koren G. Excretion of fluoxetine and its metabolite, norfluoxetine, in human breast milk. *Journal of Clinical Pharmacology* 1996; **36**: 42–7.

109. Burch KJ, Wells BG. Fluoxetine/norfluoxetine concentrations in human milk. *Pediatrics* 1992; **90**: 676–7.

110. Mammen OK, Perel JM, Rudolph G, Foglia JP, Wheeler SB: Sertraline and norsertraline levels in three breastfed infants. *Journal of Clinical Psychiatry* 1997; **58**: 100–3.

111. Wisner KL, Perel JM, Blumer J. Serum sertraline and N-desmethylsertraline levels in breast-feeding mother–infant pairs. *American Journal of Psychiatry* 1998; **155**: 690–2.

112. Altshuler LL, Burt VK, McMullen M, Hendrick V. Breastfeeding and sertraline: a 24-hour analysis. *Journal of Clinical Psychiatry* 1995; **56**: 243–5.

113. Spigset O, Carleborg L, Norstrom A, Sandlund M. Paroxetine level in breast milk. *Journal of Clinical Psychiatry* 1996; **57**: 39.

114. Stowe ZN, Cohen LS, Hostetter A, Ritchie JC, Owens MJ, Nemeroff CB: Paroxetine in human breast milk and nursing infants. *American Journal of Psychiatry* 2000; **157**: 185–9.

115. Yoshida K, Smith B, Craggs M, Kumar RC. Investigation of pharmacokinetics and of possible adverse effects in infants exposed to tricyclic antidepressants in breast-milk. *Journal of Affective Disorders* 1997; **43**: 225–37.

116. Stancer HC, Reed KL. Desipramine and 2-hydroxydesipramine in human breast milk and the nursing infant's serum. *American Journal of Psychiatry* 1986; **143**: 1597–600.

117. Sovner R, Orsulak PJ. Excretion of imipramine and desipramine in human breast milk. *American Journal of Psychiatry* 1979; **136(4A)**: 451–2.

118. Bader TF, Newman K. Amitriptyline in human breast milk and the nursing infant's serum. *American Journal of Psychiatry* 1978; **137**: 855–6.

119. Breyer-Pfaff U, Entenmann A, Gaertner HJ. Secretion of amitriptyline and metabolites into breast milk. *American Journal of Psychiatry* 1995; **152**: 812–13.

120. Brixen-Rasmussen L, Halgrener J, Jorgensen A. Amitriptyline and nortriptyline excretion in human breast milk. *Psychopharmacology Berlin* 1982; **76**: 94–5.

121. Wisner KL, Perel JM. Nortriptyline treatment of breast-feeding women. *American Journal of Psychiatry* 1996; **153**: 295.

122. Wisner KL, Perel JM. Serum nortriptyline levels in nursing mothers and their infants. *American Journal of Psychiatry* 1991; **148**: 1234–6.

123. Kemp J, Ilett KF, Booth J, Hackett LP. Excretion of doxepin and N-desmethyldoxepin in human milk. *British Journal of Clinical Pharmacology* 1985; **20**: 497–9.

124. Matheson I, Pande H, Alertsen AR. Respiratory depression caused by N-desmethyldoxepin in breast milk. *Lancet* 1985; **2**: 1124.

125. Wisner KL, Perel JM, Foglia JP. Serum clomipramine and metabolite levels in four nursing mother-infant pairs. *Journal of Clinical Psychiatry* 1995; **56**: 17–20.

126. Schimmell MS, Katz EZ, Shaag Y, Pastuszak A, Koren G. Toxic neonatal effects following maternal clomipramine therapy. *Clinical Toxicology* 1991; **29**: 479–84.

127. Buist A, Janson H. Effect of exposure to dothiepin and northiaden in breast milk on child development. *British Journal of Psychiatry* 1995; **167**: 370–3.

128. Verbeeck RK, Ross SG, McKenna EA. Excretion of trazodone in breast milk. *British Journal of Clinical Pharmacology* 1986; **22**: 367–70.

129. Ilett KF, Hackett LP, Dusci LJ *et al.* Distribution and excretion of venlafaxine and O-desmethylvenlafaxine in human milk. *British Journal of Clinical Pharmacology* 1998; **45**: 459–62.

130. Jensen PN, Olesen OV, Bertelsen A, Linnet K. Citalopram and desmethylcitalopram concentrations in breast milk and in serum of mother and infant. *Therapeutic Drug Monitoring* 1997; **19**: 236–39.

131. Spigset O, Carleborg L, Ohman R, Norstrom A. Excretion of citalopram in breast milk. *British Journal of Clinical Pharmacology* 1997; **44**: 295–8.

5

Interpersonal psychotherapy for antepartum depressed women

MARGARET G. SPINELLI

PREGNANCY

Pregnancy is sometimes described as a period of emotional crisis, but it is truly a developmental period in which a woman makes the transition from independence to motherhood.[1] Pregnancy is a complicated, life-changing experience.[2] The expectant mother's social position, status in the community, career standing and social and family relationships are all about to change. The expectant mother anticipates the quick progression from her old independence to a new lifetime of family responsibility. There will be an alteration in her role as wife, as well as a redefinition of her relationship with her own mother. To complicate this upheaval further, the new mother must begin the process of separation from her own newborn child.

The pregnant woman in the USA is burdened with the myth of perfect motherhood. And while only the rewarding aspects of motherhood once confirmed the female identity, we have now come to recognize that some antepartum women may have ambivalent or even hostile feelings towards their pregnancy and the fetus they are carrying.

The unique hormonal environment of pregnancy has significant physiological and psychological sequelae. The pregnant woman experiences a range of emotions, from elation to fear and ambivalence.[3] In addition, she must adjust to her own ever-altering body image, as well as to the reactions of others around her to her pregnancy.

While normal pregnancy results in the recognition of the above mentioned conflicts, the developmental and psychological tasks of women with high-risk pregnancies are even more cumbersome. Pre-existing maternal disorders (e.g. diabetes, hypertension and cardiovascular disease)[4] and pregnancy complications (e.g. pre-eclampsia, multiple gestation, placenta praevia and abruptio placenta) may precipitate anxiety in the pregnant mother. These factors, as well as obstetric conditions that may cause fetal compromise (e.g. uterine dysfunction, pelvic disproportion, abnormal presentation, size or development of the fetus), may affect the outcome of the pregnancy and consequently the quality of life of the mother and her infant. Medical complications and associated concerns can increase anxiety and guilt, both of which predispose the new mother to depression.

DEPRESSION IN PREGNANCY

Although the prevalence of antepartum depression is similar to the rate found among postpartum and non-childbearing women, the myth of hormonal protection during pregnancy has been incorrectly perpetuated in the literature. Whereas 10% of pregnant women fulfil the criteria for major or minor depression,[5–7] antenatal depression often remains undiagnosed because the symptoms are similar to somatic complaints of pregnancy.[8]

Depressed pregnant women are at risk for anorexia, and are more likely to use nicotine, drugs and alcohol.[9] They are also less likely to seek and obtain adequate prenatal care. Serious sequelae which emphasize the need for early intervention are increased rates of accidental injury, child abuse and child neglect.[10]

During gestation, society expects the pregnant woman to be unfailingly happy, virtually to the point of elation. The stigma of mental illness is more prominent at this well-defined time in a woman's life. Although the emphasis on puerperal depression focuses on the postpartum period, many postpartum depressed women recall the onset of depressive symptoms during the pregnancy. Factors that predispose to antepartum depression include a personal or family history of mood disorder.[11] In addition, precipitant stressors such as marital dysfunction have been identified.[11] Demographic variables such as the young age of the mother, low level of education and increased number of children increase the risk of antenatal depression.[6] Because prenatal depression is the strongest predictor of postpartum depression,[12] the time for diagnosis and treatment of the parents of children at risk[13] is before birth.

Depression during pregnancy places the entire family at risk, and specifically it interferes with the mother–child interaction. Depressed pregnant women are at increased risk of raising infants who are withdrawn, irritable and difficult to console.[9] Children of depressed mothers may also develop significant behavioral problems such as sleep and eating disorders, frequent temper tantrums and the exacerbating effects of lower socio-economic status, such as delayed language development.[14]

Because the mother is less responsive to infant cues and may provide less warmth and acceptance[15] early development is marked by insecure attachment behavior.

Preschool difficulties include poor ability in problem-solving, anger,[15] intellectual deficits,[16] impaired social functioning, and a predisposition to depression itself.[13]

The relationship between early developmental problems and maternal depressive symptoms may begin during pregnancy. Altered intrauterine climate, including changes in maternal hormones and monoamine function, may affect the newborn's neurobehavioral function. Differences in the affective behavior of infants of depressed mothers compared to controls are reflected in frontal lobe activity on EEG.[17] This may indicate state changes that predispose infants to depression during their own lifetimes.

DIAGNOSING DEPRESSION IN A PUERPERAL WOMAN

Antepartum depression often goes unnoticed because the somatic complaints that accompany pregnancy are so symptomatically similar to depression, or are attributed to the pregnancy itself. Depression during pregnancy is often associated with somatic complaints,[8] and it is important to determine whether the somatic symptoms of depression are attributable to the pregnancy, or to stress and other associated factors. Klein and Essex[8] reviewed those common complaints of pregnancy which may overlap and be confused with depressive symptoms, such as fatigue, emotional lability, food cravings or aversions, nausea and vomiting, diminished interest in sex, feeling overweight, and problems with concentration. Complaints of fatigue, anergia and hypersomnia often challenge the clinician's differential diagnosis.

Because depressive symptoms may be confused with the expected and normal complications of pregnancy, it is important to determine the duration, quality and associated cause of these depressive symptoms. A review of symptoms and mild discomforts associated with various times of gestation includes, in the first trimester, fatigue, hypersomnia, anergia, nausea, vomiting, appetite change, mood lability and frequent urination. In the second trimester, fetal movement occurs and there is an overall improvement in somatic symptoms. In the last trimester, the woman again experiences fatigue, anergia and frequent urination. Insomnia may be secondary to the movements of the baby.

TREATMENT

Antepartum depressed women remain an underdiagnosed and undertreated population in psychiatry. Consequently, no treatment guidelines exist. The task of the physician must be to achieve wellness for the mother without compromising the fetal environment. A risk/benefit assessment should be presented, and the least invasive and most effective treatment followed. The informed consent of the prospective parents must always be a central concern for the physician in the overall treatment plan.

In an attempt to offer a safe and effective treatment during pregnancy, interpersonal psychotherapy (IPT) has been adapted and modified to treat antepartum depressive symptoms (IPT-P). In the National Institute of Mental Health (NIMH) Treatment of Depression Collaborative Research Program,[18,19] IPT was shown to reduce depressive symptoms significantly and to improve psychosocial functioning.

IPT has been adapted to several clinical populations.[20] Clinical trials have demonstrated the efficacy of IPT in acute[21,22] and maintenance[23] treatment of major depression. In a pilot controlled trial with HIV-positive outpatients,[24] Markowitz and colleagues focused on the HIV-positive diagnosis as a calamitous life event. Successful treatment was also reported in both adolescent depression[25] and bulimia.[26]

The efficacy of treatment of postpartum depression with IPT has been demonstrated by Stuart.[27]

Until recently there had been no controlled clinical trials of individual psychotherapy for the depressed, pregnant woman. IPT is a non-invasive treatment of proven efficacy which represents an excellent treatment alternative in this population. It is a brief 12 to 16-week fixed end-point treatment designed to treat non-psychotic major depression.[28] The goals of IPT include decreased neurovegetative symptoms of depression and the resolution of interpersonal conflicts. Although the emphasis is on current problems and concerns, treatment also deals with past problems as they relate to the present situation and also to depression.

Treatment of the depressed pregnant woman poses an obvious dilemma for both physician and patient. Commonly, the least invasive treatments are considered, initially as well as an evaluation of the seriousness of the mood disorder. Although the benefits of efficacious psychotherapy may outweigh the risks of pharmacotherapy in appropriately diagnosed women, the seriousness of the disorder will dictate appropriate treatment. The clinician must pay heed to the reality that the risks of untreated depression on the developing fetus have not been well studied. If a mother is not eating, sleeping or attending to her prenatal care, the well-being of the fetus is clearly placed in jeopardy.

Traditionally, the use of pharmacotherapy was believed to pose an absolute risk to the developing fetus, and only supportive psychotherapy was used to treat major and minor depressions in pregnant women. The medico-legal complications of pharmacotherapy in our present environment frequently dictate the type of treatment that is employed during gestation. Treatment has often remained merely supportive until decompensation or suicidality has indicated hospitalization or urgent electroconvulsive therapy.

Recent controlled clinical treatment trials on the use of psychotropic drugs during gestation have provided new and useful information about the relative safety of certain medications during pregnancy (see Chapter 5).[29–31] However, there is still little information available to assist the clinician in assuring the expectant parent of the absolute safety of most psychopharmacological interventions.[32]

Before the recent pharmacotherapy treatment trials, electroconvulsive therapy (ECT) was generally regarded as a safe and effective treatment for certain psychiatric disorders during pregnancy. Often indicated for psychotic mood disorders, severe depression or catatonia, ECT has also been used for psychiatric emergencies, as a replacement for failed treatments, or instead of psychotropic medications during the first trimester of pregnancy.[33]

Phototherapy,[34] which is used to treat seasonal affective disorder, is a new and relatively non-invasive alternative antidepressant therapy which has proved successful in clinical settings, and has recently become the focus of a pilot controlled treatment trial at three major psychiatric centers.[34]

INTERPERSONAL PSYCHOTHERAPY

In addition to the biological changes, pregnant women have to cope with other significant stressors (e.g. a changing role in their family and in society, concerns about obstetric difficulties, and acceptance of the parental role itself). IPT[28] is designed to enable the patient to cope better with interpersonal problems associated with symptom onset. The goals of IPT include a decrease in neurovegetative symptoms of depression and a resolution of interpersonal conflicts.[28] IPT does not assume an interpersonal etiology of depression, but rather that depression occurs in an interpersonal context. It is a focused treatment which examines specific problem areas and related data in the life of the patient.

IPT takes place in three distinct phases. In the initial phase, the therapist compiles an interpersonal inventory of the patient. Psychoeducation and selection of a treatment focus are also an essential focus of this initial phase, and an important component of the early phase of treatment. The medical model is used to explain depression as a biological illness, and the major issues associated with depression are then identified. Finally, a contract or agreement is then negotiated with the patient to focus treatment on the selected problem area.

In the intermediate phase, the main task for the therapist and patient is to identify one or two of the five problem areas normally associated with depression. Klerman and colleagues[28] have described four areas, namely grief, role dispute, role transition and interpersonal deficits. IPT modified for the antepartum patient (IPT-P) has one additional area of focus, namely the complicated pregnancy.[35] Treatment issues are always focused on the present, with previous relationships only being investigated as they relate to or parallel the current relationships. The work of IPT-P begins with an emphasis on the patient's particular problem as it relates to depression. The therapist must have an account of the patient's current and past relationships, as well as the pattern of relationships as they endure over time. Beliefs, expectations and the patient's role in the relationships as well as the associated affect and interpersonal experience, complete the therapist's focus during the intermediate phase.

In, the third phase, known as termination, the patient's feelings about the termination itself as well as a discussion of the progress made in therapy and the work that has still to be done are all considered. If the patient delivers before the 16 weeks of IPT-P are completed, then either the psychotherapy is resumed after delivery or antidepressant medication may be considered. After delivery, the patient is evaluated on a monthly basis for 6 months in order to determine the status of her depression during the postnatal period. This extended period of IPT-P into early parenting enables postpartum mood and the mother–infant interaction to be evaluated.

In summary, IPT-P is a modified therapy which addresses role transition, the developmental stages of pregnancy and the interpersonal issues related to the spouse, children and the woman's parents as they affect her parenting role. It should be noted that the demands on the patient's time, the occasional need for bed rest and the delivery itself may require scheduling flexibility and occasional telephone sessions. Also, in view of the fact that there is a role transition for both the prospective mother and the father, couples' sessions may be indicated.

INITIAL PHASE

As described above, IPT-P has been adapted to treat antepartum depression. The presence of acute suicidality, psychosis or substance abuse renders the patient unsuitable for IPT-P. During the initial phase of treatment, depressive symptoms are monitored weekly and psychoeducation is started.[28] The interpersonal inventory or the roster of significant others in the patient's life provide a background for exploration of the patient's interpersonal experience. The focus of the therapy will provide the substance of the treatment contract between the patient and the therapist.

According to Klerman and colleagues,[28] the therapist should accomplish certain tasks during the initial phase of treatment. Although the initial sessions should be focused, the patient should be permitted to mention any significant complaints as well as a history of current illness, duration of symptoms and the reasons why she is presenting at this time. The patient should also undergo a physical examination by her obstetrician, and laboratory tests, including thyroid function tests.

The diagnosis should be assessed according to the DSM-IV[36] criteria. Ratings of symptom severity using standardized tests such as the Hamilton Rating Scale for Depression[37] and the Edinburgh Postnatal Depression Scale[38] should be included.

Past psychiatric history, including the time and duration of past episodes of depression, treatment modalities, interpersonal precipitants or subsequent difficulties should be recorded at this stage. The seriousness of the depression is evaluated, and the degree of suicidal intent is assessed. The risks/benefits of pharmacotherapy must also be evaluated and discussed with the patient, and she should be advised that depression is a time-limited and treatable illness.[28]

The suitability of the patient for treatment is also assessed at this time. In addition, the feasibility of attendance should be discussed and its importance emphasized, with the necessary flexibility around childbirth issues being considered. Because many women prefer to avoid medication during gestation, they may be particularly motivated to seek IPT-P intervention. Moreover, the IPT-P therapist is often a welcome support during this time of high anxiety. Many women have concerns, fears and questions, particularly if this is their first pregnancy.

Although IPT-P appears to be well suited as a non-invasive treatment for most pregnant women, it is of course not appropriate for all women. This initial phase of therapy is the appropriate time to evaluate the circumstances surrounding conception and subsequent pregnancy. For the married woman with financial, social and emotional supports in place, a planned pregnancy is of course a wonderful and welcomed event. However, for women who have no 'significant other' or who have experienced a breakup of the relationship which fostered the pregnancy, the process can be overwhelming. Even under the best of circumstances, most women experience ambivalent feelings about pregnancy, and have significant concerns about childbirth. Under difficult circumstances, the depressed woman without external support systems may ultimately be overwhelmed. The course and ultimate success of IPT-P therefore hinge on the completeness of this initial investigation.

The formal interpersonal inventory is a roster of the significant relationships in the patient's life.[28] This catalogue should be supplemented by an inquiry to determine the nature of the interactions between the patient and her significant others. During this investigation there will also be an opportunity for inquiry into her feelings towards the infant. The purpose of this inventory is to collect information which can later be used to explain and demonstrate how the patient interacts with her world.

The psychotherapy techniques that are used to collect information for the interpersonal inventory in the first phase of treatment are direct inquisition and exploration.[28] A receptive silence on the part of the therapist encourages discussion.

The focus of treatment is the principal problem area related to the patient's depressive symptoms, even though it may be neither the cause nor the result of the mood disorder. As mentioned above, the areas of focus include role dispute, grief, role transition, interpersonal deficits and complicated pregnancy.

During this initial phase the therapist should explain the rationale for interpersonal therapy, and describe the guidelines for the progress of the treatment. The patient should develop a good understanding of the theory of IPT-P and how it relates to her depression. The course, timing and duration of appointments should be explained, and the feasibility of treatment explored. The therapist's policy for broken appointments is an important point of discussion. As discussed earlier, the need for flexibility because of needed bed rest, hospitalization or problems of child care should be elucidated.

The IPT-P treatment contract depends on an understanding between the patient and the therapist that the problem area is always the central focus of the therapy. The time for establishing this contract is during these early sessions. Agreement must be reached about such issues as the time and duration of appointments. In addition, financial contract which includes a policy for broken appointments and notice of cancellation requirements must be established. The patient must be assured that all information is treated as confidential. She should also be advised of the therapy timeframe, the specific time limit should be discussed and established.

The patient must understand that she is free to discuss any topic during the treatment. She must be encouraged to take the 'sick role' and allow herself the opportunity for care that she has otherwise not received during this illness.[28,39] This may of course be difficult for a mother who has other small children at home. Nonetheless, she should be encouraged to rest whenever possible.

Depression is presented to the patient as a biological illness, this being achieved through the use of verbal and pictorial representations. Analogies are drawn to other medical illnesses such as diabetes or pneumonia.

THE MIDDLE PHASE

The therapist will come to learn that psychotherapy with a pregnant woman[40] is a unique experience. The expectant mother has both an active fantasy life and a unique capacity for insight. Physiological changes and fetal growth take a new toll on her emotional life, and the pressure to achieve a new stability or emotional equilibrium before the birth. The need to make rapid psychological changes[40] further increase the already heavy burden of pregnancy.

The middle phase of IPT-P concentrates on the process of this change as the patient develops new interpersonal skills. Both the therapist and the patient will be active in bringing feelings, issues and conflicts to these sessions. The therapy highlights the specific problem area, while issues and associated affect are also explored. The goals to be met during this middle phase of treatment include an evaluation of the patient for worsening symptoms and the possible need for adjunctive therapy, the facilitation of discussion of issues that are relevant to the identified problem area, and the identification of feelings that are associated with both the problem area and the therapeutic relationship itself. The therapist should be flexible about permitting significant others into therapy sessions, and should assist the patient in identifying conflicts in the maternal role as they relate to the central problem area.

The principal psychotherapy technique used in these middle sessions is encouragement of affective expression,[28] specifically as it relates to the problem area. Facilitation of affect is thus the major task of this phase of treatment, whereby the patient is encouraged to connect her emotional responses with the substance of the interpersonal therapy. The patient's ability to work with affect is the essential force in fostering change in psychotherapy. Direct inquiry by the therapist about the patient's feelings should be accompanied by the therapist's assistance in helping to differentiate feelings from the impulse to act them out. Discussion of painful, hostile and emotionally laden material should be encouraged by the therapist.[28]

The patient now begins actively to address feelings experienced during the preceding weeks of therapy. The therapist should give positive reinforcement to the patient's progress, remaining empathic with her affective responses. The therapist plays a less active role than in the first-phase associate sessions, and facilitates the patient's ability to discuss feelings and associating their feelings with the relevant issues. The therapist must constantly evaluate the progress of the treatment in order to determine whether the current focus of treatment should be continued. The monitoring of depressive symptoms is an ongoing process, and a formal review of symptoms should take place before each new session.

The relevance of new information should be considered, and the patient should be encouraged to focus on the issue. In the middle phase, if the patient starts to wander from the established focus in order to introduce historical material, for example, they should be redirected to the central focus and to the issues at hand. At the conclusion of the session, the therapist may provide a brief synopsis of the session, closing with an emphasis on the problem area.

It is imperative that the therapist is mindful of the new and developing relationship between patient and therapist, and that they attempt at this time to identify and understand their feelings about the patient.[28] It is also crucial to identify the patient's reactions to and feelings about this new relationship, and to encourage them to share these feelings. This is especially important if the focus of treatment is interpersonal deficits, as the patient–therapist relationship becomes the model for developing new interpersonal skills, and it can also illuminate how the patient relates to others in her life.

The interpersonal nature of the treatment means that significant others may be invited to occasional sessions. In addition, psychoeducation about depression (a frequently neglected area) can help family members to understand and facilitate the patient's recovery.

Directive techniques such as education, advice, modeling and direct help may help to solve practical problems for the patient. Young mothers in particular may need assistance in finding child care, financial aid or other critical necessities. The therapist should progress from direct interventions to encouragement of the patient's own independence in problem-solving. Direct help is useful initially.[28] However, the patient must be made aware that she is ultimately responsible for her own decisions. Direct techniques should therefore be used sparingly, to be gradually replaced by the patient's growing self-confidence and self-reliance.

As the patient develops a new sense of mastery over her feelings and actions, the therapist should help to instil a sense of competence, so that the patient can continue to develop and employ these interpersonal skills in her everyday life.

The patient should always be reminded of the brief time-frame of therapy as the treatment progresses. Self-reliance is the goal of therapy.

Problem areas

GRIEF

Pregnancy may stir up feelings about other relationships or losses. The normal grief reaction includes physical symptoms and somatic anxiety, preoccupation with the lost person, feelings of guilt and hostility, and a change in the usual patterns of behavior.[41] Bereavement may not occur with the loss, but may be delayed or postponed indefinitely as a result of the patient's coping mechanisms. Grief may be manifested during a subsequent event in the patient's life, such as a pregnancy, birth or death. Manifestations of abnormal bereavement include overreacting, the development of somatic symptoms in the bereaved person, exacerbation of preexisting physical disorders, broken relationships, repressed hostility and rage, social withdrawal, self-destructive activities and agitated depression.

In their description of the role that grief plays in IPT, Klerman and colleagues[28] described abnormal grief as either delayed or distorted grief. In a delayed grief reaction, grieving is postponed only to present later as depression. New events or losses may trigger this delayed grief. During the first-phase interpersonal inventory, the history of loss was explored in order to help explain the possible genesis of this grief, as the patient is no doubt unaware that a previous loss is somehow connected to the current depression.

Thus a distorted grief reaction may occur immediately or be postponed. The grief reaction, now inappropriate to the loss, may manifest itself in either indifference or somatic concerns. Lewis[42] has described the inhibition of mourning by pregnancy. He proposes that bereavement is extremely difficult because the pregnant woman is preoccupied with thoughts, fantasies and feelings about her new baby.[43] Therefore normal mourning is precluded. Moreover, because mourning requires a similar preoccupation with the deceased in order to free oneself from the loss, it is impossible to resume mourning at a later time. This now unresolved mourning may then be activated in pathological forms by unrelated events as depression.

A complicated grief reaction may be experienced in response to perinatal death. Mothers may blame themselves for the death of the newborn, they may feel angry about the injustice of the loss, they may yearn to regain the dead child and they may devalue their maternal competency. Denial is the powerful defense which often impedes mourning in perinatal death. Factors such as guilt, dependency on the deceased or the suddenness of the event may prevent the resolution of mourning.

In the case of perinatal loss,[44] there may be unconscious selection of a subsequent child to replace the lost child. This new child may be identified with the deceased. Efforts should be made to separate the identity of the dead child from that of the child chosen to replace the loss, and the mother must come to recognize this confusion with the deceased before the dead child's identity can be finally relinquished. Overprotection of and anxiety about the newborn may be the dominant features of her interaction with the new child. The mother must confront both her fears of another loss, and her anger that the replacement child cannot cancel the loss of the deceased. Because the mother may have had either minimal or no inter-action with the deceased, her feelings are more easily displaced from the lost child to the subsequent pregnancy. In addition, the knock to self-worth may result in eagerness to be pregnant again in order to repair the narcissistic damage. If mourning is incomplete, the subsequent child cannot be loved in its own right and will always remain an unsatisfactory substitute for the dead child.

A woman with a history of one or more induced or spontaneous abortions is also at risk for mood changes during pregnancy, particularly if she was ambivalent about a previous pregnancy or termination. When she ultimately has a successful pregnancy and delivery, she may still continue to feel guilty, and have heightened concerns about her infant's health and well-being.

The task of the IPT-P therapist is to facilitate expression of the mother's grief through empathic and non-judgmental encouragement, and to share her feelings of sadness and loss. The context of grief must be shared in the wishes, fantasies and hopes of a child who will never be. Termination of treatment will be crucial, and will highlight how completely the loss has been resolved.[44]

ROLE TRANSITION

Pregnancy is a time of developmental upheaval that is similar in impact to the onset of adolescence or the passage into menopause.[45] The woman's self-image is reorganized as she begins to adapt to her new role as mother. This adaptation is completed with the psychological separation of the child from the mother.

A woman with a satisfying career may have difficulty in changing from her old work habits and lifestyle. With the arrival of her child and the responsibilities involved, she may indeed come to resent the intrusion of the infant. If she has invested strongly in her body image, she may become distressed by the changing shape of her body. She may also fear disruption of the bond she has formed with her partner. These issues may cause the expectant mother to become ambivalent or even resentful about the inevitable changes that will occur in all aspects of her life.

The new role of mother is associated with a necessary loss of independence. Klerman and colleagues[28] describes the difficulties in coping, which may manifest as loss of familiar social supports, management of associated emotions (e.g. anger or fear) the need for a new reper-toire of social skills, and diminished self-esteem.

Treatment strategies for a role transition are similar to treatment strategies for grief, in that the tasks involved in mastering the role transition can only be achieved if the woman has completed the tasks of her former role.

The patient must also separate from her former role before she can successfully move on to her new role. The therapist should assist the patient in evaluating the old role, which may well be idealized as a result of the anxiety associated with the new role, the need for security and comfort causing her to maintain a hold on her old role. The benefits of the former role should be delineated and the affective expression of its loss encouraged.[28] Because a lack of mastery of the new role may generate anxiety, the therapist must facilitate the patient's ability to master the tasks that are necessary to her new role as a mother. Although many skills may be handed down from her own mother, mothering may also be learned in prepared childbirth and/or parenting classes. The new mother must also be encouraged to develop new social skills by forming relationships with other new mothers and/or parent groups.

New social supports are established when the woman forms her own network of friends who are themselves parents of young children. She should also be encouraged to attend parenting classes as a way to ease her apprehension and she should be encouraged to include her partner in these activities.

INTERPERSONAL DEFICITS

If the patient is socially impoverished, with few if any lasting background relationships and a history of extreme social isolation, then personality deficits must be considered as the treatment focus.[28]

The challenge and goal of the treatment will be to minimize the patient's social isolation.[28] Because there is an absence of strong current relationships, old or past relationships must become the focus of her treatment. The tasks involved in handling the problem of interpersonal deficits have been described by Klerman and colleagues.[28]

These socially impoverished patients require a more complete personal inventory that include any past romantic relationships or childhood friends. The best and worst aspects of each relationship are explored, and eventually more recent relationships are examined. Often the parental relationship of the woman provides the springboard for exploring her lifelong pattern of interactions. The pattern of the patient's role in her own family often helps to explain how she perceives herself in the world. For example, if she has few or no close friends, this may well be a response to rejection or criticism.

If the patient has difficulty in expressing anger, she may 'act out' her anger outside treatment. Such patients can be taught appropriate means of expression through the model of the therapist–patient relationship.[28] This provides the most direct data about the patient. Solving problems, negotiating treatment contracts and co-operating with the therapist provide a useful model for the patient with regard to developing future relationships. Participation in role play may be an important modality in these patients. Use of the therapeutic relationship is a very powerful tool, particularly in this problem area. The relationship between the therapist and patient should serve as a model for treatment because it is a 'here-and-now' example of interpersonal difficulties. Once the therapeutic alliance is established, the patient should be encouraged to express her feelings about the therapist.[28] The transference relationship is used as an instrument for modeling and role play. However, in contrast to dynamic psychotherapy, there is no interpretation of the transference by the therapist.[28]

INTERPERSONAL ROLE DISPUTE

Klerman and colleagues[28] define a role dispute as one in which two people in a relationship have conflicting expectations. A typical example is the pregnant woman who expects to stop work to become a 'full-time mother' after her child is born. However, because of a fall in her husband's earnings, she finds that she must return to work. The role dispute must occur in the context of depression. Disputes contribute to the patient's poor self-esteem, causing her to feel both powerless and out of control. In addition, the possible loss of the relationship itself may pose a threat. If the couple has poor communication skills, then they are likely to reach an impasse that renders them incapable of conflict resolution.[28]

The cognitive impairment present in depression predisposes the patient to feelings of failure and guilt for both problems in her environment and difficulties in her relationships. When completing the interpersonal inventory, the therapist should explore the patient's relationship changes both before and after the onset of depression.

The goals and strategies of treatment should be determined, with the patient being encouraged to play an active role in the design of the planned strategy. The therapist should help to illuminate any current dispute, and design plans for a program to help modify the patient's communication and expectations. It is not the therapist's task to salvage a relationship if the patient is unenthusiastic about this. The therapist must follow the patient's lead and explore a desirable and realistic outcome. Klerman and colleagues[28] advise that the stages of role dispute should be determined before active treatment begins.[28]

The role of the IPT-P therapist is to foster an understanding of role expectations, to master negotiations, and to aid in the resolution of conflict. Questions should be posed. For example, what are the factors in the dispute? What are the values and expectations? What does each party want from the relationship? Are these desires realistic? What is the patient's capacity for personal change? What are the possibilities for change in the relationship?

It is important to explore parallels of current problems in the patient's former relationships. The patient should always be encouraged to express anger, as well as feelings of hurt and fear.

DISORDERS OF THE MOTHER–INFANT RELATIONSHIP

Although the concept of a role dispute between mother and infant may seem unlikely, if not peculiar, mother–infant relationship disorders are adapted to the role dispute problem category. Hostile feelings towards the infant may occur in an unwanted pregnancy or in other difficult circumstances surrounding the pregnancy.[46] The antenatal period is an excellent time to explore and resolve these feelings.

Disorders of the mother–infant bond range from delayed attachment to infanticide.[47] Approximately 10% of new mothers will experience a delayed attachment to their infant. A further 1% will have negative or hostile thoughts about their newborn, and whereas child abuse is also on the continuum of poor attachment, infanticide occurs in 1 in 50 000 births.

Although the bond with the infant may not form immediately, most bonds will strengthen during the weeks after delivery. Mother–infant attachment disorders are most often described in the postpartum period, but they can be detected and explored during gestation so as to facilitate the resolution of hostile feelings before delivery.

Obsessional intrusive thoughts about the infant may also arise during gestation.[48] Although feelings of rejection are more common in unwanted pregnancies, they may also occur in pregnancies where, for example, an amniocentesis has revealed a congenital anomaly or genetic defect. The mother's guilt, anger or feelings of failure about this serve to generate hostile feelings towards the baby, and she may feel trapped if she is beyond the point of possible termination. The patient must therefore be assisted in resolving her sadness and anger.

Delayed attachment can have significant sequelae, such as failure to thrive, impaired emotional and cognitive development and difficulty in developing relationships.[48] In his review of infanticide, Resnick states that neonaticide (murder of a newborn in the first 24 h after birth) occurs in young, unmarried mothers without evidence of psychosis.[49]

It has been this author's experience that young unmarried mothers who commit neonaticide do in fact have serious psychiatric illnesses including dissociative states and often transient states of psychoses. These women are profoundly depressed, and are so detached from the fetus that they deny their own pregnancies. If psychiatric symptoms are detected in the prenatal period, infanticide may be prevented.

COMPLICATED PREGNANCY

Complicated pregnancy includes the presence of major life events such as a serious illness, obstetrical difficulties, the death of a loved one or a previous perinatal loss. For example, an unwanted pregnancy may be the result of rape. Even a successful conception after a period of infertility may complicate the pregnancy.

The transition to motherhood may be further burdened by concurrent life events such as a move to a new house or a change in job status. Distressing events such as bereavement, job loss, negative results of fetal diagnostic tests or a threatened miscarriage can provoke anxiety, grief, rejection and loss – all at a time when happiness and fulfilment should be the normal expectations. Conflicting feelings must be integrated, and the mother should be enabled to work towards their resolution, while at the same time sustaining the hopefulness of pregnancy.

Conflicted pregnancy refers to an unplanned, untimely or overvalued pregnancy.[40] Overvalued pregnancies are those which result after prolonged if not extraordinary efforts to conceive. Such efforts might involve infertility treatment or *in-vitro* fertilization. This also includes pregnancies that occur after a previous stillbirth, habitual spontaneous abortions or perinatal death. Ambivalence is manifested as the mother-to-be vacillates between hopefulness and distrust, elation and detachment, idealization and nihilism. Such patients may become overanxious parents – the kind who will monitor the infant's every move and breath.

Unsupported women – those who find themselves alone after divorce, abandonment or the death of a partner – are also highly distressed. They lack the feeling that they can control their own destinies. Their grief, fear, guilt, resentment, sadness and fragility conflict with the common expectations of a happy pregnancy. These negative feelings must be disentangled and resolved before the birth of a child who may otherwise be forced to bear the brunt of unresolved 'baggage'. The mother may even feel that the newborn is responsible for the breakup with the partner, and such feelings may be unconsciously conveyed to the child.

An independent woman with an unplanned pregnancy must evaluate her single identity and determine the relationship within which she wishes to raise her new child. This decision may well involve moral, emotional and financial considerations as well as the possible complication of career demands. A fragile relationship could go into crisis, and even a well-established marriage could suddenly experience conflict. Some partners when faced with the dilemma of an unplanned pregnancy will accept the situation, but only with considerable ambivalence.

An untimely pregnancy may be one in which a very young mother's adolescence is interrupted, or in which an older mother-to-be is concerned about the interruption to her established lifestyle or the statistical increase in the risk of birth defects with age.

The pregnancy itself may be 'wrong.' A 'wrong' pregnancy results from rape or incest and presents complications at many different levels. Will the baby be normal? How will the family endure? What about internalized feelings of blame and badness? If the woman continues with the pregnancy, she has the additional burden of differentiating between the baby and the rape of which the baby will always be a reminder.

In a complicated pregnancy, the woman and perhaps also her partner may lack the ability to parent adequately because of their own lack of proper nurturance or adequate mothering.

Concurrent illness may take the form of psychiatric disorders, chronic medical illness or obstetrical complications. In general, the woman is significantly more anxious during pregnancy than she is in her prepregnant state. She becomes increasingly introspective and preoccupied with the pregnancy, and may also have heightened dependency needs.[50]

During pregnancy, psychiatric disorders may be exacerbated or conversely, the woman may experience a period of increased well-being. If a disorder is exacerbated, treatment dilemmas may occur.

Iancu has stated that 0.5–1.0 in 1000 women will develop severe and intractable nausea and vomiting during the first trimester of pregnancy.[51] Hyperemesis gravidarum is characterized by dehydration, weight loss, electrolyte imbalance, ketosis and even liver or renal damage (see Chapter 9). Although several organic and functional causes of vomiting during pregnancy have been described, it has been suggested that immaturity or lack of coping skills may contribute to the etiology. Poor study methodology has resulted in a significant lack of knowledge of psychological and physiological causes.[50] Early psychological intervention may contribute to the well-being of these women.

For the most part, infectious diseases do not seriously affect the pregnant woman or her fetus. However, there are some infectious diseases which have serious or even life-threatening consequences for the pregnant woman. Rubella (German measles) contracted during the first 4 months of gestation may result in congenital defects or even fetal death. Infants who survive a mother's rubella during pregnancy have prolonged active viral infections.

Another serious infection is autoimmune deficiency in HIV-positive women. Although there seems to be little placental transmission of the virus, transmission via breast-milk is common. These women must be educated about the infectious transmission of the virus and cautioned against breastfeeding. In addition, women with the later stages of AIDS may be in need of bereavement counseling and assistance with plans to care for their children.[52]

Another issue of longstanding concern is the influence of diabetes mellitus, which places a significant physical burden on the pregnant woman. The diabetes may be pre-existing or it may have been precipitated by the pregnancy.[52] Complications of diabetes may include disturbed water balance, hypertension or pre-eclampsia, macrosomia an excessively large infant), stillbirth or neonatal death. These pregnant women must deal with both their own anger at being cheated of a normal pregnancy and their consequent fears about the outcome of the pregnancy and delivery.

The causes of vaginal bleeding are varied. Placenta praevia is the premature separation of an abnormally implanted placenta, with consequent hemorrhage.[4] The seriousness of placenta praevia is determined by the position of the placenta and the covering of the cervical opening. Such factors will determine the appropriate treatment, which ranges from bed rest to elective termination by Cesarean section. Bleeding accompanied by pain may indicate abruptio placenta, which necessitates emergency delivery.

Bed rest takes a large toll on the emotional health of the mother. It may be ordered because of premature contractions, or because of multiple births. The consequences of bed rest, including the lack of exercise, possible loss of a career, concern about fetal well-being and the limited outlets for anxiety may all contribute to increased feelings of depression.

Clearly the emotional consequences of giving birth to a defective child can be devastating.[53] Fetal anomalies may be detected by the use of amniocentesis accompanied by genetic counseling. The emotional trauma of losing a wanted pregnancy or adapting to life with a child with a defect is often overwhelming. The couple may feel responsible, regard themselves as defective in some way and consequently suffer a blow to their self-esteem. The initial reaction to the child is one of shock and disbelief, followed by anger, and finally grief and/or depression.

Selective termination may be sought if the mother has a multiple pregnancy. This may be undertaken if one or more of the fetuses is abnormal, or if continuation of the pregnancy poses a serious risk to the mother's well-being or to the pregnancy itself. This situation is most often encountered in previously infertile women who now have multiple gestations due to ovulation induction.[53]

TERMINATION OF TREATMENT

The termination of treatment for the pregnant mother can be complicated. If she has given birth before the end of treatment, she is accompanied by her baby to the final sessions. The patient now faces the new task of ending her relationship with the therapist.[28] The emphasis must now be focused on the patient's newly developed sense of confidence and her newly discovered ability to deal with issues which had previously been managed with the help of the therapist.

It is not unusual for depressive symptoms to return in the final days of therapy. The patient should be encouraged to explore any recurrent feelings of hopelessness or helplessness, and the therapist should explain that these feelings are merely a consequence of the termination.[28] It is vital for the patient to realize that the task of termination is really her responsibility. Although her condition has improved with the help of the psychotherapist, in all likelihood she will not regress in the therapist's absence. The therapist should explore the patient's feelings and concerns about the end of treatment. The patient's successes should be reiterated, and she should be congratulated. Areas of potential concern should be discussed, and contingency plans for potential problem-solving should be outlined.

SUMMARY

An open-trial pilot study on the modification of IPT for depressed antepartum women (IPT-P) assessed the possibility that IPT-P would be effective in the treatment of antenatal depression.[35] A total of 13 antepartum depressed women who met DSM-III-R criteria for a major depressive episode received 16 weekly sessions of IPT-P.

End-point analysis demonstrated a significant decrease in mean depression scores over the course of treatment for all of the subjects who entered the study.[35] Of the 10 women available at 3 months postpartum, none reported depressive symptoms. This study served as a basis for a controlled clinical trial involving 50 women who were randomized to either IPT-P or a parenting education control condition. Funded by the National Institute for Mental Health, this study provides the opportunity to determine a hierarchy of treatment guidelines for antepartum depression in women who might otherwise require medication.

This chapter has included guidelines for conducting IPT-P, a discussion of the different phases of treatment, and modifications relating to the specific concerns of the antepartum woman. The developmental stages of pregnancy, particularly role transition as the patient approaches delivery, have been addressed. If IPT-P is found to be an effective treatment for depression in a controlled clinical trial, treatment guidelines may be established for antepartum depression. Sessions which extend into the postpartum period may provide an excellent opportunity for monitoring the mother–infant interaction and correlating this relationship with depressive symptoms. The study of antepartum women is a potentially fruitful area of research in a previously underserved population. Because prenatal depression may predict the onset of postpartum depression,[12] the optimal time to diagnose depression is during pregnancy in order to provide secondary prevention by treating the parents of children at risk.

The study described above provides an opportunity to test a central method of delivering care, to determine the outcome of mothers and infants who are victims of untreated mental illness, to establish guidelines for treating psychiatrically ill pregnant women, and to educate our colleagues in psychiatry and obstetrics on these issues.

REFERENCES

1. Benedek T. Parenthood as a developmental phase: a contribution to the libido theory. *Journal of the American Psychanalytical Association* 1959; **7**: 389–576.
2. Zajicek E. The experience of being pregnant. In:Wolind S, Zajicek E (eds) *Pregnancy: a psychological and social study*. London: Academic Press, 1984: 31–56.
3. Carr ML. Normal and medically complicated pregnancies. In: Stewart DE, Stotland ND (eds) *Psychological aspects of women's health*. Washington, DC: American Psychiatric Association Press, 1993, 15–35.
4. Willson JR, Carrington ER, Ledger WJ. *Obstetrics and gynecology*, 7th edn. St Louis, MO: CV Mosby Company, 1983.
5. O'Hara M, Zekoski EM, Philipps LH *et al*. Controlled prospective study of postpartum mood disorders: comparison of childbearing and non-childbearing women. *Journal of Abnormal Psychology* 1990; **99**: 3–15.
6. Gotlib IH, Whiffen VE, Mount JH. Prevalence rates and demographic characteristics associated with depression in pregnancy and the postpartum. *Journal of Consulting and Clinical Psychology* 1989; **57**: 269–74.
7. Kumar R, Robson KM. A prospective study of emotional disorders in childbearing women. *British Journal of Psychiatry* 1984; **144**: 35–47.
8. Klein MH, Essex MJ. Pregnant or depressed? The effect of overlap between symptoms of depression and somatic complaints of pregnancy on rates of major depression in the second trimester. *Depression* 1994; **2**: 1165–7.
9. Zuckerman B, Bauchner H, Parker S *et al*. Maternal depressive symptoms during pregnancy, and new born irritability. *Developmental and Behavioral Pediatrics* 1990; **114**: 190–4.
10. Scott D. Early identification of maternal depression as a strategy in the prevention of child abuse. *Child Abuse and Neglect* 1992; **16**: 345–58.
11. Dimitrovsky L, Perez-Hishberg M, Itskowitz R. Depression during and following pregnancy: quality of family relationships. *Journal of Psychology* 1986; **12**: 213–18.
12. Graff LA, Dyck DG, Schallow JR. Predicting postpartum depressive symptoms and structural modeling analysis. *Perceptual and Motor Skills* 1991; **73**: 1137–8.
13. Weissman MM, Gammon GD, John K *et al*. Children of depressed parents: increased psychopathology and early onset of major depression. *Archives of General Psychiatry* 1987; **44**: 847–53.
14. Murray L. The impact of postnatal depression on infant development. *Journal of Child Psychology and Psychiatry* 1992; **35**: 343–61.
15. Biringen Z, Robison J. Emotional availability in mother–child interaction: a reconceptualization for research. *American Journal of Orthopsychiatry* 1991; **61**: 258–71.
16. Cogill SR, Caplan HL, Heather A *et al*. Impact of maternal postnatal depression on cognitive development of young children. *British Medical Journal* 1986; **292**: 1165–7.
17. Dawson G, Klinger LG, Panagiotides H *et al*. Frontal lobe activity and affective behavior of infants of mothers with depressive symptoms. *Child Development* 1992; **63**: 725–37.
18. Weissman MM, Rounsaville BJ, Chevron E. Training psychotherapists to participate in psychotherapy outcome studies: identifying and dealing with the research requirements. *American Journal of Psychiatry* 1982; **139**: 1442–6.
19. Elkin I, Shea MT, Watkins JT *et al*. NIMH treatment of depression collaborative research program: general effectiveness of treatments. *Archives of General Psychiatry* 1989; **46**: 971–82.
20. Klerman GL, Weissman MM. *New applications of interpersonal psychotherapy*. Washington, DC: American Psychiatric Association Press, 1993.
21. Weissman MM, Prusoff BA, Dimascio A *et al*. The efficacy of drugs and psychotherapy in the treatment of acute depressive episodes. *American Journal of Psychiatry* 1979; **136**: 555–8.

22. Sloane RB, Staples FR, Schneider LS. Interpersonal therapy versus nortriptyline for depression in the elderly. In: Burrows GD, Norman TR, Dennerstein L (eds) *Clinical and pharmacological studies in psychiatric disorders. Biological psychiatry. New prospects* London: John Libbey, 1985: 344–46.

23. Kupfer DT, Frank E. The advantage of early treatment intervention in recurrent depression. *Archives of General Psychiatry* 1989; **46**: 771–5.

24. Markowitz JC, Klerman GL, Perry SW *et al*. Interpersonal psychotherapy of depressed HIV-positive outpatients. *Hospital and Community Psychiatry* 1992; **43**: 885–90.

25. Mufson L, Moreau D, Weissman MM *et al*. *Interpersonal psychotherapy for depressed adolescents.* New York: The Guilford Press, 1993.

26. Agras WS. Nonpharmacologic treatments of bulimia nervosa. *Journal of Clinical Psychiatry* 1991; **52** (Supplement 10): 29–33.

27. Stuart S: Treatment of postpartum depression with interpersonal psychotherapy. *Archives of General Psychiatry* 1995; **52**: 75–6.

28. Klerman GL, Weissman MM, Rounsaville BH *et al*. *Interpersonal psychotherapy of depression*. New York: Basic Books, 1984.

29. Misri S, Sivertz K. Tricyclic drugs in pregnancy and lactation: a preliminary report. *International Journal of Psychiatry in Medicine* 1991; **21**: 157–72.

30. Pastuszak A, Schick-Boschetto B, Zuber C *et al*. Pregnancy outcome following first-trimester exposure to fluoxetine. *Journal of the American Medical Association* 1993; **269**: 2246–8.

31. Jacobson, SJ, Jones K, Johnson K *et al*. Prospective multicenter study of pregnancy outcome after lithium exposure. *Lancet* 1992; **39**: 530–3.

32. Nulman I, Rovet J, Stewart DE *et al*. Neurodevelopment of children exposed *in utero* to antidepressant drugs. *New England Journal of Medicine* 1997; **6**: 258–62.

33. Stewart DE, Robinson GE. Psychotropic drugs and electroconvulsive therapy during pregnancy and lactation. In: Stewart DE, Stotland NL (eds) *Psychological aspects of women's health.* Washington, DC: American Psychiatric Association Press, 1993, 71–95.

34. Terman M, Terman JS, Quitkin FM *et al*. Light therapy for seasonal affective disorder. *Neuropsychopharmacology* 1989; **2**: 1–22.

35. Spinelli M. Interpersonal psychotherapy for depressed antepartum women: a pilot study. *American Journal of Psychiatry* 1997; **154**: 1028–30.

36. American Psychiatric Association. *Diagnostic and statistical manual of mental disorders*, 4th edn. Washington, DC: American Psychiatric Association Press, 1994.

37. Hamilton MA. Rating scale for depression. *Journal of Neurololgy, Neurosurgery and Psychiatry* 1960; **23**: 56–62.

38. Harris B, Huckle P, Thomas R *et al*. The use of rating scales to identify postnatal depression. *British Journal of Psychiatry* 1989; **154**: 813–17.

39. Parsons T. Illness and the role of the physician: a sociological perspective. *Journal of Orthopsychiatry* 1951; **21**: 452–60.

40. Raphael-Leff J. Psychotherapy and pregnancy. *Journal of Reproductive and Infertility Psychology* 1990; **8**: 119–35.

41. Lindenmann E: Symptomatology and management of acute grief. *American Journal of Psychiatry* 1944; **101**: 141–8.

42. Lewis E. Inhibition of mourning by pregnancy: psychopathology and management. *British Medical Journal* 1979; **2**: 27–8.

43. Lewis E, Casement P. The inhibition of mourning by pregnancy: a case study. *Psychoanalytical Psychotherapy* 1986; **2**: 45–52.

44. Leon IG. Short-term psychotherapy for perinatal loss. *Psychotherapy* 1987; **24**: 186–95.

45. Trad PV. On becoming a mother: in the throes of developmental transformation. *Psychoanalytical Psychology* 1990; **7**: 341–61.

46. St Andre M. Psychotherapy during pregnancy: opportunities and challenges. *American Journal of Psychotherapy* 1993; **47**: 372–590.
47. Robinson GE, Stewart DE. Postpartum disorders. In: Stewart DE, Stotland NL (eds) *Psychological aspects of women's health*. Washington, DC: American Psychiatric Association Press, 1993, 115–38.
48. Brockington I, Cox-Roper A. The nosology of puerperal mental illness. In: Kumar R, Brockington IF (eds) *Motherhood and mental illness*. Vol. 2. London: Wright, 1988, 1–17.
49. Resnick PJ. Murder of the newborn: a psychiatric review of neonaticide. *American Journal of Psychiatry* 1970; **126**: 1414–20.
50. Miller LJ. Psychiatric disorders during pregnancy. In: Stewart DE, Stotland NL (eds) *Psychological aspects of women's health care*. Washington, DC: American Psychiatric Association Press, 1993, 55–70.
51. Iancu J. Psychiatric aspects of hyperemesis gravidarum. *Psychotherapy Psychosomatics* 1994; **61**: 143–9.
52. Devinsky O, Bartlik B. Psychiatric disorders and pregnancy. In: Devinsky O, Feldmann E, Hainline B. (eds) *Advances in neurology: neurological complications of pregnancy. Vol. 64*. New York: Raven Press, 1994, 215–30.
53. Robinson GE, Wisner KL. Fetal Anomalies. In: Stewart DE, Stotland NL (eds) *Psychological aspects of women's health*. Washington, DC: American Psychiatric Association Press, 1993, 37–55.

6

The treatment of bipolar disorder during pregnancy

LORI L. DAVIS, STACY SHANNON, ROGER G. DRAKE AND FREDERICK PETTY

INTRODUCTION

A number of factors must be evaluated in order to determine the safety of any medication that is being considered for use during pregnancy. All psychotropic medications diffuse readily across the placenta. No psychotropic medication has been approved by the Food and Drug Administration (FDA) for use during pregnancy, and pregnant women have tradition-ally been excluded from pharmacologic research. Numerous studies have shown a high relapse rate in psychiatric patients whose medications were discontinued. When deciding whether or not to treat a psychiatric patient during pregnancy, the guiding principle is to weigh the risks of fetal exposure to a psychotropic medication against the risks to both the mother and the fetus of not treating a psychiatric illness. Patients with bipolar disorder are at significant risk of relapse if untreated, particularly following abrupt discontinuation of lithium.[1] Untreated bipolar illness with recurrence of mania may result in progression of the disorder. Another risk is disease chronicity and treatment resistance.

The natural course of bipolar illness during pregnancy is not well defined, but several patterns in the course of bipolar illness of women are suggested by retrospective and prospec-tive investigations. Bipolar women have a higher rate of rapid cycling, more depressive episodes, and more mixed (as opposed to pure) mania episodes compared to bipolar men.[2] The literature indicates that untreated bipolar women have a significantly higher rate of relapse within the first 3 months postpartum compared to those using non-lithium mood stabilizers.[2-5] The risk of bipolar relapse after delivery is estimated to be 20–50%, and this risk is substantially reduced with postpartum prophylactic treatment.[5] Less is known about the risk of relapse during pregnancy for untreated bipolar illness.

The need for long-term treatment of bipolar illness is well established. However, the type and timing of treatment during pregnancy are not well defined. Each patient must be assessed for the risks and benefits of an individually tailored treatment plan. This chapter will review the teratogenic risks of commonly used mood stabilizers in the treatment of bipolar disorder.

LITHIUM

Lithium is a well-established and effective acute and prophylactic treatment for bipolar I disorder. Reports of its soothing effects on mood date back to the second century AD, although it was not until 1954 that the first controlled study of the antimanic effects of lithium in human subjects was completed in Europe. The FDA approved lithium for the treatment of acute mania in 1970, and for maintenance therapy in 1974. Lithium is classified as an FDA Pregnancy Category D drug. This category carries the warning that 'there is evidence of human fetal risk, but the potential benefits from the use of the drug in pregnant women may be acceptable despite its potential risks.'[6] The risks of lithium therapy for treating bipolar disorder during pregnancy fall into six categories:

1 maternal toxicity;
2 morphological teratogenicity;
3 behavioral teratogenicity;
4 fetal and neonatal toxicity;
5 carcinogenicity and mutagenicity; and
6 other effects.

The teratogenic effects of lithium in premammalian organisms were recognized and studied during the last century. Reports of birth defects in children of lithium-treated mothers first began to appear in the late 1960s. Early reports indicated that lithium was associated with a high risk for a specific cardiovascular system defect, namely Ebstein's anomaly.[7] However, recent studies indicated that lithium exposure during cardiogenesis may be associated with congenital heart defects, but the risk is not as high as was initially estimated.[8]

Maternal toxicity

Lithium has a relatively narrow therapeutic index. A therapeutic response is achieved with serum concentrations of 0.5–1.5 mEq/L when measured 12 h after the last dose. Early signs of toxicity may begin to emerge even at doses within this therapeutic range. The severity and number of signs and symptoms of lithium toxicity correlate closely with the serum levels. This relationship also exists during pregnancy. Symptoms of lithium toxicity include difficulty in concentrating, sluggishness, drowsiness, coarse tremor, muscle twitches, dysarthria, loss of appetite, nausea, vomiting, diarrhea, lethargy, confusion and ataxia.[5] Unfortunately, the side-effects of lithium toxicity may not receive early recognition because they are mistaken for common gestational syndromes, which also include nausea, vomiting, fluid retention, and weight gain. Diuretic therapy and sodium-restricted diets are often used to limit the fluid retention that is commonly experienced during pregnancy. As a further complication, both treatment regimens promote lithium retention, which causes rapidly escalating serum lithium levels and corresponding toxicity.

Medication pharmacokinetics are altered during pregnancy, leading to lowered lithium levels caused by a higher volume of distribution and increased renal clearance.[9] The glomerular filtration rate (GFR) increases by 30–50% and the plasma volume increases by approximately 50%

by the third trimester.[9] There is a cumulative retention of sodium because lithium is excreted entirely by renal elimination. Pregnancy-associated physiological changes may result in decreased serum lithium concentrations. Lithium concentrations may quickly rise in the mother postpartum as GFR and plasma volumes return to normal pre-pregnancy levels, potentiating possible lithium toxicity. Thus it is very important to monitor closely the late pregnant and postpartum female and her offspring for signs and symptoms of toxicity.[10]

Lithium dosing should be adjusted on the basis of frequently observed measurements of serum lithium concentrations. Serum lithium concentrations should be determined at least once monthly during pregnancy and weekly during the final month of pregnancy. Ten days prior to delivery lithium should be tapered to achieve a dose that is approximately 30% lower than the pregnant dose by delivery in order to minimize the risks of lithium toxicity to both the mother and the newborn. Lithium therapy should not be abruptly lowered in dose or discontinued. It should be tapered over a number of days and carefully monitored to ensure therapeutic serum concentrations and avoid relapse in the postpartum period.[3,5] In addition, maternal thyroid function should be monitored regularly. Thyroxine should be given if necessary to prevent a hypothyroid state in the mother and the fetus receiving none because thyroxine does not cross the placenta.

Morphologic teratogenicity

Morphologic teratogenicity is defined as an identifiable major or minor anatomic abnormality.[11] The teratogenic potential of lithium is a widely debated topic, and many studies have been conducted in an attempt to assess lithium's teratogenic potential. Preclinical studies showed that maternal exposure to lithium during embryogenesis was associated with increased frequencies of intrauterine death and malformations. It is difficult to extrapolate these results to humans because the doses shown to produce fetal damage in animals were given at lithium concentrations nine times higher than the usual human therapeutic doses. The findings of studies in which rodents were exposed to as much as nine times the usual human dose were compatible with continued maternal health, unimpaired fertility, and litters with the background frequency of congenital anomalies.[7] Lithium did not appear to have a high teratogenic potential in experimental animals at normal human therapeutic doses. Even at high doses, the fetal damage was typically species-specific (e.g. cleft palate in mice). In no instance in any species was lithium associated with signs of selective developmental toxicity. No cardiovascular defects were reported.[8]

As mentioned above, the first reports of congenital anomalies among children born to mothers treated with lithium during gestation began to appear in the late 1960s. The International Register of Lithium Babies was started in 1970 in order to receive and archive reports of pregnancies exposed to lithium in the first trimester, regardless of outcome. Initial reports from this register suggested that lithium exposure was associated with a higher incidence of all congenital anomalies. The frequency of congenital cardiovascular defects was five times the expected rate, and the rate of Ebstein's anomaly was approximately 400 times the general population background rate.[12] Ebstein's anomaly is a congenital cardiac malformation in which malattachment of the tricuspid leaflets leads to tricuspid insufficiency, right ventricular dilation and occasionally a ventricular septal defect. Ebstein's anomaly is diagnosed in 1 in 20 000 births in the general population. Of the 225 cases of infants exposed to lithium in at least the first trimester of pregnancy in the Lithium Register study, congenital anomalies were reported in 25 children (11.1%), cardiovascular defects in 18 children (8.0%), and six (2.7%) had Ebstein's anomaly. However, these were registry data, which are confounded by reporting bias (voluntary case-reporting, and possible overestimates of the prevalence of adverse outcomes), inclusion of pregnancies exposed to polydrug therapy regimens, and lack of an appropriate control group. Nevertheless, clinical practice was guided for over 25 years by the registry data.

More conservative estimates of the teratogenic potential of lithium are based on two cohort studies and four case–control studies conducted with appropriate controls. Kallen and Tandberg[13] linked records of women with manic-depressive illness with the Swedish birth registry, and identified 59 infants born to mothers treated with lithium early in pregnancy. A comparison group of patients with bipolar illness not treated with lithium during pregnancy included 228 infants. In the lithium-treated cohort, 4 infants (6.8%) had congenital heart disease, but none of them had Ebstein's anomaly. In the control cohort that was not exposed to lithium, 2 infants (0.9%) had cardiac malformations, corresponding to the background rate in the general population. Lithium-exposed infants had 7.7-fold more congenital heart disease than the control group. Congenital anomalies of all types were increased in frequency (12%) in the lithium-treated cohort compared to controls (4%). In a prospective study, 148 women who were treated with lithium during the first trimester of pregnancy, and were identified after consulting a teratogen information center, were matched with appropriate controls.[14] Four of 106 infants (4%) in the lithium cohort had a major congenital anomaly, compared to 3 of 123 infants (2%) in the control cohort. There was one cardiac malformation in each cohort (0.9% of the lithium cohort and 0.8% of the control cohort). Neither of these findings was statistically significant, but it may be clinically significant that the one cardiac malformation in the lithium-exposed group was Ebstein's anomaly. Four case–control studies analyzed the association of lithium exposure with Ebstein's anomaly.[8] Among cases with Ebstein's anomaly and also among normal controls the frequency of exposure to lithium was analyzed. Among 208 children with Ebstein's anomaly, none were exposed to lithium during embryonic development. In the control group of children with some type of birth defect other than Ebstein's anomaly, 2 of 398 children were found to have mothers who had been treated with lithium. Each of these studies had a power of 97% or higher to be able to detect the 400-fold increase in the risk of Ebstein's anomaly that the original Lithium Register data suggested.

Lithium may have teratogenic potential when given during the first trimester of pregnancy, but the risk of major cardiac anomalies does not appear to be the 400-fold increased rate first reported. Down's syndrome, clubfoot, meningomyelocele, thyroid abnormalities[15] and renal malformations have been reported with lithium exposure during pregnancy,[16] but a causal relationship with lithium exposure seems unlikely. Lithium exposure during cardiogenesis may be associated with an increased risk of Ebstein's anomaly, but the risk is probably .05–.10%.

Bipolar women of childbearing age need to be counseled about these increased risks of birth defects as a result of early lithium exposure to the fetus, and about the importance of contraception to avoid an unplanned pregnancy. If lithium exposure occurs during embryogenesis, Doppler flow analysis of the fetal tricuspid valve is warranted.

Behavioral teratogenicity

Behavioral teratogenicity is defined as enduring changes of higher cortical function, associated with alterations in neurotransmitter or neuroreceptor functioning.[8] Few follow-up studies of children exposed to lithium *in utero* are published. The postnatal development at 5 years of age or older, as reported by mothers, of 60 of the original Lithium Register children in Scandinavia born without malformations was compared with that of 57 of their siblings who were not exposed to lithium during gestation. Both groups showed signs of mild developmental delay, but there were no significant differences in development between these sibling groups. Weaknesses of the study include the developmental 'assessment' by the mothers and the small study size. Thus the possibility of late developmental abnormalities due to gestational lithium exposure cannot be excluded, but the findings do suggest that if abnormalities are present they are not conspicuous.[17]

Fetal and neonatal toxicity

Lithium readily crosses the placenta, and serum concentrations rapidly achieve equilibrium in maternal and fetal circulations. Fetal toxicity is related to cumulative daily doses of lithium and to transient peaks in lithium concentration.[18] Even transient pulses of high serum lithium concentrations can impair fetal development in laboratory animals.[19] It is recommended that lithium should be given in three to five equal multiple daily doses of no more than 300 mg per dose if possible, and maternal serum lithium concentrations should be maintained at the lowest possible effective levels.[7]

Neonatal lithium toxicity may present in a variety of ways. These syndromes are not distinctive, and may be diagnosed as non-specific transitory neonatal distress.[7] Clinical features of neonatal lithium toxicity include cyanosis, lethargy, hypotonia ('floppy baby' syndrome), poor gag and suck reflexes, cardiac arrhythmias, cardiomegaly, transient hypothyroidism and neonatal goiter, impaired respiration and transient nephrogenic diabetes. Therapeutic, toxic and even subtherapeutic peripartum serum lithium concentrations have been associated with symptoms of neonatal toxicity. Neonatal toxicity has been reported to occur at serum lithium concentrations as low as 0.35 mEq/L and as high as 1.1 mEq/L.[18] Therefore, serum lithium concentrations cannot be used as a indicator of neonatal toxicity or safety.

Infants who develop lithium toxicity require adequate oxygenation, airway maintenance and temperature control. Infant serum lithium levels, electrolytes, hydration and nutritional status should be monitored. Neonatal lithium elimination half-life is 68–96 h. The neonatal side-effects of lithium toxicity are usually self-limiting and resolve without complication within 1–2 weeks.[20] However, cardiac arrhythmia and goiter may persist for a longer period of time. Lithium toxicity in neonates and mothers may be minimized by gradually tapering the dose down over the 10–day period immediately prior to delivery. The target-dosing regimen is approximately 30% lower than the highest dose given during pregnancy.

Carcinogenicity and mutagenicity

It is not known whether lithium is carcinogenic or mutagenic,[15] but it is highly unlikely to be so.[21]

Other effects

Conflicting reports have been published regarding the use of lithium during pregnancy and premature deliveries or large-for-gestational-age infants. Premature deliveries are postulated to be related to increased production of prostaglandins resulting from lithium blockade of the phosphoinositol pathway.[22] Large-for-gestational-age infants are postulated to be due to an 'insulin-like' effect of lithium on carbohydrate metabolism.[14] The Lithium Register babies were 2.5 times more likely to have been premature than the general population. A preponderance of large-for-gestational-age babies was also found among the Registry infants. A similar increase in premature births in lithium-treated mothers was found in a controlled cohort study, although no differences in infant birth weight were found.[23] Another cohort study found no differences between lithium-treated mothers and those not treated with lithium, except for a small but statistically significant increase in birth weight among infants whose mothers used lithium during gestation.[14]

Lithium and lactation

The concentration of lithium in breast-milk is approximately 30–50% of the mother's serum level.[24] At concentrations that produce no toxic effects in an adult, neonates may be at increased risk of toxicity for several reasons. They are very sensitive to changes in electrolyte and fluid balance. Moreover, neonatal renal function is not fully developed, resulting in a long half-life for lithium (68–96 h) in the neonate. Transitory neonatal disturbances of fluid and electrolyte balances due to diarrhea and vomiting may further escalate serum lithium concentrations. Lithium toxicity in infants from breast-milk, particularly in association with dehydration or infection,[25] has been reported to include lethargy, cyanosis, hypotonia and electrocardiogram abnormalities. The American Academy of Pediatrics has recommended that mothers who are being treated with lithium should not breastfeed their infants.

VALPROATE

Before 1981, the use of valproate (also called valproic acid, VPA, Depakote or Depakene) during pregnancy was not considered to be a risk factor for congenital anomalies. VPA is one of the anticonvulsants of choice for controlling seizures in women of childbearing age, and during pregnancy. VPA was known to be a potent animal teratogen, but only one unconfirmed case of birth defects in a VPA-exposed human fetus was published between 1969 and 1976. This case was also exposed to two other anticonvulsants. Other cases published before and after 1980 reported healthy full-term infants that were exposed to VPA *in utero*. The first confirmed report of congenital defects in an infant exposed to VPA during gestation was published in 1980.[26] The mother had taken 1000 mg of VPA daily throughout gestation, and the infant was growth-retarded, with facial dysmorphism and with heart and limb defects. The child died 19 days after birth. Similar abnormalities in infants exposed to VPA during gestation were reported in several subsequent studies and case reports.

Maternal and fetal VPA pharmacokinetics

VPA readily crosses the placenta, and with higher fetal concentrations than maternal levels. Pregnancy can have a significant effect on the maternal clearance of VPA. The blood level: dose ratio for VPA begins to decrease in the second trimester and continues to decline until delivery. The change in this ratio is thought to be due to hypoalbuminemia and increased free fatty acids in the maternal blood that partially displace the drug from maternal binding sites. Both of these mechanisms result in the accumulation of more VPA in the fetus than in the mother.[26,27] Pharmacokinetic studies indicate that the clearance of VPA and its metabolites from the fetal compartment is slower than that from the maternal compartment. Moreover, the half-life of VPA in a newborn is increased by about four times the adult half-life to 43–47 h because of decreased glucuronidation.[26]

The findings of pharmacokinetic studies of VPA in pregnant sheep after both maternal and fetal intravenous bolus administration parallel observations in humans.[27]

Morphologic teratogenicity

Prenatal VPA exposure has been associated with major and minor congenital anomalies, intrauterine growth retardation, hyperbilirubinemia, hepatoxicity (which may be fatal) and fetal/neonatal distress. A plethora of minor anomalies are observed in infants who have been exposed prenatally to various anti-epileptic drugs. However, VPA-associated anomalies are clearly distinct from those associated with other anticonvulsants, and they constitute a 'fetal valproate syndrome (FVS).'[28] FVS is characterized by neural-tube defects, craniofacial anomalies, digit and limb defects, urogenital malformations, retarded psychomotor development and low birth weight. Other congenital anomalies associated with FVS include congenital heart disease, cleft lip and palate, and abdominal wall defects. Facies associated with FVS include trigonocephaly, tall forehead with bifrontal narrowing, epicanthic folds, infraorbital groove, medial deficiency of eyebrows, flat nasal bridge, broad nasal root, anteverted nares, shallow philtrum, long upper lip with thin vermilion, thick lower lip and small, down-turned mouth.

The most serious congenital anomalies associated with VPA exposure are neural-tube defects. The risk of such defects due to prenatal VPA exposure is 1–2%.[26] Exposure to VPA between days 17 and 30 after fertilization must occur for the drug to be considered a cause of neural-tube defects. VPA increases the risk for spina bifida tenfold.[29] Spina bifida was diagnosed prenatally in six of 92 pregnancies that were exposed to VPA during embryogenesis. Of these six pregnancies, five were exposed to VPA monotherapy and one to a combination of VPA and carbamazapine. Fetuses with spina bifida had higher maternal serum levels (73 µg/mL) of the drug than unaffected infant's (44 µg/mL).[30]

The frequency of congenital heart defects among infants exposed to VPA during organogenesis is approximately four times the background rate in the general population, and oral clefts occur about five times more frequently.[28] Liver toxicity was reported in three infants after *in utero* exposure to VPA, all of whom had physical signs of FVS at birth but normal liver function tests. One to two months after birth the infants presented with enlarged livers and liver function tests revealed a cholestatic-type hyperbilirubinemia. Liver biopsy demonstrated fibrosis with progressive liver necrosis.[26]

Behavioral teratogenicity

Among 40 children exposed *in utero* to either phenobarbitone, phenytoin or VPA, children exposed to VPA exhibited hyperexcitability and neurological dysfunction at 6 years of age.[29] This suggests that VPA may cause immediate and long-term cerebral dysfunction in addition to spina bifida and congenital heart disease.

CARBAMAZEPINE

Carbamazepine (CBZ) is metabolized in the liver via arene oxidation to CBZ-10, 11–epoxide (CBZ-E) by cytochrome P-450. CBZ-E is thought to be responsible for the teratogenicity of CBZ.[31] CBZ crosses the placenta rapidly, and is not metabolized by it. CBZ-E is found in cord blood, probably due to fetal liver metabolism of CBZ and/or the direct transfer of maternal CBZ-E to the fetus.[32] During pregnancy the conversion of CBZ to CBZ-E is increased by raised levels of microsomal oxidation. However, the next step of metabolism, namely hydrolysis of CBZ-E to carbamazepine-diol, is not proportionately increased.[33] This implies a disproportionally higher fetal exposure to CBZ-E, especially if CBZ doses/schedules are increased so as to maintain therapeutic levels.

Preclinical studies of CBZ or CBZ-E in pregnant laboratory animals indicated an increased frequency of a spectrum of congenital anomalies, including umbilical hernias, hydronephrotic kidneys, dilated cerebral ventricles, cleft palate, hypoplastic atria and skeletal defects.[31]

However, not all animal studies have shown that CBZ is embryotoxic.[34]

CBZ is an alternative treatment for bipolar mania. However, research on pregnancy outcome after exposure to CBZ in early pregnancy has been conducted on epileptic women treated with the drug. Malformation rates in the offspring of epileptic mothers, independent of anticonvulsant use, are about threefold higher than in the general population. However, Nulman and colleagues[35] found equal incidences of major malformations among non-medicated epileptic mothers and those treated with CBZ or phenytoin during the pregnancy. The incidence of minor anomalies (e.g. craniofacial and digital anomalies) was higher in the group of infants whose mothers were treated with anticonvulsants during pregnancy. Epilepsy and anticonvulsant use during pregnancy have independent effects on the developing embryo and fetus, perhaps contributing synergistically to the occurrence of major congenital anomalies.

CBZ was the drug of choice for treating epilepsy during pregnancy for several decades. However, in the 1980s it was discovered that this drug was associated with an increased risk of spina bifida and other congenital anomalies, including craniofacial dysmorphology (short nose, long philtrum, upslanting palpebral fissures, hypertelorism, high arched or cleft palate and epicanthal folds), fingernail hypoplasia and developmental delay.[36] Spina bifida occurs in 0.5–1.0% of infants who were exposed to CBZ during the first trimester,[37] whereas the risk of spina bifida in the general population is 0.03% (3 in 10 000). Polydrug therapy during pregnancy increases the risk of congenital anomalies. Neurobehavioral studies of infants exposed to CBZ prenatally have yielded conflicting results and were poorly controlled. A recent study found negligible differences in the neurobehavioral outcome of children who had been exposed to CBZ prenatally compared to those who had not. However, drug-exposed children had a decreased average head circumference compared to controls.[38]

NEUROLEPTICS

A more comprehensive review of neuroleptic use during pregnancy is presented in Chapter 11 and elsewhere.[3,39,40] Neuroleptics are often used to treat severe cases of bipolar illness. Newer antipsychotic medications, such as olanzapine and risperidone, are also used to treat bipolar disorder. More data are available for low-potency neuroleptics because these agents have been used for longer periods of time. The use of high-potency antipsychotics during pregnancy is recommended because they have fewer autonomic, sedative and cardiovascular side-effects. Prospective and retrospective investigations indicate that antipsychotic agents do not increase the frequency of congenital malformations compared to the general population. However, untreated psychotic illness itself may be a risk factor for poor pregnancy outcome. Reversible neonatal toxicity (extrapyramidal symptoms and cholestatic jaundice) has been reported in neonates of mothers treated with neuroleptics.

OTHER MEDICATIONS

Other medications that are used to treat bipolar illness include benzodiazepines for mania and antidepressants for the depressed phase. Treatment recommendations for antidepressant use during pregnancy are given in Chapter 4, and benzodiazepine treatment is reviewed in Chapters 7 and 8.

NON-PHARMACOLOGIC TREATMENT

Cognitive-behavioral therapy, family therapy, group therapy, interpersonal therapy, psycho-dynamic therapy, and psychoeducation have been used to treat bipolar patients. Most studies have analyzed psychotherapy's augmentation of pharmacologic therapy.[41] The psychoeducative approach combined with cognitive–behavioral therapy seem to be successful, but more controlled investigations are needed to confirm the efficacy of this approach. Non-pharmacologic psychotherapeutic approaches would be extremely useful in the female patient with bipolar illness during the first trimester, in order to avoid the teratogenic risks of medications, if effective. Alternatively, non-pharmacologic therapies could be supplemented with lower doses of pharmacotherapy to augment the response and ensure maintenance stabilization of the bipolar disease during pregnancy.

Another treatment option is electroconvulsive therapy (ECT). It is an effective treatment modality that was not shown to be harmful in more than 300 pregnancies treated with ECT, but it is probably under-used for treatment of the psychiatrically ill pregnant patient.

TREATMENT GUIDELINES AND RECOMMENDATIONS

It is necessary to treat bipolar illness in order to avoid relapse and the psychosocial devastation that mania frequently causes in a patient's life. Therefore it is not a question of whether or not to treat a pregnant bipolar patient, but rather of how to do so. The treatment regimen must consider the individual patient, her past psychiatric history, the number, severity and frequency of manic episodes, her past response to various treatments, and her personal preference. It is important that the patient is informed about the risks and benefits of treatment both for her and for her unborn baby.

The ideal approach is treatment planning prior to conception, and avoidance of medication during the critical stage of organogenesis of the embryo. Abrupt discontinuation of any medication is contraindicated in bipolar illness because of the high risk of relapse. Instead, the current medication dose should be tapered down and possibly discontinued prior to conception. Discontinuation of medication is a decision that the doctor and patient must make jointly. A patient with well-controlled bipolar illness and long interepisode euthymia may choose to avoid psychotropic medication during the first trimester. Unfortunately, conception may not occur for months or even years, particularly among older women. Thus complete discontinuation of medication prior to pregnancy is not considered to be prudent. The physician should therefore consider switching to the least teratogenic maintenance treatment, and should then employ the lowest possible dose until conception is confirmed. Medication options include lithium, high-potency neuroleptics, and finally, CBZ for lithium non-responders. VPA should be avoided in women who are planning to become pregnant, because it has the highest teratogenic potential of any mood stabilizer. In addition, anticonvulsants should not be used in a polytherapy regimen because of their possible synergistic teratogenic effects.

If clinical signs of deterioration occur after discontinuing lithium, a high-potency antipsychotic such as haloperidol is an excellent treatment alternative to resuming lithium therapy. The efficacy of high-potency neuroleptics in bipolar prophylaxis is not clearly established, but they are not associated with an increased frequency of congenital anomalies. High-potency benzodiazepines, such as lorazepam, may be used alone or in combination with a high-potency neuroleptic in a pregnant manic patient. If necessary, lithium therapy may be resumed during the second and third trimesters. The risk of birth defects would not be increased with lithium used during the latter two trimesters, but pregnancy complications (e.g. polyhydramarios, diabetes insipidus and fetal goiter) may occur.

Lithium must be continued in women who have very severe forms of bipolar disorder with multiple episodes. Such patients are at an unacceptably high-risk of decompensation-associated morbidity if lithium is discontinued. For this special group of patients, lithium therapy prior to and throughout the pregnancy is the treatment of choice. Reproductive risk counseling should be provided, and the increased risk of congenital heart defects in the infant should be discussed. Prenatal diagnosis screening and options should also form part of the consent. Briefly, high-resolution ultrasound and fetal echocardiography and Doppler flow studies may be performed at gestational weeks 16–18 to screen for congenital anomalies.

Treatment planning prior to pregnancy is rarely an option. For women who become pregnant while on lithium therapy without preconception planning, similar general guidelines should be followed. It is important to minimize first-trimester exposure to lithium, and to provide appropriate counseling to help the mother to make informed decisions about the pregnancy should a birth defect be discovered during prenatal diagnoses. The aid of a medical geneticist should be enlisted in prenatal counseling, especially if a birth defect is discovered.

If lithium prophylaxis is used during pregnancy, the dose should be tapered to 30% of the highest dose during gestation at the time of delivery. Tapering should begin 10 days prior to the estimated date of delivery. The risks of peripartum maternal and infant lithium toxicity will be minimized by fluid shifts during puerperium. Lithium should not be discontinued, as bipolar mothers are highly susceptible to relapse during the postpartum period. If lithium is discontinued during pregnancy, it should be resumed immediately after delivery in order to avoid postpartum relapse.

As disscussed earlier, VPA is a human teratogen that causes serious neural-tube defects in 1–2% of infants who are exposed prenatally to the drug. It should therefore be avoided either as monotherapy or as a component of poly therapy.

In summary, safe pharmacotherapeutic treatment of bipolar illness is possible during pregnancy, and pregnant mothers with this disorder should be reassured that the benefits of treatment outweigh the risks in most cases. The risks are optimally managed with preconceptional counseling and therapeutic regimen management. Cognitive-behavioral, supportive, psychoeducative and family therapy can augment the treatment during the sometimes vulnerable periods of pharmacotherapy interruption or dose minimization during pregnancy.

REFERENCES

1. Suppes T, Baldessarini RJ, Faedda GL, Tohen M. Risk of recurrence following discontinuation of lithium treatment in bipolar disorder. *Archives of General Psychiatry* 1991; **48**: 1082–8.
2. Leibenluft E. Women with bipolar illness: clinical and research issues. *American Journal of Psychiatry* 1996; **153**: 163–73.
3. Altshuler LL, Cohen L, Szuba MP, Burt VK, Gitlin M, Mintz J. Pharmacologic management of psychiatric illness during pregnancy: dilemmas and guidelines. *American Journal of Psychiatry* 1996; **153**: 592–606.
4. Cohen LS, Sichel DA, Roberston LM, Heckscher E, Rosenbaum JF. Postpartum prophylaxis for women with bipolar disorder. *American Journal of Psychiatry* 1995; **152**: 1641–5.
5. Viguera AL, Honacs R, Cohen LS, Tondo L, Murray A, Baldessarini RJ. Risk of recurrence of bipolar disorder in pregnant and non-pregnant women after discontinuing lithium maintenance. *American Journal of Psychiatry* 2000; **157**: 179–184.

6. Fact and Comparisons, Inc. *Drug facts and comparisons. FDA pregnancy categories*. St Louis, MO: 1996.

7. Weinstein MR. Lithium Treatment of women during pregnancy and in the post-delivery period. In: Johnson FN (ed.) *Handbook of lithium therapy*. Lancaster: MTP Press, 1980: 421–9.

8. Cohen LS, Friedman JM, Jefferson JW, Johnson EM, Weiner ML. A re-evaluation of risk of *in utero* exposure to lithium. *Journal of American Medical Association* 1994; **271**: 146–50.

9. Little BB. Pharmacokinetics during pregnancy: evidence based maternal dose formulation. *Obstetrics and Gynecology* 1999; **93**: 858–68.

10. Yonkers KA, Little BB, March D. Lithium during pregnancy: drug effects and therapeutic implications. *CNS Drugs* 1998; **4**: 261–9.

11. Miller LJ. Psychiatric medication during pregnancy: understanding and minimizing risks. *Psychiatric Annals* 1994; **24**: 69–75.

12. Weinstein NM. The International Register of Lithium Babies. *Drug Information Journal* 1976; **10**: 94–100.

13. Kallen B, Tandberg A. Lithium and pregnancy: a cohort study on manic-depressive women. *Acta Psychiatrica Scandinavica* 1983; **68**: 134–9.

14. Jacobson SJ, Jones K, Johnson K *et al*. Prospective multicentre study of pregnancy outcome after lithium exposure during first trimester. *Lancet* 1992; **339**: 530–3.

15. McEvoy GK (ed.) *Lithium drug monograph. American hospital formulary service drug information*. Bethesda, MD: American Society of Health-System Pharmacists, Inc, 1996.

16. Eikmeier G. Fetal malformations under lithium treatment. *European Journal of Psychiatry* 1996; **11**: 376–7.

17. Schou M. Lithium treatment during pregnancy, delivery, and lactation: an update. *Journal of Clinical Psychiatry* 1990; **51**: 410–13.

18. Ananth J. Lithium during pregnancy and lactation. *Lithium* 1993; **4**: 231–7.

19. Goldfield M, Weinstein MR. Lithium in pregnancy: a review with recommendations. *American Journal of Psychiatry* 1971; **127**: 888–93.

20. Perry PJ, Alexander B, Liskow BI (eds) *Psychotropic drug handbook*, 7th edn. Washington, DC: American Psychiatric Association Press, 1997.

21. Leonard A, Hantson P, Gerber GB. Mutagenicity, carcinogenicity, and teratogenicity of lithium compounds (abstract). *Mutation Research* 1995; **339**: 131–7.

22. Nishiwaki T, Tanaka K, Sekiya S. Acute lithium intoxication in pregnancy (letter). *International Journal of Gynecology and Obstetrics* 1996; **52**: 191–2.

23. Troyer WA, Pereira GR, Lannon RA, Belik J, Yoder MC. Association of maternal lithium exposure and premature delivery. *Journal of Perinatology* 1993; **13**: 123–7.

24. Kuller JA, Katz VL, McMahon MJ, Wells SR, Bashford RA. Pharmacologic treatment of psychiatric disease in pregnancy and lactation: fetal and neonatal effects. *Obstetrics and Gynecology* 1996; **87**: 789–94.

25. Maitra R, Menkes DB. Psychotropic drugs and lactation. *New Zealand Medical Journal* 1996; **109**: 217–219.

26. Briggs GG, Freeman RK, Yaffe SJ. *A reference guide to fetal and neonatal risk: drugs in pregnancy and lactation*. Baltimore: MD: Williams and Wilkins: 1994.

27. Gordon JD, Riggs KN, Rurak DW *et al*. The pharmacokinetics of valproic acid in pregnant sheep after maternal and fetal intravenous bolus administration. *Drug Metabolism and Disposition* 1995; **23**: 1303–9.

28. Clayton-Smith J, Donnai D. Fetal valproate syndrome. *Journal of Medical Genetics* 1995; **32**: 724–7.

29. Koch S, Jager-Roman E, Losche G *et al*. Antiepileptic drug treatment in pregnancy: drug side-effects in the neonate and neurological outcome. *Acta Paediatrica* 1996; **85**: 739–46.

30. Omtzigt JG, Nau H, Los FJ *et al*. The disposition of valproate and its metabolites in the late first trimester and early second trimester of pregnancy in maternal serum, urine, and amniotic fluid:

effect of dose, co-medication, and the presence of spinal bifida. *European Journal of Clinical Pharmacology* 1992; **43**: 381–8.

31. Bennett GD, Amore BM, Finnell RH *et al*. Teratogenicity of carbamazepine-10, 11-epoxide and oxcarbamazepine in the SWV mouse. *Journal of Pharmacology and Experimental Therapeutics* 1996; **279**: 1237–42.

32. Pienimaki P, Lampela E, Hakkola J, Arvela P, Raunio H, Vahakangas K. Pharmacokinetics of oxcarbamazepine and carbamazepine in human placenta. *Epilepsia* 1997; **38**: 309–16.

33. Bernus I, Hooper WD, Dickinson RG, Eadie MJ. Effects of pregnancy on various pathways of human antiepileptic drug metabolism. *Clinical Neuropharmacology* 1997; **20**: 13–21.

34. Hansen DK, Dial SL, Terry KK, Grafton TF. *In vitro* embryotoxicity of carbamazepine and carbamazepine-10, 11-epoxide. *Teratology* 1996; **54**: 45–51.

35. Nulman I, Scolnik D, Chitayat D, Farkas LD, Karen G. Findings in children exposed *in utero* to phenytoin and carbamazepine monotherapy: independent effects of epilepsy and medications. *American Journal of Medical Genetics* 1997; **68**: 18–24.

36. Ornoy A, Cohen E. Outcome of children born to epileptic mothers treated with carbamazepine during pregnancy. *Archives of Disease in Childhood*, 1996; **75**: 517–20.

37. Rosa F. Spina bifida in infants of women treated with carbamazepine during pregnancy. *New England Journal of Medicine* 1991; **324**: 674–7.

38. Scolnik D, Nulman I, Rovet J *et al*. Neurodevelopment of children exposed *in utero* to phenytoin and carbamazepine monotherapy. *Journal of American Medical Association* 1994; **271**: 767–70.

39. Wisner KL, Perel JM. Psychopharmacological treatment during pregnancy and lactation. In: Jensvold MF, Halbreich U, Hamilton JA (eds) *Psychopharmacology and women: sex, gender, and hormones*. Washington, DC: American Psychiatric Association Press; 1996: 191–224.

40. Trixler M, Tenyi T. Antipsychotic use in pregnancy. What are the best treatment options? *Drug Safety Concepts* 1997; **6**: 403–10.

41. Colom F, Vieta E, Martinez A, Jorquera A, Gasto C. What is the role of psychotherapy in the treatment of bipolar disorder? *Psychotherapy and Psychosomatics* 1998; **67**: 3–9.

7

Panic disorder

DANA MARCH AND KIMBERLY A. YONKERS

INTRODUCTION

Panic disorder, also known as DaCosta's syndrome and hyperventilation syndrome, is a type of anxiety disorder that can be complicated by agoraphobia. Panic disorder occurs in approximately 2% of the general population, although in psychiatric settings, it represents the primary diagnosis in 1 of every 10–20 patients.[1-3] As with most other anxiety disorders, panic disorder predominantly affects women.[4] Furthermore, women are more likely to have a chronic course with lower remission and higher relapse rates.[5] Thus it is likely that a patient with panic disorder will be a woman. The unique physiological and hormonal changes of the female life cycle, particularly those that occur during pregnancy, add an additional dimension to psychiatric disorders, and panic disorder is no exception. In this chapter we shall review extant research on the epidemiology and course of panic disorder, with or without agoraphobia, in pregnant women from conception to the postpartum period. Biological and psychological effects are addressed, and current risk–benefit assessments of effective treatments are discussed. Directives to practitioners and areas for further study are also suggested.

DIAGNOSIS OF PANIC DISORDER

Essential to a DSM-IV diagnosis of panic disorder is the recurrence of unprecipitated panic attacks, which lead to persistent concerns about subsequent attacks or their implications, or a change in behavior for at least 1 month's duration.[6] Occasionally referred to as 'anxiety attacks', panic attacks have an abrupt onset with a crescendo-like pattern over the course of

Table 7.1 *DSM-IV panic attack symptoms**

Cognitive symptoms	Somatic symptoms	
Depersonalization and/or derealization	Shortness of breath	Chills and/or hot flushes
Fear of losing control and/or going crazy	Choking sensation	Dizziness and/or lightheadedness
Fear of dying	Chest pain and/or	Palpitations
Paresthesias	discomfort	Nausea and/or abdominal
	Tremulousness	discomfort
	Sweating	

* A diagnosis of panic disorder requires the presence of at least four of the above symptoms.
Adapted from American Psychiatric Association. *Diagnostic and statistical manual of mental disorders*, 4th edn. Washington, DC: American Psychiatric Association, 1994.

several minutes, and manifest themselves in a variety of cognitions and somatic sensations (see Table 7.1). The frequency of panic attacks varies widely among patients. Similarly, there is considerable variation in the constellation of symptoms for each attack. Often patients experience clusters of symptoms, such as cardiovascular symptoms (e.g. heart palpitations, chest pain and paresthesias) or cognitive symptoms (e.g. the conviction that a catastrophic event, including death, will imminently occur).[7] Patients who have several panic attacks and who suffer from worry or develop a change in behavior typically experience more impairment and thus a more malignant course. Patients often suffer from attacks precipitated by stressors or traumatic events. Technically, these attacks do not qualify for a diagnosis of panic disorder because they are not unexpected. Plausibly, patients who do not qualify for a diagnosis of panic disorder may experience functional impairment as extensive as those who meet the DSM-IV criteria. However, research does not clearly differentiate between prognoses.[8–10]

Several general medical conditions commonly occur alongside panic disorder. Both hyperventilation and sleep deprivation commonly induce or worsen panic attacks. Panic attacks are also frequent in patients who suffer from chest pain that is not associated with coronary artery disease or mitral valve prolapse.[11] Conversely, many patients with panic disorder also have mitral valve prolapse.[12] Patients with hyperthyroidism or who experience hot flushes (medical conditions that are more likely to occur in women) frequently have panic attacks. It has also been proposed that physical sensations, such as those caused by medical illnesses that affect the autonomic nervous system, may form somatic triggers that give rise to catastrophic thoughts and the subsequent development of panic.[13] In addition, the use of caffeine, alcohol, cannabis, cocaine and even cold preparations can induce or worsen panic attacks.

COURSE DURING PREGNANCY

There are compelling theoretical reasons to believe that panic attacks may either improve or worsen during pregnancy. On the one hand, progesterone may have anxiolytic properties, either by itself or by virtue of some of its metabolites[14,15] that function as agonists at the GABA-benzodiazepine receptor. On the other hand, respiratory mechanics change during pregnancy and may increase the propensity to panic. Pregnant women often take smaller breaths with less respiratory excursion. This occurs because progesterone induces mild hyperventilation,[16] but also because the pelvic and abdominal contents can compress the diaphragm. In the former case, panic attacks would decrease, whereas in the latter, mechanical changes may predispose pregnant women to an increase in panic.

Although there has been a deficit of corroborating data, the medical community has maintained that pregnancy buffers against psychiatric disorders[17,18] particularly panic disorder.[19] Contrarily, recent data indicate that women, especially those with a previous history of affective instability, may have a heightened susceptibility to psychiatric disorders during pregnancy and the postpartum period.[20–23] Research over the past decade on the course of panic disorder during pregnancy has revealed several patterns. An initial case study of three women reported a marked improvement in panic symptoms during pregnancy, and postulated that the attenuation of symptoms might be due to pregnancy-induced blunting of the sympatho-adrenal response to physiologic stimuli, effects on benzodiazepine receptors, or improvement in psychological functioning.[24] However, further investigation revealed that although the majority of women experienced a decrease in panic symptoms during their pregnancy, there was significant variation both between and within patients.[25] Most recently, Cohen and colleagues[20] shed light on the variable impact of pregnancy on the clinical course of panic disorder in women with pregravid diagnoses. Retrospective evaluation of symptoms across three trimesters and the extent to which severity predicted course during pregnancy revealed an insignificant change or improvement in clinical status in 77% of women, while 20% of the cohort experienced an increase in the severity of their panic symptoms. Those who improved had relatively mild symptoms, and those who deteriorated clinically had more severe symptoms. Thus women with mild pregravid panic symptoms are likely to experience symptomatic attenuation, while worsening may occur in women with severe illness. The same study also examined the rates of successful discontinuation from prophylactic antipanic pharmacotherapy. The data revealed a dichotomous effect on the impact of pregnancy on the course of panic disorder. Nine of 17 women who attempted to discontinue antipanic medication prior to conception failed. Six of these women attempted to discontinue pharmacotherapy after documentation of pregnancy, and only three were successful. The fact that some women are able to discontinue pharmacotherapy successfully after conception supports the hypothesis that pregnancy has a variable impact on the clinical course of the illness, with some women experiencing a salutary effect. Conversely, some women evince more severe panic symptoms, and for this subgroup of patients, discontinuing pharmacotherapy is less plausible. However, little is known about the clinical course of moderate pregravid panic symptoms during pregnancy – moderate symptoms could either worsen or attenuate during pregnancy (see Figure 7.1).

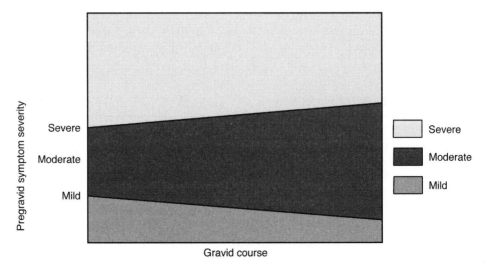

Figure 7.1 *Pregravid symptom severity and gravid course.*[20]

PANIC WITH AGORAPHOBIA

A number of patients* who suffer from panic disorder also experience anxiety associated with fear of being in a place from which escape may be difficult or help unavailable. This condition, known as agoraphobia, often causes those afflicted by it to become phobically avoidant of potentially problematic places such as motor vehicles or crowded shopping malls, or to endure these sites only with severe distress and discomfort. In extreme cases, patients will not leave the house without a trusted companion, a situation which renders them virtually housebound. Patients who suffer from panic with agoraphobia have a less promising prognosis than those who suffer from uncomplicated panic.[13,28] However, it is not known whether pregnant women are more likely to suffer from panic disorder with agoraphobia than from uncomplicated panic. It is also still unclear whether or not the gravid course of panic with agoraphobia differs from the non-gravid course of the disorder.

TREATMENT

In general, panic disorder treated on an outpatient basis rarely requires hospitalization, and panic disorder during pregnancy is no exception. In the same way that pregravid symptom severity functions as a predictor of the clinical course of panic disorder during pregnancy, symptom severity during pregnancy should function as a guideline for the treatment prescribed. Treating physicians should consider that panic-free patients are not necessarily recovered patients; the absence of panic attacks during treatment is not indicative of symptom remission and/or successful treatment discontinuation. In fact, relapse rates are high in patients suffering from panic disorder who discontinue pharmacotherapy.[29] Furthermore, findings from a recent study that examined medication prescribed and patients' ability to discontinue treatment indicate that pregnancy does *not* increase the likelihood of successful discontinuation of pharmacologic treatment.[20] Therefore women with more severe panic symptoms may be at risk for symptomatic persistence that warrants maintenance treatment.

Non-pharmacologic treatment

Psychotherapy has been the predominant psychiatric treatment for patients suffering from panic disorder. However, it has proved difficult to define psychotherapeutic aspects clearly, and only recently has the efficacy of various modalities been formally evaluated.[7] Several forms of psychotherapy are known to be effective in the treatment of panic disorder: psychodynamic psychotherapy, cognitive–behavioral therapy, and group therapy.

Psychodynamic treatment of panic disorder is based on the notion that subconscious processes mediate the disorder, and that illuminating these processes can therefore catalyze symptom remission.[30,31] This modality typically requires more time than cognitive–behavioral therapy to achieve treatment goals, although several authors have found no difference.[32–34]

Cognitive–behavioral therapy (CBT) has been well studied and established as an effective treatment for panic disorder.[7] Several controlled studies have demonstrated that it is superior to other non-pharmacological treatments.[35] Typically, treatment lasts for between 3 and 6 months, and involves psychoeducation, continuous panic monitoring, breathing retraining, cognitive restructuring and exposure to fear cues.[7] The patient is educated about their illness

---

* Reports of the incidence of panic with agoraphobia are variable, ranging from 7% in women[26] to as high as 33–50%.[27]

and treatment procedure, while practitioners carefully monitor their symptoms. Treatment providers guide the exploration of both catastrophic and negative thoughts, as well as fears of various bodily sensations. The patient completes assignments that enable them to identify and correct negative thinking and dysfunctionally avoidant behaviors. They may be instructed to expose themselves gradually to phobic places or items in a process known as 'graded exposure'. In addition, patients are also taught to control or manage panic attacks by relaxation and deep-breathing exercises.* Typically, group therapy assumes a cognitive-behavioral framework.

There is little to no risk involved in these particular treatment modalities, and while some women with mild pregravid panic symptoms may experience symptom relief, others with more severe symptoms may not benefit significantly from cognitive–behavioral therapy alone. There is also a need to define more clearly the effective components of CBT and the duration of treatment. A substantial number of pregnant women, especially those with moderate to severe panic symptoms, often require some intervening medication treatment, either alone or in conjunction with psychotherapy.[35,36]

Pharmacologic treatment

Two broad classes of medications are effective pharmacologic treatments for panic disorder. The first class consists of benzodiazepine anxiolytics, and the second class consists of antidepressants, including tricyclic antidepressants (TCAs), selective serotonin reuptake inhibitors (SSRIs), monoamine oxidase inhibitors (MAOIs) and others (see Table 7.2). The efficacy of the latter classes of medications in the treatment of panic disorder will be briefly evaluated here, although Chapter 4 describes the effects of pregnancy on treatments with and teratogenicity of the various classes of antidepressants. The efficacy and teratogenicity of benzodiazepines are a primary focus of this chapter.

Selective serotonin reuptake inhibitors
Selective serotonin reuptake inhibitors (SSRIs) have been found to be effective in the treatment of panic disorder (sertraline and paroxetine are FDA-approved for the treatment of panic disorder), although relatively few data are available on the teratogenicity of compounds in this class. The largest available body of data on teratogenicity exists for fluoxetine (see Chapter 4), although risks may vary even among compounds in the same class. In addition, the initial treatment response may take as long as 4 weeks, and a full response typically requires 8–12 weeks of treatment. Bearing in mind that individual cases should be evaluated and treated appropriately, physicians should consider these points when prescribing SSRIs to pregnant women with panic disorder.

Tricyclic antidepressants
Tricyclic antidepressants (TCAs) have also been shown to be effective in the treatment of panic disorder.[37] As with SSRIs, a reduction is phobic avoidance has been demonstrated with TCA therapy, although specific phobias actually respond less well. The length of time required to respond to TCAs is comparable to that for SSRIs (i.e. initial response in 4 weeks and full response in 8–12 weeks), so the treatment guidelines vis-à-vis temporal concerns also apply. The side-effect profile of TCAs is dissimilar to that of SSRIs. TCAs are associated with more anticholinergic effects, namely dry mouth, constipation, and difficulty in urinating. Pregnant women typically have problems with constipation, and the side-effects associated with TCAs can therefore worsen this complication of pregnancy.

* A number of self-help books and tapes that describe these techniques are available at bookstores.

Table 7.2 *Antidepressant treatments for panic disorder*

Group	Generic name	Trade name	Standard dose (mg/day)
TCAs	Amitriptyline	Elavil and others	150–300
	Clomipramine	Anafranil	100–250
	Desipramine	Norpramin and others	150–300
	Doxepin	Sinequan and others	150–300
	Imipramine	Tofranil	150–300
	Nortriptyline	Pamelor and others	75–200
SSRIs	Fluoxetine	Prozac	5–80
	Fluvoxamine	Luvox	50–300
	Paroxetine	Paxil	10–50
	Sertraline	Zoloft	50–200
MAOIs	Phenelzine	Nardil	45–90
	Tranylcypromine	Parnate	30–70
Other	Venlafaxine	Effexor	37.5–225

Adapted from Schatzberg AF, Cole JO, *Manual of clinical psychopharmacology*, 2nd edn. 1992, Washington, DC: American Psychiatric Association Press, 1992 and American Psychiatric Association. Practice guideline for the treatment of patients with panic disorder. Work Group on Panic Disorder. *American Journal of Psychiatry* 1998; **155 (Supplement 5)**: 1–34.

Monoamine oxidase inhibitors

Monoamine oxidase inhibitors (MAOIs) are broad-range agents that are effective in the treatment of panic disorder.[37] However, they are associated with serious potential adverse hyperthermic and hypertensive reactions if they are used in conjunction with food or other compounds that contain high levels of either tyramine or serotonin. Given the seriousness of these reactions, which can be lethal, MAOIs should not be used in pregnancy except under the most selective circumstances (see Chapter 4). New compounds in this class, which are reversible inhibitors of monoamine oxidase (RIMAs), have neither the anticholinergic properties nor the dietary restrictions of MAOIs. However, no data on the teratogenicity of these compounds are yet available.

Benzodiazepines

Among the most widely prescribed drugs, benzodiazepine anxiolytics are common and effective treatments for anxiety disorders, particularly panic disorder, due to their rapid and effective onset of action.[37] Benzodiazepines are lipophilic, undissociated molecular agents that readily penetrate membranes. These properties enable these drugs to function pharmacokinetically by promoting binding to the gamma-aminobutyric acid (GABA)–benzodiazepine cell-membrane-receptor complex, which increases its affinity and augments the inhibitory activity of the neurotransmitter GABA. This inhibitory activity is thought to be the source of the tranquilizing, myorelaxing and anticonvulsant properties of benzodiazepines, as it raises the threshold of neuronal firing and thereby modulates the neurotransmission of serotonin, dopamine and norepinepherine.[38]

Several classes of benzodiazepines exist (see Table 7.3), including those with long half-lives (20–60 h) and active metabolites, known as the 2–keto group.[39] Members of this class include chlordiazepoxide, clonazepam, clorazepate, diazepam and prazepam. The 3–hydroxy group is composed of compounds such as lorazepam and oxazepam, which have shorter half-lives (9–14 h) and no active metabolites. These compounds are cleared via phase-two conjugated metabolism in the liver. A third group, the triazolo compounds, includes alprazolam and triazolam. The half-lives of these compounds have a broad range, from several to 14 h, and

Table 7.3 *Benzodiazepine treatments for panic disorder*

Group	Generic name	Trade name	Standard dose (mg/day)
2-Keto	Chlordiazepoxide	Librium	20–80
	Clonazepam	Klonapin	1–4
	Clorazepate	Tranxene	15–60
	Diazepam	Valium	10–40
	Prazepam	Centrax	20–80
3-Hydroxy	Lorazepam	Ativan	2–8
	Oxazepam	Serax	30–70
	Temazepam	Restoril	7.5–30
Triazolo	Alprazolam	Xanax	2–8
	Triazolam	Halcion	0.125–0.5

Adapted from Schatzberg AF, Cole JO, *Manual of clinical psychopharmacology*, 2nd edn. Washington, DC: American Psychiatric Association Press, 1992.

Table 7.4 *Benzodiazepine withdrawal symptoms*

Anxiety	Sleeplessness
Tremulousness	Palpitations
Sweating	Headache
Abdominal pain and/or discomfort	Mild systolic hypertension
Photosensitivity	Audiosensitivity
Craving	Seizures

Adapted from Kaplan HI, Sadock BJ. *Pocket handbook of clinical psychiatry*. Baltimore, MD: Williams & Wilkins, 1990.

are oxidized to active metabolites. Along with anxiolytic properties, these medications have sedative properties and can cause anterograde amnesia. There is also potential for abuse and dependence in a subgroup of patients, and all patients who remain on these medications for a substantial period of time experience withdrawal symptoms if treatment is discontinued abruptly. Abrupt withdrawal manifests itself in the form of the re-emergence of anxiety symptoms, but can include other effects, such as insomnia and even seizures (see Table 7.4).

There are gender differences in the metabolism of benzodiazepines. Compounds from the 3–hydroxy group undergo conjugative metabolism, and their levels can be slightly lower in women than in men. Some evidence also suggests that the rate of clearance of a member of the 2–keto group, namely chlordiazepoxide, is slower in women. The results of similar research on diazepam are equivocal – some researchers have found lower sustained plasma levels in women, while others have found no significant difference.[40]

There is great concern about maternal exposure to medications, particularly during the first trimester of pregnancy. Approximately one-third of pregnant women take psychotropic medications during pregnancy, and 37% of them take benzodiazepines.[41] However, alterations of both drug pharmacokinetics and plasma levels during pregnancy complicate dosing.[42] Gravid processes that are known to decrease the bioavailability and thus increase the dose requirement of drug include (but are not limited to) decreases in gastrointestinal motility and the secretion of gastric acids, the expansion of plasma volume (although the total plasma clearance remains unchanged), and a change in the ratio of drug to drug metabolites.[42] Furthermore, processes that are likely to increase the drug requirement include changes in plasma protein-binding with a relative decrease in plasma proteins, decreases in plasma protein affinity for the drug, and an increase in cardiac output, which increases hepatic metabolism and renal blood flow. It may be difficult to predict what change in dosage will be required during pregnancy for compounds that are not primarily renally excreted.

Benzodiazepines exhibit a rapid placental transfer with significant uptake of the drug during both early and late pregnancy. The changes in placental structures and uterine circulation during pregnancy are conducive to greater placental passage in late pregnancy. The disposition of diazepam in women during late pregnancy changes with the terminal half-life in gravid women, and thus increases to twice that of controls.[43] These changes give rise to the three potential fetal effects associated with medication use during pregnancy, namely morphological teratogenicity, neonatal toxicity and postnatal behavioral sequelae,[44] Information concerning the use of benzodiazepines is thus organized in this manner. However, it should be noted when considering these effects that the risk of untreated psychiatric disorders may affect feto-placental integrity and fetal CNS development.[45]

Although it is clinically maintained that benzodiazepines are probably not teratogenic, these compounds can disturb the development of the fetal central nervous system during several key developmental processes, namely organogenesis, early differentiation of neural anlagen after neural tube closure, and biochemical differentiation of the fetal brain.[46] There have been a number of studies and individual case reports concerning the use of benzodiazepines during pregnancy. However, the data regarding both morphological and behavioral teratogenicity, as well as postnatal development, are inconsistent.[47] The teratogenic effects of specific benzodiazepines have been outlined by the Teratogen Information System (TERIS),[48] in which Friedman and Polifka compiled epidemiological and other data to evaluate the magnitude of teratogenic risks following gestational exposure to various pharmacological agents (see Table 7.5). The most ubiquitous teratologic data are available for diazepam (see Table 7.6), although alprazolam is a similar compound. St Clair and Schirmer[49] found no significant difference in the number of malformations between children exposed to alprazolam during the first trimester and their controls. Chlordiazepoxide is the second most widely evaluated benzodiazepine (see Table 7.7, p.144). Although there are patterns in extant data on the teratogenicity of benzodiazepines, more case–control epidemiological studies are needed.

Morphological teratogenicity

Morphological teratogenicity, also known as organ malformation, is associated with fetal drug exposure during the first 12 weeks of gestation.[42] As a frame of reference, the baseline incidence of congenital malformations in the USA is 2.0–2.5%.[42] An excellent meta-analysis of extant cohort and case–control studies by Dolovich and colleagues[50] revealed several concrete findings concerning benzodiazepine use in the first trimester of pregnancy and morphological teratogenicity. Pooled (case–control and cohort) data showed no association between fetal exposure to benzodiazepines and the risk of major malformations or oral cleft, although analyses of case–control studies alone revealed a significantly increased risk for either major malformations or oral cleft. Altshuler and colleagues[44] analyzed extant data and determined that although first-trimester exposure to benzodiazepines may increase the risk for congenital anomalies, such as oral cleft (from 0.06–0.7%), the absolute risk remains low.

Neonatal toxicity

Neonatal toxicity, often referred to as perinatal syndrome, encompasses a wide range of physical and behavioral symptoms that are noted shortly after birth. These symptoms, which are presumably related to fetal exposure to pharmacological agents during the third trimester of pregnancy or at the time of parturition, are limited in duration, lasting from hours to months

Table 7.5 *Evaluation of benzodiazepine teratogenicity based on available epidemiological data*

Benzodiazepine	Class	Magnitude of teratogenic risk factor gestational exposure	Quality and quantity of data on which risk estimate is based	Comments
Alprazolam (Xanax)	Triazolo	Unlikely	Fair	Therapeutic doses during pregnancy are unlikely to pose a substantial risk, but data are insufficient to conclude that there is no risk
Chlordiazepoxide (Librium)	2-keto	Unlikely	Fair to good	Neonatal withdrawal symptoms are similar to those with other benzodiazepines
Diazepam (Valium)	2-keto	Minimal	Good	
Flurazepam	2-keto	Unlikely	Limited	
Lorazepam (Ativan)	3-hydroxy	Undetermined	Limited	No epidemiological studies of congenital anomalies in infants whose mothers used lorazepam during pregnancy have been conducted as of 1999
Temazepam	3-hydroxy	Undetermined	Very limited	

Adapted from Friedman JM, Polifka JE. *The teratogen information system.* Washington, DC: The University of Washington, 1999.

Table 7.6 *Human epidemiological studies of malformations associated with first-trimester fetal exposure to diazepam*

Author(s)	Year(s)	n	Association with anomaly	Comments
Jick *et al.*	1981	150	None[*]	
Crombie *et al.*	1975	150	None[*]	
Aselton *et al.*	1985	60	None[*]	
Czeizel *et al.*	1988	417	None[*]	
Bracken and Holford	1981	1427	Yes; 3 times more frequent[*]	
Restrepo *et al.*	1990	222	Yes; 8 times more frequent[*]	
Rosenburg	1983	611	None[†]	
Saxen	1975	194	None[†]	
Czeizel	1988	1201	None[†]	
Shiono and Mills	1984	854	None[†]	
Rothman *et al.*	1979	383	Yes[‡]	
Bracken and Holford	1981	390	Yes[‡]; see comments	Data re-analyzed by Bracken; no significance found
Zierler and Rothman	1985	298	None[‡]	Anomalies: ventricular septal defects, conotruncal malformations
Tikkanen and Heinonen	1991, 1992	150	None[‡]	
Laegrid *et al.*	1992	17	Yes[§]; see comments	Weight normal by 10 months; head circumference still smaller than expected by 18 months (Laegrid *et al.*, 1992)

[*] Various congenital anomalies.
[†] Oral cleft, cleft lip.
[‡] Cardiovascular malformations.
[§] Birth weight and head circumference.
Adapted from Friedman JM, Polifka JE. *The teratogen information system*. Washinjgton, DC: The University of Washington, 1999.

after birth.[42,47] Because the fetus has a lower hepatic excretion rate than that of the mother, drug concentrations are higher than the therapeutic concentrations, and fetal tolerance of pharmacologic compounds administered during the last trimester is reduced.[38] McElhatton studied infants who had been exposed to benzodiazepines during the third trimester and/or at the time of birth, and found that some of them exhibited marked withdrawal symptoms, ranging from mild sedation, hypotonia and reluctance to suck, to apnoeic spells, cyanosis and impaired metabolic response to cold stress. Thus exposure during late third trimester and labor appears to be associated with much higher risks to the neonate.[47] However, it should be noted that while some studies may find statistically significant increases in the risks for fetal malformations after exposure to benzodiazepines, the absolute risk of anomalies remains relatively small.[44]

POSTNATAL BEHAVIORAL SEQUELAE

Postnatal behavioral sequelae, or behavioral teratogenicity, refers to the potential for long-term neurobehavioral abnormalities in children following *in utero* exposure to pharmacological

Table 7.7 *Human epidemiological studies of malformations associated with fetal exposure to chlordiazepoxide*

Author(s)	Year(s)	n	Association with anomaly	Comments
Crombie *et al.*	1975	38	No greater than expected[*]	
Kullander and Kallen	1976	98	No greater than expected[*]	
Heinonen *et al.*	1977	89	No greater than expected[*]	
Milkovich and van den Berg	1974	35	Yes; see comments[*]	Congenital anomalies loosely defined; no specificity of the anomalies present in the children was found
Bracken and Holford	1981	1427	None[*]	
Rothman *et al.*	1979	390	None[†]	
Czeizel	1988	1201	None[‡]	
Milkovich and van den Berg	1974	175	No greater than expected[*]	Cohort study
Heinonen *et al.*	1977	740	No greater than expected[*]	Cohort study

[*] Various congenital anomalies
[†] Cardiac malformations
[‡] Oral cleft, cleft lip
Adapted from Friedman JM, Polifka JE. *The teratogen information system.* Washington, DC: The University of Washington, 1999.

agents.[51,52] A prospective study conducted by Viggedal and colleagues suggests that prenatal exposure to benzodiazepines may cause a general delay in mental development up to 18 months of age. Specifically, the mean development quotients (DQ) and general development quotients (GQ) of infants prenatally exposed to benzodiazepines on all subscales of the Griffiths' Developmental Scale* were consistently lower than those of paired controls, respectively, at 5 months (102.4, SD = 12.6; 108.3, SD = 8.7; P = NS), 10 months (99.3, SD = 5.2; 109.5, SD = 6.7; $P < 0.001$), and 18 months (101.7, SD = 7.9; 107.6, SD = 8.3; $P < 0.05$).[55] A caveat to these data is the possibility that comorbid illnesses (e.g. epilepsy) confound the results and therefore bias the analyses. Furthermore, Viggedal and colleagues did not specify the benzodiazepine compounds to which children were exposed. Beyond the age of 18 months, the data are more promising.[47] In a controlled study that analyzed the statistical relationships between prescription data of pregnant mothers and evaluations of their children's subsequent behavior in school, no significant difference was found between the two groups and their controls.[56] In a study of 550 children who were followed for various times up to the age of 4 years, there was no increase in malformation rate or in adverse effects on either neurobehavioral development or IQ. It was not possible to establish a direct cause–effect relationship with prenatal benzodiazepine exposure for children in whom developmental deficits persisted.[47]

POSTPARTUM COURSE OF PANIC DISORDER

Little is known about the course of panic disorder during the postpartum period, although it is widely known that women have a heightened vulnerability to the development and relapse

* The developmental scale[53,54] provides mental ages, a general developmental quotient, and developmental quotients for locomotor, personal–social behavior, hearing and speech, eye–hand coordination and performance subscales.

of mood and anxiety disorders. To date, only three articles that focus primarily on the postpartum course of panic disorder have been published. Both Altshuler and colleagues[57] and Cohen and colleagues[20] further emphasize that women have a heightened vulnerability to relapse of panic disorder during the postpartum period, although there are no published data which solely address panic disorder with postpartum onset. In order to evaluate and treat effectively women suffering from postpartum panic disorder, more research is needed in this area, including both epidemiological and case–control studies.

TREATMENT DIRECTIVES

Because recent research suggests that the variation in the course of panic disorder during pregnancy is predicted by pregravid symptom severity, the latter should be retrospectively assessed prior to treatment during pregnancy. Likewise, gravid panic symptom severity should be closely monitored. Pharmacotherapy should be prescribed only if the patient's symptom severity warrants such measures. With regard to fetal exposure to benzodiazepines, level 2 ultrasonography should be used to rule out visible forms of oral cleft until more research is reported.[50]

LACTATION

Small amounts of benzodiazepines, including diazepam and several other benzodiazepine-like molecules, occur naturally in the milk of mothers who are non-users of benzodiazepine anxiolytics. They are thought to have either dietary or endogenous biosynthetic origins, although a direct relationship has not been established.[58] Benzodiazepines ingested by nursing mothers appear in human milk, but only relatively high clinical doses might be expected to have an effect on the neonate.* In newborns, particularly premature infants, elimination of benzodiazepines is less rapid relative to the immaturity of the hepatic systems that metabolize pharmacotherapeutic compounds. In general, therefore, high single doses and repeated and prolonged administration should be avoided.[43] It should be noted that no psychotropics have been approved by the Food and Drug Administration for use during lactation.

SUMMARY

In conclusion, pregnancy has a variable impact on the course of panic disorder. As evidenced by extant data collected from case–control and epidemiological studies alike, pregravid symptom severity currently functions as the most accurate predictor of the gravid course of the disorder. Under the tenet that panic disorder if left untreated during pregnancy is probably teratogenic to fetuses and has an equally deleterious effect on neonates, gravid symptom severity should be utilized by practitioners as a compass for directing treatment during pregnancy. Due to the dearth of literature and data currently available, additional research is required to define more clearly the effects of pregnancy on the course, prognoses and the safest and most efficacious treatments of the disorder.

---

* Clonazepam, clorazepate, diazepam, lorazepam, midazolam, nitrazepam and oxazepam are the only benzodiazepine anxiolytics for which data on excretion into human breast-milk are currently available.[47]

Acknowledgments

Financial assistance for the research described in this chapter was provided in part by a Fellowship from the Stanley Foundation (DM) and the University of Texas Southwestern Medical Center at Dallas (DM and KAY). Additional assistance was provided by the Department of Psychiatry, Yale University School of Medicine (DM and KAY).

REFERENCES

1. Barrett JE, Barrett JA, Oxman TE, Gerber PD. The prevalence of psychiatric disorders in primary care practice. *Archives of General Psychiatry* 1988; **45**: 1100–6.
2. Kirmayer LJ, Robbins JM, Dworkind M, Yaffe MJ. Somatization and the recognition of depression and anxiety in primary care. *American Journal of Psychiatry* 1993; **150**: 734–41.
3. Rouillon F. Epidemiology of panic disorder. *Encephale* 1996; **22**: 25–34.
4. Roth M, Argyle N. Anxiety, panic and phobic disorders: an overview. *Journal of Psychiatric Research* 1988; **22** (Supplement 1): 33–54.
5. Yonkers KA, Zlotnick C, Allsworth J, Warshaw M, Shea T, Keller MB. Is the course of panic disorder the same in women and men? *American Journal of Psychiatry* 1998; **155**: 596–602.
6. American Psychiatric Association. *Diagnostic and statistical manual of mental disorders (DSM-IV)*, 4th edn. Washington, DC: American Psychiatric Association, 1994: 886.
7. American Psychiatric Association. Practice guidelines for the treatment of patients with panic disorder. Work group on panic disorder. *American Journal of Psychiatry* 1998; **155** (Supplement 5): 1–34.
8. Chambless DL, Mason J. Sex, sex-role stereotyping and agoraphobia. *Behaviour Research and Therapy* 1986; **24**: 231–5.
9. Stein MB, Schmidt PJ, Rubinow DR, Uhde TW. Panic disorder and the menstrual cycle: Panic disorder patients, healthy control subjects, and patients with premenstrual syndrome. *American Journal of Psychiatry* 1989; **146**: 1299–303.
10. Cook BL, Noyes R, Garvey MJ, Beach V, Sobotka J, Chandry D. Anxiety and the menstrual cycle in panic disorder. *Journal of Affective Disorders* 1990; **19**: 221–6.
11. Carney RM, Freedland KE, Ludbrook PA, Saunders RD, Jaffe AS. Major depression, panic disorder, and mitral valve prolapse in patients who complain of chest pain. *American Journal of Medicine* 1990; **89**: 757–60.
12. Crowe R. Mitral valve prolapse and panic disorder. *Psychiatric Clinics of North America* 1985; **8**: 63–71.
13. Yonkers K, Pratt L, Vitali A *et al*. Unique features of panic disorder in women. *Biological Psychiatry* 1993; **33**: 148A.
14. Freeman EW, Purdy RH, Coutifaris C, Rickels K, Paul SM. Anxiolytic metabolites of progesterone: correlation with mood and performance measures following oral progesterone administration to healthy female volunteers. *Neuroendocrinology* 1993; **58**: 478–84.
15. Majewska MD, Harrison NL, Schwartz RD, Parker JL, Paul SM. Steroid metabolites are barbiturate-like modulators of the GABA receptor. *Science* 1986; **232**: 1004–7.
16. Klein DF. False suffocation alarms and spontaneous panic: subsuming the CO_2 hypersensitivity theory. *Archives of General Psychiatry* 1993; **50**: 306–17.
17. Kendell RE, Wainwright S, Hailey A, Shannon B. The influence of childbirth on psychiatric morbidity. *Psychological Medicine* 1976; **6**: 297–302.
18. Zajicek E. Psychiatric problems during pregnancy. In: Wolkind S, Wolkind ZE (eds) *Pregnancy: a psychological and social study*, London: Academic Press, 1981: 57–73.

19. George DT, Ladenheim JA, Nutt DJ. Effect of pregnancy on panic attacks. *American Journal of Psychiatry* 1987; **144**: 1078–9.
20. Cohen LS, Sichel DA, Dimmock JA, Rosenbaum JF. Impact of pregnancy on panic disorder: a case series. *Journal of Clinical Psychiatry* 1994; **55**: 284–8.
21. Cohen LS, Sichel DA, Faraone SV, Robertson LM, Dimmock JA, Rosenbuam JF. Course of panic disorder during pregnancy and the puerperium: a preliminary study. *Biological Psychiatry* 1996; **39**: 950–4.
22. Cohen LS, Sichel DA, Dimmock JA, Rosenbaum JF. Postpartum course in women with pre-existing panic disorder. *Journal of Clinical Psychiatry* 1994; **55**: 289–92.
23. Altshuler LL, Hendrick V, Cohen LS. Course of mood and anxiety disorders during pregnancy and the postpartum period. *Journal of Clinical Psychiatry* 1998; **59** (Supplement 2): 29–33.
24. George DT, Ladenheim JA, Nutt DJ. Effect of pregnancy on panic attacks. *American Journal of Psychiatry* 1987; **144**: 1078–9.
25. Villeponteaux VA, Lydaird RB, Laraia MT, Stuart GW, Ballenger JC. The effects of pregnancy on pre-existing panic disorder. *Journal of Clinical Psychiatry* 1992; **53**: 201–3.
26. Robins LN, Helzer JE, Weissman MM *et al*. Lifetime prevalence of specific disorders in three sites. *Archives of General Psychiatry* 1984; **41**: 949–58.
27. Weissman MM, Bland RC, Canino GJ *et al*. The cross-national epidemiology of panic disorder. *Archives of General Psychiatry* 1997; **54**: 305–9.
28. Keller MB, Yonkers KA, Warshaw MG *et al*. Remission and relapse in subjects with panic disorder and panic with agoraphobia. *Journal of Nervous and Mental Disease* 1994; **182**: 290–6.
29. Pollack MH, Smoller JW. The longitudinal course and outcome of panic disorder. *Psychiatric Clinics of North America* 1995; **18**: 785–801.
30. Milrod B, Busch F, Cooper A, Shapiro T *et al*. *Manual of panic-focused psychodynamic psychotherapy*, Washington, DC: American Psychiatric Association Press, 1997.
31. Kohut H. Thoughts on narcissism and narcissistic rage. *Psychoanalytical Study of the Child* 1972; **27**: 360–400.
32. Bash M. *Doing brief Psychotherapy*. New York: Basic Books, 1995.
33. Gray J. The neuropsychiatry of anxiety. *British Journal of Psychology* 1978; **69**: 472–83.
34. Sifneos P. The current status of individual short-term dynamic psychotherapy and its future: an overview. *American Journal of Psychotherapy* 1984; **38**: 472–83.
35. Goldberg C. Cognitive–behavioral therapy for panic: effectiveness and limitations. *Psychiatric Quarterly* 1998; **69**: 23–44.
36. Cohen LS, Sichel DA, Dimmock JA, Rosenbaum JF. Impact of pregnancy on panic disorder: a case series. *Journal of Clinical Psychiatry* 1994; **55**: 284–8.
37. Yonkers KA, Kando JC, Cole JO, Blumenthal S. Gender differences in pharmacokinetics and pharmacodynamics of psychotropic medication. *American Journal of Psychiatry* 1992; **149**: 587–95.
38. Hernández Alvarez LA, Márquez Orozco MC, Márquez Orozco A, Hicks Gomez JJ. Teratologic effects of benzodiazepines. *Ginecologia Y Obstetricia De Mexico* 1991; **59**: 195–201.
39. Schatzberg AF, Cole JO. *Manual of Clinical Psychopharmacology*, 2nd edn. Washington, DC: American Psychiatric Press, 1992: 294.
40. Yonkers KA, Hamilton J. Sex differences in pharmokinetics of psychotropic medications. Part II. Effects on selected psychotropic. In: Jensvold MJ, Halbreich U, Hamilton JA (eds) *Psychopharmacology of women: sex, gender and hormonal considerations. Vol. 1.* Washington, DC: American Psychiatric Association, 1995.
41. Lanczik M, Knoche M, Fritze J. Psychopharmacotherapy during pregnancy and lactation. 1. Pregnancy. *Nervenarzt* 1998; **69**: 1–9.
42. Altshuler LL, Cohen L, Szuba MP, Burt VK, Gitlin M, Mintz J. Pharmacologic management of psychiatric illness during pregnancy: dilemmas and guidelines. *American Journal of Psychiatry* 1996; **153**: 592–606.

43. Olive G, Rey E. Benzodiazepines and pregnancy. Transplacental passage, labor and lactation. *Encephale* 1983; **9** (Supplement 2): 87B-96B.
44. Altshuler LL, Cohen L, Szuba MP, Burt VK, Gitlin M, Mintz J. Pharmacologic management of psychiatric illness during pregnancy: dilemmas and guidelines. *American Journal of Psychiatry* 1996; **153**: 592–606.
45. Cohen LS, Rosenbaum JF. Psychotropic drug use during pregnancy: weighing the risks. *Journal of Clinical Psychiatry* 1998; **59** (Supplement 2): 18–28.
46. Weber LW. Benzodiazepines in pregnancy – academic debate or teratogenic risk? *Biological research in pregnancy and perinatology* 1985; **6**: 151–67.
47. McElhatton PR. The effects of benzodiazepine use during pregnancy and lactation. *Reproductive Toxicology* 1994; **8**: 461–75.
48. Friedman J, Polifka J. *Teratogenic effects of drugs: a resource of clinicians (TERIS)* Baltimore, MD: Johns Hopkins University Press, 2000.
49. St Clair SM, Schirmer RG. First-trimester exposure to alprazolam. *Obstetrics and Gynecology* 1992; **80**: 843–6.
50. Dolovich LR, Addis A, Vaillancourt JM, Power JD, Koren G, Einarson TR. Benzodiazepine use in pregnancy and major malformations or oral cleft: meta-analysis of cohort and case–control studies. *British Medical Journal* 1998; **317**: 839–43.
51. Vernadakis A, Parker KK. Drugs and the developing central nervous system. *Pharmacology and Therapeutics* 1980; **11**: 593–647.
52. Vorhees CV, Brunner RL, Butcher RE. Psychotropic drugs as behavioral teratogens. *Science* 1979; **205**: 1220–5.
53. Griffiths R. *The abilities of babies: a study in mental measurement*. London: University of London Press, 1954.
54. Griffiths R. *The abilities of young children*. London: Child Development Research Centre, 1970.
55. Viggedal G, Hagberg BS, Laegreid L, Aronsson M. Mental development in late infancy after prenatal exposure to benzodiazepines – a prospective study. *Journal of Child Psychology and Psychiatry and Allied Disciplines* 1993; **34**: 295–305.
56. Stika L, Elisová K, Honzáková L *et al*. Effects of drug administration in pregnancy on children's school behaviour. *Pharmaceutisch Weekblad Scientific Edition* 1990; **12**: 252–5.
57. Altshuler LL, Szuba MP. Course of psychiatric disorders in pregnancy. Dilemmas in pharmacologic management. *Neurological Clinics* 1994; **12**: 613–35.
58. Peña C, Medina JH, Piva M, Diaz LE, Danilowicz C, Paladini AC. Naturally occurring benzodiazepines in human milk. *Biochemical and Biophysical Research Communications* 1991; **175**: 1042–50.

8

Obsessive-compulsive disorder during pregnancy and postpartum

MARGARET ALTEMUS

INTRODUCTION

Obsessive-compulsive disorder (OCD) is an anxiety disorder characterized by intrusive recurrent thoughts and ritualized, repetitive behaviors that are experienced as irrational or excessive. OCD affects 1–3% of the population across a wide variety of cultures.[1] This disorder usually first appears during childhood, adolescence or early adulthood and it almost always has a chronic course.[2,3] OCD can cause marked distress and severe impairment of social and occupational functioning. Although the disorder often has an earlier age of onset in boys,[4] the prevalence of the illness in adulthood is similar in men and women. OCD is distinguished from other anxiety disorders and major depression by a selective response to serotonin reuptake inhibiting antidepressants.[5]

Most patients perform compulsions in order to relieve temporarily the anxiety associated with obsessive thoughts. For example, handwashing provides relief from obsessions about contamination, and checking provides relief from fears of potentially dangerous errors. Other patients describe urges to perform compulsions such as tapping or symmetrical arranging, which are not accompanied by clear obsessive fears. Rather, performance of the rituals relieves a sensation that things are not 'just right'. Factor analysis studies have identified the following four categories of obsessions and compulsions: contamination fears with washing rituals; intrusive, violent and dangerous thoughts with exaggerated harm avoidance; hoarding; and ritualistic symmetry or arranging compulsions. Excessive doubts and checking commonly occur across these categories.[6] From an ethological perspective, each of the four categories of symptoms can be regarded as exaggerations of behaviors which are adaptive for survival. This has led to a conceptualization of the illness as the emergence of phylogenetically more primitive instincts which exist in all humans but are normally suppressed.[7]

CLINICAL FEATURES

Longitudinal course

For over 30 years, clinicians have reported an increased incidence of obsessive-compulsive disorder in association with pregnancy.[8,9] However, because OCD is a relatively prevalent disorder and pregnancy is common, it is possible that the onset of OCD in association with pregnancy is a coincidental event. No controlled epidemiological studies have been conducted to determine whether there is in fact an increased risk of OCD onset during pregnancy or postpartum. In addition, no prospective studies of OCD symptoms have been conducted with pregnant women, so it is unclear when in the course of pregnancy or the postpartum period OCD may tend to develop. Retrospective accounts of symptom onset are well known to be unreliable, but currently these are the only form of data available. Recent retrospective studies have reported the onset of OCD associated with pregnancy in 16–52% of women with OCD who have had children. In one retrospective survey of 59 women with OCD who had children, 23 women (39%) described the onset of their OCD specifically as occurring during pregnancy.[10] Interestingly, in this study, for the women with OCD who had never had children, the most common ages of onset of OCD were 13–15 years of age, coinciding with the onset of puberty. In another retrospective study of mothers with OCD, 6 of 39 women (18%) reported onset during pregnancy, and a larger proportion, 8 women (30%), reported onset of illness postpartum.[11] In a third study,[12] 5 of 31 mothers (16%) with OCD reported onset of the illness during pregnancy, and none of the 31 mothers had experienced a postpartum onset of OCD. Although OCD is usually a chronic disorder, and many women with onset of OCD in association with pregnancy have chronic symptoms,[13] in a few reported cases, pregnancy-associated OCD remitted postpartum.[14–16]

In addition to onset of OCD during pregnancy, some evidence suggests that pre-existing OCD may be exacerbated during pregnancy, although the retrospective surveys and case reports of OCD symptom response to pregnancy have produced conflicting results.[12,17] In one survey, no changes in OCD symptoms occurred with pregnancy in 20 of 29 women (69%) with OCD who became pregnant, while 5/29 (17%) reported symptom worsening during pregnancy and 4/29 (14%) reported improvement.[12] In the same study, in the postpartum period, symptom exacerbation was reported in 7/24 (29%) of women with pre-existing OCD.

Tics and Tourette's Syndrome often occur in association with OCD in the general population, although this comorbidity is more common in men with OCD than women with OCD. There has been extremely little study to date of tics during pregnancy, but the available data indicates that tics tend to remain stable during pregnancy.[18] In contrast, Syndenham's chorea, another childhood-onset movement disorder which has high comorbidity with OCD, often recurs during pregnancy.[19]

In an attempt to begin to clarify the time-course of OCD exacerbation associated with pregnancy, two small prospective studies were conducted in the Intramural Research Program at the National Institute of Mental Health (NIMH). The first study examined the onset of OCD in an unselected population of healthy pregnant women. A total of 100 healthy women with no current Axis I psychiatric disorders were evaluated in the third trimester of pregnancy and 6 weeks, 16 weeks and 1 year postpartum. Six (6%) of the women experienced the onset of OCD during pregnancy. For four of these women, this was the initial presentation of OCD, and the other two women had previous transient symptoms of OCD in association with a previous pregnancy. In contrast, no new cases of OCD occurred during the first year postpartum in the remaining 94 subjects. Three of the six women who developed OCD during pregnancy had complete remission of their OCD symptoms by 1 year postpartum without treatment, and two showed marked improvement in their OCD symptoms over the following year. The sixth woman, who had the most severe OCD symptoms, began treatment with a serotonin reuptake inhibitor at 3 months postpartum, which led to marked resolution of her symptoms.

In addition to the six women who developed OCD during pregnancy, a large proportion of women in the study (25 of 94; 26%) had subclinical degrees of OCD during pregnancy. In total, 19 (76%) of these women reported that their symptoms were exaggerated during pregnancy, two (8%) felt that the subclinical OCD symptoms improved during pregnancy, and four (16%) felt that the symptoms remained unchanged compared to the period before the pregnancy. In the postpartum follow-up, 13 of 25 women (52%) had resolution of subclinical OCD symptoms, 5 of 25 women (20%) experienced worsening of their symptoms, but still did not meet the criteria for obsessive-compulsive disorder, and in 7 of 25 women (28%) the degree of subclinical OCD symptoms remained unchanged.

Finally, two of our cases and one in the literature[15] reported a return of symptoms with subsequent pregnancies, so women with a history of pregnancy-related OCD should be followed closely during subsequent pregnancies.

The second prospective study examined the course of symptoms during pregnancy and the first year postpartum in 13 women with a pre-existing diagnosis of chronic OCD prior to pregnancy. Nine of the 13 women (69%) described the OCD symptoms during pregnancy as more severe than their pre-pregnancy symptoms, one woman (8%) felt that the symptom severity had remained unchanged during pregnancy, and three (23%) felt that their symptoms improved during pregnancy. Following pregnancy, five of these women started taking psychotropic medication immediately, with an improvement in their symptoms. Of the remaining eight women who did not receive pharmacotherapy postpartum, two felt worse at 5 weeks postpartum, three felt the same and three felt better, indicating that there is no clear effect of completion of pregnancy on the course of the disorder.

The conflicting findings of the studies reviewed above may reflect not only the unreliability of restrospective accounts but also the heterogeneous nature of OCD. This disorder is likely to result from a variety of etiologic processes, including genetic, traumatic, environmental, immunologic and hormonal factors, in different combinations. Some of these forms of OCD may be more responsive to reproductive events than others.

Symptom profile

It is noteworthy that all cases of new-onset OCD during pregnancy in our case series, and all of those reported in the literature to date, describe contamination obsessions and cleaning rituals and/or intrusive violent thoughts of harming the infant.[11,13-17] Intrusive violent thoughts can also occur in women with postpartum psychosis. However, in postpartum psychosis, infanticide is egosyntonic and is perceived as a way to 'save' the infant from danger. In women with OCD, the intrusive images of harming the infant are very disturbing and egodystonic. This is an important differential diagnosis, since women with postpartum psychosis are at real risk of harming their infant. Conversely, it is important to reassure mothers with OCD and their partners that intrusive violent thoughts associated with OCD are not acted out.

The specific nature of OCD symptoms that present during pregnancy suggests that such symptoms during pregnancy may represent an exaggeration of the biological mechanisms which produce normal 'nesting behaviors' and intrusive thoughts of danger during pregnancy. Healthy pregnant women commonly report fearing that harm will come to their baby, and they also commonly experience increased urges to clean and organize the house, particularly towards the end of pregnancy.

Actual nest-building behaviors are seen during pregnancy in a wide variety of animal species, and provide evidence that the hormonal changes of pregnancy drive nesting behaviors. Nest-building during pregnancy in animals involves a range of behaviors, including plucking hair, collecting other materials and arranging them. The expression of nest-building behavior during pregnancy in birds and mammals appears to be dependent on estrogen, progesterone, prolactin and oxytocin.[20–23] Close study of this phenomenon in rabbits has shown that the specific sequence of behaviors is linked to specific hormonal changes across pregnancy.[20] Digging of a space for the nest occurs while both estradiol and progesterone levels are high. Later, as progesterone levels decline, pregnant rabbits begin to collect and arrange straw for the nest. Finally, when progesterone levels have ceased falling, and estrogen levels are still high, the pregnant rabbits begin to pluck their own hair and use it to build the nest.

Comorbidity

We found that all eight women who developed new-onset OCD during pregnancy in our NIMH longitudinal study reported a history of subjectively severe premenstrual mood changes. This association between pregnancy-related OCD and premenstrual dysphoria suggests that women who develop OCD during pregnancy and the postpartum period are particularly sensitive to fluxes in gonadal steroids which occur across the menstrual cycle and during pregnancy.

In addition, in the one retrospective study which examined depression comorbidity, a large proportion of women who developed OCD prior to pregnancy (9/24; 37%) reported postpartum depression.[12] Another case series described 15 women who presented with new-onset OCD during the first 4 weeks postpartum,[13] and nine of these 15 women (60%) had comorbid major depression. In our NIMH longitudinal study of healthy women, two of the six women who developed OCD during pregnancy (33%) also had a postpartum depression. To date, there has been little examination of the inverse phenomenon, namely the frequency of obsessive features in postpartum depression. It is unclear why OCD in the postpartum period seems to be strongly associated with comorbid depression. This may represent similar biological processes predisposing to OCD and depression, or an interaction between the stress of OCD symptoms and the physical and emotional fatigue and family stress associated with infant care, all contributing to induction of a depressive illness.

Effect of lactation on OCD

There are no published data examining the effect of lactation on OCD. Preliminary data from our pilot longitudinal study at NIMH and available case reports suggest that lactation may improve subclinical OCD symptoms which are common during pregnancy (see Table 8.1), but that it is not particularly helpful for women with the full syndrome (see Table 8.2). The

Table 8.1 *Effect of lactation on subclinical OCD symptoms (16 weeks postpartum compared to third trimester of pregnancy)*

| | Number of subjects | |
	Breastfeeding	Bottle-feeding
Improved	12	1
Worse	2	3
No change	4	3

Table 8.2 *Effect of lactation on DSM-III-R OCD symptoms (OCD symptom change in medication-free women with OCD: 6 weeks postpartum compared to third trimester of pregnancy)*

| | Number of subjects | |
	Breastfeeding	Bottle-feeding
Improved	3	0
Worse	0	2
No change	3	0

lack of a clear beneficial effect of lactation on OCD symptom severity contrasts with reports that lactation has a protective effect against panic in many,[24,25] but not all[26,27] studies. One factor that potentially contributes to the differential effect of lactation on panic symptoms but not on OCD symptoms is that central GABA levels appear to be increased during lactation. Elevated GABA levels have been found in the cerebrospinal fluid and in the bed nucleus of the stria terminalis and substantia nigra in lactating sheep[28,29] and in the cerebrospinal fluid of lactating rats.[30] Since agents such as benzodiazepines which enhance GABA transmission are effective treatment agents for panic, but not for OCD, this endocrinological feature of lactation may only have beneficial effects for patients with panic disorder.

TREATMENT

Early detection and treatment of OCD during pregnancy and the postpartum period is important not only for care of the mother, but also to minimize disruption and conflict within the family and to protect against preoccupations and avoidance rituals which could impair mother–infant bonding.[31] Possible physical harm to the fetus could occur if a woman develops restrictive eating rituals, if she has avoidance behaviors, procrastination or exaggerated fears which prevent her from obtaining adequate prenatal care, or if she develops severe comorbid depression with a risk of suicidality. In the postpartum period, severe OCD could also result in restrictive infant-feeding rituals, excessive bathing or avoidance of bathing, or neglect of the infant due to irrational fears of causing harm to him or her.

Two effective treatment strategies for obsessive-compulsive disorder have been identified, namely behavior therapy and pharmacologic treatment.[32]

Women with OCD who are planning a pregnancy should gain experience in using behavioral techniques to control their symptoms, and have a good working relationship with a behavioral therapist who can work with them during and prior to the pregnancy, as attempts are made to reduce medication dosages. Behavior therapy, based on exposure and response prevention, and often combined with some cognitive techniques, can be a very effective treatment for OCD. However, a substantial proportion of OCD patients are too anxious or otherwise unwilling to participate in the treatment protocols. Moreover, in many areas of the USA behavior therapists who are trained in the treatment of OCD are not available. However, a number of instructional books are now available to help patients and clinicians to design and carry out a program of exposure and response prevention.[33–36] Although there have been no studies to date of behavioral treatments during pregnancy and postpartum, there is little reason to believe that the efficacy of this treatment would be impaired by pregnancy.

Serotonin reuptake inhibitors (e.g. anafranil, fluoxetine, sertraline, paroxetine, fluvoxamine, citalopram) are the current first-line pharmacological treatment for obsessive-compulsive disorder, but most patients show only a partial response to these agents, and 25% of patients show no response.[5] Low-dose neuroleptics have been shown to be an effective augmentation agent for a subgroup of OCD patients treated with serotonin reuptake inhibitors,[37] but no other psychopharmacological treatments have been shown to be beneficial in controlled trials.[38-41] No specific additional treatments have been identified for women who develop OCD during pregnancy or postpartum.

Multiple case reports have described a good response to serotonin reuptake inhibitors in women with new-onset pregnancy-related OCD who receive the medication postpartum.[11,13-15] However, Sichel and colleagues reported that only 4 of 15 patients showed complete resolution of symptoms with continued pharmacologic treatment when assessed at 1 year postpartum. The rest of the subjects in her study had mild degrees of residual symptoms,[13] an outcome that is typical of non-pregnancy-related OCD.

The risks and benefits of the use of pharmacologic treatment during pregnancy must be weighed in each individual case. Decisions will vary greatly among patients and their practitioners. Although serotonin reuptake inhibitors and neuroleptics have not been approved by the FDA for administration during pregnancy, psychotropic medications are increasingly being used during pregnancy. Reviews of the available limited data concerning fetal exposure to antidepressants and antipsychotics indicate that they have relatively low teratogenic potential, and, to date there is little evidence of neurobehavioral sequelae postnatally.[42-44] For several drugs, particularly fluoxetine, a relatively large amount of safety data has been collected. In addition, several studies of small numbers of infants exposed to antidepressant medications through breast-milk indicate that most such infants will have minimal levels of medication in their blood.[45]

It is most advisable to prepare prior to pregnancy so that the use of medication can be minimized without severe relapse of the illness. If possible, the medication dose should be tapered down slowly prior to pregnancy, in order to determine the lowest dose which maintains symptoms at a tolerable level. OCD commonly recurs on discontinuation of medication[46,47] so patients should anticipate intensification of symptoms if they try to taper down their medication dosage. Many patients may be willing to tolerate a higher level of symptoms during pregnancy in order to reduce fetal exposure to pharmacologic agents. It is also a good idea to plan pregnancy for a time when other life stresses are minimized.

It is unclear what proportion of cases of pregnancy-related OCD resolve without any treatment at all. In our study in which healthy subjects were recruited to participate in an infant feeding study, three of the six women with a new onset of OCD during pregnancy had complete remission of symptoms without treatment. A similar course has been described by others in case reports.[16]

PATHOPHYSIOLOGY

Worsening of OCD during pregnancy or the postpartum period may arise from the stress of pregnancy and caring for a new infant. Pregnancy and the postpartum period can be a time of marital, financial, and occupational stress, and women typically experience moderate to severe sleep disruption during the later stages of pregnancy[48] and while caring for a newborn. However, a variety of lines of evidence indicate that the hormonal changes of pregnancy contribute to symptom exacerbation. Pregnancy causes steep rises in circulating levels of estrogens (estradiol, estriol and estrone), progesterone and androgenic steroid hormones, as well as rises in multiple hypothalamic and placental peptide hormones, including prolactin, oxytocin and corticotropin releasing hormone. Subsequently, there is a dramatic decrease in all of the steroid hormones and placental peptides within a few days after delivery. Prolactin and oxytocin secretion continues to be elevated in women who lactate postpartum. There is no evidence that women with pregnancy-related OCD have abnormal changes in circulating hormones during pregnancy or postpartum. Instead, these women appear to react to the normal hormonal changes during pregnancy with new onset or worsening of OCD symptoms. Differential sensitivity to reproductive hormones may be mediated through differences in gonadal steroid and peptide receptors, differences in intracellular cofactors which mediate the action of hormone-bound steroid receptors on gene transcription, or differences in the target systems (e.g. serotonin or vasopressin) which are modified by reproductive hormones.

Several findings in addition to the observation of OCD onset during pregnancy suggest that gonadal steroids provoke OCD symptoms. Recent reports have described OCD occurring in association with polycystic ovary disease[49] and congenital adrenal hyperplasia,[50] two disorders in which there is elevated production of gonadal steroids and androgenic adrenal steroids. Increases in OCD symptoms have also been described during the luteal phase of the menstrual cycle, when levels of estrogen, progesterone and androgenic hormones are also elevated.[12,51] Moreover, two published case studies and four case reports have described a reduction in OCD symptoms during treatment with drugs that antagonize gonadal steroids. Casas and colleagues[52] conducted an open study with cyproterone acetate, an androgen synthesis inhibitor and androgen receptor antagonist which also suppresses luteinizing-hormone release, in five female patients with severe OCD symptoms. These patients experienced a marked improvement with a gradual re-emergence of obsessive-compulsive symptoms after 3–6 months of treatment. Leonard and Swedo[53] reported two childhood cases of OCD that were successfully treated with a combination of spironolactone, an androgen-receptor antagonist, and testolactone, an aromatase inhibitor. An 8–year-old boy had a remission lasting for 6 months and a 15–year-old boy experienced a moderate improvement throughout a 10–week trial. More recently, Weiss and colleagues[49] and Eriksson[54] described two additional cases of OCD improvement in response to cyproterone acetate treatment. Chouinard and colleagues[55] reported beneficial effects of aminoglutethamide, a drug which globally inhibits steroid biosynthesis, in a treatment-resistant OCD patient.

Unfortunately, the gonadal steroid treatment regimens in these treatment trials and the reproductive events associated with symptom exacerbation have relatively non-specific and complex effects on gonadal steroid systems. This has made it difficult to identify which particular steroids or steroid receptors have the most important role in mediating the effects of gonadal steroids on OCD. The results of one recent study suggest that gonadal steroid exacerbation of OCD is not mediated by androgen receptors. Treatment of 8 OCD patients with flutamide, a selective competitive antagonist of the androgen receptor, was not beneficial.[56] However, minimal improvement in OCD symptoms was noted in a group of patients with a primary diagnosis of Tourette's syndrome after flutamide treatment.[57] These data suggest that any effects of gonadal steroids in exacerbating OCD symptoms are more likely to be mediated via estrogen receptors or receptor-independent mechanisms.

Gonadal steroids can affect brain systems implicated in OCD through multiple mechanisms, including alterations in neurotransmitter and neuropeptide signaling efficiency, neuronal excitability, neural structure and synaptic plasticity.[58] Classical gonadal steroid receptors have been identified in the striatum, a brain area identified as dysfunctional in OCD by imaging and neuropathological studies, and also in the raphe nucleus, the primary output nucleus for serotonergic neurons.[59] In addition, gonadal steroids are also known to have a rapid affect on neuronal function through receptor-independent mechanisms, including regulation of ion channels, uncoupling of G-protein second-messenger systems, phosphorylation of transcription factors, and modification of neurotransmitter synthesis and metabolism as well as neurotransmitter-receptor structure.[60,61] Finally, gonadal steroids also modulate a variety of immune function parameters,[62] so pregnancy may alter the course of cases of OCD resulting from an autoimmune pathology.[63]

Estrogen

Preclinical data indicate that estrogen modulates a number of neurochemical systems which have been implicated in the pathophysiology of OCD.

First, studies in animals have shown that estrogen administration has profound, region-specific effects on serotonergic function. A major hypothesis of OCD is that the illness is caused by a relative deficiency of serotonin. This hypothesis is primarily based on the selective efficacy in OCD of serotonin reuptake inhibitor treatment.[5] Chronic administration of serotonin reuptake inhibitors increases the efficiency of serotonergic neurotransmission.[64] To date, 14 serotonin receptor subtypes have been identified, some of which may have separate and opposing actions with regard to anxiety. Activation of the $5HT_3$ postsynaptic receptor appears to produce anxiogenic effects, while activation of $5HT_{1A}$ and possible $5HT_{2C}$ postsynaptic receptors appears to have more anxiolytic effects. Reported effects of estrogen treatment on serotonergic systems include reduced metabolism by inhibition of monoamine oxidase,[65] increased tryptophan hydroxylase mRNA expression in the dorsal raphe,[66] increased serotonin transporter mRNA expression in the dorsal raphe,[67] increased density of serotonin transporter binding in multiple other brain areas,[67,68] increased density of $5HT_{2A}$ receptor binding in the dorsal raphe and several cortical and limbic areas,[69] and increased serotonin levels in the dorsal raphe.

Second, estradiol potentiates dopamine activity in the striatum[70] and has region-specific effects on striatal D_2 dopamine-receptor binding.[71] Augmentation of serotonin reuptake inhibitor treatment with dopamine antagonists appears to be useful for a subset of OCD patients,[37] thus implicating dopaminergic pathways in the illness. Estrogen also inhibits the activity of a major dopamine-metabolizing enzyme, namely catechol-o-methyl-transferase (COMT).[72–74] COMT has a common genetic polymorphism, causing a fourfold reduction in enzyme activity. The low-activity form of the enzyme has been associated with an increased risk of OCD,[75] suggesting that enzyme inhibition by estrogen may also increase the risk of developing OCD.

Third, estrogen exacerbation of OCD may also involve activation of oxytocin and vasopressin systems. High levels of the neuropeptides oxytocin and vasopressin have been linked to OCD, although the evidence from different studies is conflicting.[76–78] Oxytocin receptors are profoundly upregulated by estrogen[79] and estrogen also enhances the expression of vasopressin in limbic areas, including the amygdala and the bed nucleus of the stria terminalis.[80,81] Although peripheral levels of oxytocin increase during pregnancy, spinal fluid sampling and microdialysis studies suggest that central levels do not increase until the onset of labor.[28,82–84]

Although anecdotal evidence suggests that estrogen may exacerbate OCD symptoms, in healthy controls and other clinical conditions estrogen appears to blunt anxiety. Subclinical anxiety symptoms are reduced in postmenopausal women who are given estrogen replacement therapy[85,86] and estrogen appears to blunt autonomic (heart rate and blood pressure) responses to stress in postmenopausal women.[87] Estrogen also has anxiolytic effects in a number of animal models of anxiety and fear.[88–91] In addition, it enhances the anxiolytic effects of several compounds, including diazepam infused into the central gray matter, and intraventricularly administered oxytocin.[79] The findings of depression treatment studies, although conflicting, generally support an antidepressant effect of estrogen administration.[92,93]

Progesterone

Increases in the levels of circulating progesterone and some metabolites of progesterone during pregnancy will facilitate transmission at $GABA_A$ receptors, similar to the effect of benzodiazepines which act at an adjacent site within the $GABA_A$-receptor complex. Although not all progesterone metabolites are anxiolytic, progesterone is metabolized to several compounds that have anxiolytic effects, including pregnenolone sulfate and allopregnanolone, both in the adrenal gland and locally in the brain.[94]

Worsening of OCD during pregnancy contrasts sharply with reports of improvement of panic during pregnancy in some[24,25] but not all[26,27] studies, and an increase in panic symptoms immediately postpartum.[24,25,26,95]. As in lactation, the differential course of these two disorders during pregnancy may reflect the divergent response of the two illnesses to benzodiazepine treatment. In addition to progesterone-mediated increased sensitivity to GABA agonists during pregnancy, increased cerebrospinal fluid GABA levels have been described in sheep during pregnancy.[96]

Although a reduction in fear behaviors in response to progesterone has been attributed to potentiation of $GABA_A$ receptors, progesterone effects may also involve co-modulation with estrogen of other neurotransmitter and neuropeptide systems. Neurosteroids have also been shown to modulate dopamine release from striatal neurons, which could be postulated to play a role in changes in OCD symptoms during pregnancy. In addition, Klein and colleagues have proposed that high levels of progesterone during pregnancy increase the respiratory rate and lower pCO_2 levels, so that patients are protected from triggering a 'suffocation alarm' which could play a role in generating panic attacks in some cases.[24]

Autoimmunity

Recent evidence suggests that some cases of OCD are autoimmune in etiology, and may represent a variant form of Sydenham's chorea, with similar inflammatory damage to basal ganglia.[64] Sydenham's chorea occurs in approximately 10% of patients with rheumatic fever. Rheumatic fever is caused by antibodies to Group A streptococcus bacteria which cross-react with tissues of the heart, joints and other tissues, including the basal ganglia. Several studies have found a 70–90% incidence of obsessive-compulsive symptoms in patients with Sydenham's chorea.[97,98] Imaging studies have implicated the basal ganglia as a primary site of dysfunction in OCD[99] as well as Sydenham's chorea and multiple cases of OCD have been documented to result from discrete, traumatic basal ganglia lesions in adulthood.[100]

Pregnancy may unmask a pre-existing potential for autoimmune chorea and OCD, or promote a recurrence of chorea and OCD which was transiently manifested in childhood. Chorea which appears during pregnancy (chorea gravidarum) is a rare disorder that is estimated to occur in 1 in 140 000 pregnancies.[101] The strongest risk factors for this disorder are a history of Sydenham's Chorea[19] in childhood and the presence of antiphospholipid and anticardiolipin antibodies,[102,103] which are often a feature of systemic lupus erythematosus. There is a very high incidence of OCD in Sydenham's chorea,[97,98] again suggesting a pathophysiological association between inflammatory chorea and OCD. Chorea gravidarum can begin in the first trimester of pregnancy and resolve within 2–3 months in patients with a history of Sydenham's chorea or it may appear later in pregnancy and progressively worsen until delivery in patients with antiphospholipid antibodies.[19,104] It has been suggested that the chorea during pregnancy results from an interaction of antiphospholipid antibodies with the vascular endothelium of the basal ganglia, resulting in reversible focal ischemia.[104–106] Further support for this model comes from evidence that chorea responds to high-dose glucocorticoid treatment. Both antiphospholipid antibody-mediated chorea and rheumatic fever-associated chorea[107,108] have also been reported to occur in association with oral contraceptive use. One report noted that an estrogen-based birth control pill exacerbated the chorea, but a progesterone-only pill was well tolerated.[107] At this point there are no additional recommended treatments when OCD occurs during pregnancy in a woman who has a history of Syndenham's chorea or lupus.

Alterations in thyroid autoimmunity may also contribute to increases in OCD and generalized anxiety during pregnancy and the postpartum period. Antithyroid antibodies are present in 10–20% of women of childbearing age. Although these antibodies are usually nonpathologic, studies have shown that titers become markedly elevated postpartum,[109] and that women with antithyroid antibodies are at greatly increased risk of autoimmune thyroiditis, with an increase in thyroid hormone production during the first few months postpartum (often associated with anxiety) and subsequent hypothyroidism (often associated with depression).[109]

SUMMARY

Pregnancy and the postpartum period do appear to be associated with the onset of OCD and possibly the exacerbation of pre-existing OCD. There is no evidence that lactation affects OCD symptom severity, but it may reduce subclinical OCD symptoms which develop during pregnancy. Pregnancy associated OCD is often characterized by comorbid major depression, intrusive violent thoughts, contamination obsessions, and a good response to treatment with serotonin-reuptake inhibitors.

Unfortunately, most of these data were obtained from retrospective surveys and case reports. Controlled prospective studies need to be conducted in order to assess accurately the risk of new-onset OCD during pregnancy, the typical course of pre-existing OCD during pregnancy and the postpartum period, the effect of lactation on symptom severity, the risk of recurrence with subsequent pregnancies, and the response to pharmacologic and behavioral treatments. There is no evidence that women with OCD have reduced fertility, so most women with OCD can be expected to carry a pregnancy to term at some time in their lives. In order to make rational decisions about family planning and to plan for psychiatric treatment during pregnancy and postpartum, it is essential that well-controlled prospective phenomenological and treatment studies are carried out.

In contrast to women with OCD, women with panic disorder often appear to improve during pregnancy and lactation, although again there are no prospective data, and the findings of retrospective studies and case reports are conflicting. To date, there are no data on the effects of pregnancy on post-traumatic stress disorder or generalized anxiety disorder. Further research may help to define the subtypes of OCD, panic disorder and generalized anxiety which respond differentially to pregnancy. Finally, identification of the physiological processes underlying these effects of reproductive hormone fluxes on OCD should provide us with a better understanding of the pathophysiology of OCD, and potentially suggest new treatment approaches.

REFERENCES

1. Weissman MM, Bland RC, Canino GJ et al. The cross-national epidemiology of obsessive-compulsive disorder. *Journal of Clinical Psychiatry* 1994; **55** (Supplement): 5–10.
2. Rasmussen SA, Eisen JL. The epidemiology and differential diagnosis of obsessive-compulsive disorder. *Journal of Clinical Psychiatry* 1992; **53**: 4–10.
3. Demal U, Lenz G, Mayrhofer A, Zapotoczky HG, Zitterl W. Obsessive-compulsive disorder and depression. A retrospective study on course and interaction. *Psychopathology* 1993; **26**: 45–50.

4. Swedo SE, Leonard HL, Rapoport JL. Childhood-onset obsessive-compulsive disorder. *Psychiatric Clinics of North America* 1992; **15**: 767–75.

5. Greist JH, Jefferson JW, Kobak KA, Katzelnick DJ, Serlin RC. Efficacy and tolerability of serotonin transport inhibitors in obsessive-compulsive disorder. *Archives of General Psychiatry* 1995; **52**: 53–60.

6. Leckman JF, Grice DE, Boardman J *et al*. Symptoms of obsessive-compulsive disorder. *American Journal of Psychiatry* 1997; **154**: 911–17.

7. Swedo S. Rituals and releasers: an ethological model of obsessive-compulsive disorder. In: Rapoport J (eds) *Obsessive-compulsive disorder in children and adolescents* Washington, DC: American Psychiatric Association Press, 1989: 269–88.

8. Ingram IM. Obsessional illness in mental hospital patients. *Journal of Mental Science* 1961; **107**: 382–402.

9. Pollitt J. Obsessional states. *British Journal of Psychiatry* 1975; **9**: 133–40.

10. Nezeroglu F, Anemone R, Yaryura-Tobia J. Onset of obsessive-compulsive disorder in pregnancy. *American Journal of Psychiatry* 1992; **149**: 947–50.

11. Buttolph ML, Holland A. Obsessive-compulsive disorder in pregnancy and childbirth. In: Jenike M, Baer L, Minichiello WE (eds) *Obsessive-compulsive disorders. Theory and management.* Chicago: Yearbook Medical Publishers, 1990: 89–95.

12. Williams KE, Koran LM. Obsessive-compulsive disorder in pregnancy, the puerperium and the premenstrum. *Journal of Clinical Psychiatry* 1997; **58**: 330–4.

13. Sichel DA, Cohen LS, Dimmock JA, Rosenbaum JF. Postpartum obsessive-compulsive disorder: a case series. *Journal of Clinical Psychiatry* 1993; **54**: 156–9.

14. Chemlow D, Halfin VP. Pregnancy complicated by obsessive-compulsive disorder. *Journal of Maternal-Fetal Medicine* 1997; **6**: 31–4.

15. Hertzberg T, Leo RJ, Kim KY. Recurrent obsessive-compulsive disorder associated with pregnancy and childbirth. *Psychosomatics* 1997; **38**: 386–8.

16. Iancu I, Lepkifker E, Dannon P, Kotler M. Obsessive-compulsive disorder limited to pregnancy. *Psychotherapy and Psychosomatics* 1995; **64**: 109–12.

17. Brandt KR, Mackenzie TB. Obsessive-compulsive disorder exacerbated during pregnancy: a case report. *International Journal of Psychiatry in Medicine* 1987; **17**: 361–6.

18. Rogers JD, Fahn S. Movement disorders and pregnancy. *Advances in Neurology* 1004; **64**: 163–78.

19. Willson P, Preece AA. Chorea gravidarum. *Archives of Internal Medicine* 1932; **49**: 471–533.

20. Gonzalez-Mariscal G, Cuamatzl E, Rosenblatt JS. Hormones and external factors: are they 'on/off' signals for maternal nest-building in rabbits? *Hormones and Behavior* 1998; **33**: 1–8.

21. Boulton MI, Wickens A, Brown D, Goode JA, Gilbert CL. Prostaglandin F_2 alpha-induced nest-building in pseudopregnant pigs. II. Space restriction stress does not influence secretion of oxytocin, prolactin, oestradiol or progesterone. *Physiology and Behavior* 1997; **62**: 1079–85.

22. Schneider JE, Lynch CB. Investigation of a common physiological mechanism underlying progesterone-induced and maternal nesting in mice, *Mus musculus. Journal of Comparative Psychology* 1984; **98**: 165–76.

23. Kofuji H, Kanda M, Oishi T. Breeding cycles and fecal gonadal steroids in the brown dipper *Cincius pallasil. General and Comparative Endocrinology* 1993; **91**: 216–23.

24. Klein DF, Skrobala AM, Garfinkel RS. Preliminary look at the effects of pregnancy on the course of panic disorder. *Anxiety* 1995; **1**: 227–32.

25. Cowley DS, Roy-Byrne PP. Panic disorder during pregnancy. *Journal of Psychosomatic Obstetrics and Gynecology* 1989; **10**: 193–210.

26. Cohen LS, Sichel DA, Faraone SV, Robertson LM, Dimmock JA, Rosenbaum JF. Course of panic disorder during pregnancy and the puerperium: a preliminary study. *Biological Psychiatry* 1996; **39**: 950–4.

27. Northcott CJ, Stein MB. Panic disorder in pregnancy. *Journal of Clinical Psychiatry* 1994; **55**: 539–42.
28. Kendrick KM, Keverne EB, Hinton MR, Goode JA. Oxytocin, amino acid and monoamine release in the region of the medial preoptic area and bed nucleus of the stria terminalis of the sheep during parturition and suckling. *Brain Research* 1992; **569**: 199–209.
29. Kendrick KM, Keverne EB, Chapman C, Baldwin BA. Intracranial dialysis measurement of oxytocin, monoamine and uric acid release from the olfactory bulb and substantia nigra of sheep during parturition, suckling, separation from lambs and eating. *Brain Research* 1988; **439**: 1–10.
30. Quereshi GA, Hansen S, Sodersten P. Offspring control of cerebrospinal fluid GABA concentrations in lactating rats. *Neuroscience Letters* 1987; **75**: 85–8.
31. Weinberg MK, Troick EZ. The impact of maternal psychiatric illness on infant development. *Journal of Clinical Psychiatry* 1998; **59** (Supplement 2): 553–61.
32. Kobak KA, Greist JH, Jefferson JW, Katzeinick DJ, Henk HJ. Behavioral versus pharmacological treatments of obsessive-compulsive disorder: a meta-analysis. *Psychopharmacology* 1998; **136**: 205–16.
33. Baer L, Rapaport J. *Getting control: overcoming your obsessions and compulsions*. New York: Plume, 1992.
34. Foa EB, Wilson R, Barlow DH. *Stop obsessing! How to overcome your obsessions and compulsions*. New York: Bantam, 1991.
35. Steketee G, White K. *When once is not enough*. Oakland, CA: New Harbringer, 1990.
36. Steketee GS. *Treatment of obsessive–compulsive disorder*. New York: Guilford Press, 1996.
37. McDougle CJ, Goodman WK, Leckman JF, Lee NC, Heninger GR, Price LH. Haloperidol addition in fluvoxamine-refractory obsessive-compulsive disorder: a double-blind, placebo-controlled study in patients with and without tics. *Archives of General Psychiatry* 1994; **51**: 302–8.
38. McDougle CJ, Goodman WK, Leckman JF *et al*. Limited therapeutic effect of addition of buspirone in fluvoxamine-refractory obsessive compulsive disorder. *American Journal of Psychiatry* 1993; **150**: 647–9.
39. Pigott TA, L'Heureux F, Hill JL, Rubenstein C, Bernstein SE, Hill JL, Murphy DL. A double-blind, placebo-controlled study of trazodone in patients with obsessive-compulsive disorder. *Journal of Clinical Psychopharmacology* 1992; **12**: 156–62.
40. Grady TA, Pigott TA, L'Heureux F *et al*. Double-blind study of adjuvant buspirone for fluoxetine-treated patients with obsessive-compulsive disorder. *American Journal of Psychiatry* 1993; **150**: 819–21.
41. Jenike MA, Baer L, Minichiello WE, Rauch SL, Buttolph ML. Placebo-controlled trial of fluoxetine and phenelzine for obsessive-compulsive disorder. *American Journal of Psychiatry* 1997; **154**: 1261–4.
42. Altschuler LL, Cohen LS, Szuba MP *et al*. Phamacologic management of psychiatric illness during pregnancy: dilemmas and guidelines. *American Journal of Psychiatry* 1996; **153**: 592–606.
43. Nulman I, Rovet J, Stewart D, Wolin J, Gardner H, Theis J, Kulin N, Koren G. Neurodevelopment of children exposed *in utero* to antidepressant drugs. *New England Journal of Medicine* 1997; **336**: 258–62.
44. Cohen LS, Rosenbaum JF. Psychotropic drug use during pregnancy: weighing the risks. *Journal of Clinical Psychiatry* 1988; **59** (Supplement 2): 18–28.
45. Llewellyn A, Stowe ZN. Psychotropic medications in lactation. *Journal of Clinical Psychiatry* 1998; **59**: 41–52.
46. Leonard HL, Swedo SE, Lenane MC *et al*. A double-blind desipramine substitution during long-term clomipramine treatment in children and adolescents with obsessive-compulsive disorder. *Archives of General Psychiatry* 1991; **48**: 922–7.
47. Pato MT, Zohar-Kadouch R, Zohar J, Murphy DL. Return of symptoms after discontinuation of clomipramine in patients with obsessive-compulsive disorder. *Amercian Journal of Psychiatry* 1988; **145**: 1521–5.

48. Brunner DP, Munch M, Biedermann D, Huch R, Huch A, Borbely AA. Changes in sleep and sleep electroencephalogram during pregnancy. *Sleep* 1994; **17**: 576–82.
49. Weiss M, Baerg E, Wisebord S, Temple J. The influence of gonadal hormones on periodicity of obsessive-compulsive disorder. *Canadian Journal of Psychiatry* 1995; **40**: 205–7.
50. Jacobs AR, Edelheit PB, Coleman AE, Herzog AG. Late-onset congenital adrenal hyperplasia: a treatable cause of anxiety. *Biological Psychiatry* 1999; **46**: 856–9.
51. Rasmussen SA, Eisen JL. Epidemiology of obsessive-compulsive disorder. *Journal of Clinical Psychiatry* 1990; **51**: 10–13.
52. Casas M, Alvarez E, Duro P *et al*. Anti-androgenic treatment of obsessive-compulsive neurosis. *Acta Psychiatrica Scandinavica* 1986; **73**: 221–2.
53. Leonard HL. Drug treatment of obsessive-compulsive disorder. In: Rapoport JL (ed.) *Obsessive-compulsive disorder in children and adolescents*. Washington, DC: American Psychiatric Association Press; 1989: 217–36.
54. Eriksson T. Anti-androgenic agent cyproterone acetate cured a woman of severe sexual obsessions (letter). *British Journal of Psychiatry* 1998; **173**: 351.
55. Chouinard G, Belanger MC, Beauclair L, Sultan S, Pearson-Murphy BE. Potentiation of fluoxetine by aminoglutethimide, an adrenal steroid suppressant, in obsessive-compulsive disorder resistant to SSRIs: a case report. *Progress in Neuro-psychopharmacology and Biological Psychiatry* 1996; **20**: 1067–79.
56. Altemus M, Greenberg BD, Keuler D, Jacobson K, Murphy DL. Open trial of flutamide for treatment of obsessive-compulsive disorder. *Journal of Clinical Psychiatry* 1999;**60**: 442–5.
57. Peterson BD, Zhang H, Anderson GM, Leckman JF. A double-blind, placebo-controlled, crossover trial of an antiandrogen in the treatment of Tourette's syndrome. *Journal of Clinical Psychopharmacology* 1998; **18**: 324–31.
58. McEwen BS, Alves SE, Bulloch K, Weiland N. Ovarian steroids and the brain: implications for cognition and aging. *Neurology* 1997; **48**: S8–15.
59. Simerly RB, Chang C, Muramatsu M, Swanson LW. Distribution of androgen and estrogen receptor mRNA-containing cells in the rat brain: an *in situ* hybridization study. *Journal of Comparative Neurology* 1990; **294**: 76–95.
60. Watters JJ, Campbell JS, Cunningham MJ, Krebs EG, Dorsa DM. Rapid membrane effects of steroids in neuroblastoma cells: effects of estrogen on mitogen-activated protein kinase signalling cascade and c-fos immediate early gene transcription. *Endocrinology* 1997; **138**: 4030–3.
61. Wong M, Thompson TL, Moss RL. Non-genomic actions of estrogen in the brain: Physiological significance and cellular mechanisms. *Critical Reviews in Neurobiology* 1996; **10**: 189–203.
62. Whitacre C, Reingold S, O'Leary P. A gender gap in autoimmunity. *Science* 1999; **283**: 1277–8.
63. Swedo SE, Leonard HL, Garvey M *et al*. Pediatric autoimmune neuropsychiatric disorders associated with streptococcal infections: clinical description of the first 50 cases. *American Journal of Psychiatry* 1998; **155**: 264–71.
64. elMansari M, Bouchard C, Blier P. Alteration of serotonin release in the guinea pig orbito-frontal cortex by selective serotonin reuptake inhibitors. Relevance to treatment of obsessive-compulsive disorder. *Neuropsychopharmacology* 1995; **13**: 117–27.
65. Luine VN, Rhodes J. Gonadal hormone regulation of MAO and other enzymes in hypothalamic areas. *Neuroendocrinology* 1983; **36**: 235–41.
66. Pecins-Thompson M, Brown NA, Kohama SG, Bethea CL. Ovarian steroid regulation of tryptophan hydroxylase mRNA expression in rhesus macaques. *Journal of Neuroscience* 1996; **16**: 7021–9.
67. McQueen JK, Wilson H, Fink G. Estradiol-17β increases serotonin transporter (SERT) mRNA levels and the density of SERT-binding sites in female rat brain. *Brain Research and Molecular Brain Research* 1997; **45**: 13–23.

68. Attali G, Weizman A, Gil-Ad I, Rehavi M. Opposite modulatory effects of ovarian hormones on rat brain dopamine and serotonin transporters. *Brain Research* 1997; **756**: 153–9.

69. Sumner BEH, Fink G. Estrogen increases the density of 5–hydroxytryptamine$_{2A}$ receptors in cerebral cortex and nucleus accumbens in the female rat. *Journal of Steroid Biochemistry and Molecular Biology* 1995; **54**: 15–20.

70. Castner SA, Xiao L, Becker JB. Sex differences in striatal dopamine: *in vivo* microdialysis and behavioral studies. *Brain Research* 1993; **610**: 127–34.

71. Bazzett TJ, Becker JB. Sex differences in the rapid and acute effects of estrogen on striatal D$_2$ dopamine-receptor binding. *Brain Research* 1994; **637**: 163–72.

72. Ladosky W, Schneider HT. Changes in hypothalamic catechol-O-methyltransferase during sexual differentiation of the brain. *British Journal of Medical and Biological Research* 1981; **14**: 409–12.

73. Timmers RJM, Graneman JCM, Lambert JGD, vanOordt PGWJ. *General and Comparative Endocrinology* 1988; **72**: 190–203.

74. Cone RI, Gavis GA, Goy RW. Effects of ovarian steroids on serotonin metabolism within grossly dissected and microdissected brain regions of the ovariectomized rat. *Brain Research Bulletin* 1981; **7**: 639–44.

75. Karayiorgou M, Altemus M, Galke BL *et al*. Genotype determining low catechol-O-methyltransferase activity as a risk factor for obsessive-compulsive disorder. *Proceedings of the National Academy of Science of the USA* 1997; **94**: 4572–5.

76. Altemus M, Pigott T, Kalogeras KT *et al*. Abnormalities in the regulation of vasopressin and corticotropin-releasing factor secretion in obsessive-compulsive disorder. *Archives of General Psychiatry* 1992; **49**: 9–20.

77. Leckman JF, Goodman WK, North WG *et al*. The role of central oxytocin in obsessive-compulsive disorder and related normal behavior. *Psychoneuroendocrinology* 1994; **19**: 723–49.

78. Altemus M, Jacobson KR, Kling MA *et al*. Normal CSF oxytocin and NPY levels in OCD. *Biological Psychiatry* 1999; **45**: 615–19.

79. McCarthy MM. Estrogen modulation of oxytocin and its relation to behavior. In: Ivell R, Russell J (eds) *Oxytocin*. New York: Plenum, 1995: 235–45.

80. DeVries GJ, Wang Z, Bullock NA. Sex differences in the effects of testosterone and its metabolites on vasopressin messenger RNA levels in the bed nucleus of the stria terminalis of rats. *Journal of Neuroscience* 1994; **14**: 1789–94.

81. Miller MA, DeVries GJ, al-Shamma HA, Dorsa DM. Decline of vasopressin immunoreactivity and mRNA levels in the bed nucleus of the stria terminalis following castration. *Journal of Neuroscience* 1992; **12**: 2881–7.

82. Takagi T, Tanizawa O, Otsuki Y, Sugita N, Haruta M, Yamaji K. Oxytocin in the cerebrospinal fluid and plasma of pregnant and nonpregnant subjects. *Hormone and Metabolic Research* 1985; **17**: 308–01.

83. Takeda S, Kuwabara Y, Mizuno M. Effects of pregnancy and labor on oxytocin levels in human plasma and cerebrospinal fluid. *Acta Endocrinologica Japonica* 1985; **32**: 875–80.

84. Kendrick KM, Keverne EB, Chapman C, Baldwin BA. Intracranial dialysis measurement of oxytocin, monoamine and uric acid release from the olfactory bulb and substantia nigra of sheep during parturition, suckling, separation from lambs and eating. *Brain Research* 1988; **439**: 1–10.

85. Ditkoff EC, Crary WG, Cristo M, Lobo RA. Estrogen improves psychological function in asymptomatic postmenopausal women. *Obstetrics and Gynecology* 1991; **78**: 991–5.

86. Wiklund I, Karlberg J, Mattsson LA. Quality of life of postmenopausal women on a regimen of transdermal estradiol therapy: a double-blind, placebo-controlled study. *American Journal of Obstetrics and Gynecology* 1993; **168**: 824–30.

87. Lindheim SR, Legro RS, Bernstein L *et al*. Behavioral stress responses in premenopausal and postmenopausal women and the effects of estrogen. *American Journal of Obstetrics and Gynecology* 1992; **167**: 1831–6.

88. Diaz-Veliz G, Urresta F, Dussaubat N, Mora S. Effects of estradiol replacement in ovariectomized rats on conditioned avoidance responses and other behaviors. *Physiology and Behavior* 1991; **50**: 61–5.

89. McCarthy M. Estrogen modulation of oxytocin and its relation to behavior. *Advances in Experimental Medical and Biology* 1995; **395**: 235–45.

90. Farr SA, Flood JF, Scherrer JF, Kaiser FE, Taylor GT, Morley JE. Effect of ovarian steroids on footshock avoidance learning and retention in female mice. *Physiology and Behavior* 1995; **58**: 715–23.

91. Altemus M, Conrad CD, Dolan S, McEwen BS. Estrogen reduces fear conditioning: differential effects on context vs. tone conditioning (abstract). *Biological Psychiatry* 1998; **43**: 14S.

92. Gregoire A, Kumar R, Everitt B, Henderson A, Studd J. Transdermal oestrogen for treatment of severe postnatal depression. *Lancet* 1996; **347**: 930–3.

93. Zweifel JE, O'Brien WH. A meta-analysis of the effect of hormone replacement therapy upon depressed mood. *Psychoneuroendocrinology* 1997; **22**: 189–212.

94. Robel P, Baulieu EE. Neurosteroids: biosynthesis and function. *Critical Reviews in Neurobiology* 1995; **9**: 383–94.

95. Sholomskas DE, Wickamaratne PJ, Dogolo L *et al.* Postpartum onset of panic disorder: a coincidental event? *Journal of Clinical Psychiatry* 1993; **54**: 476–80.

96. Kendrick KM, Keverne EB, Chapman C, Baldwin BA. Microdialysis measurement of oxytocin, aspartate, gamma-aminobutyric acid and glutamate release from the olfactory bulb of the sheep during vagino-cervical stimulation. *Brain Research* 1988; **442**: 171–4.

97. Swedo SE, Rapoport JL, Cheslow DL. High prevalence of obsessive-compulsive symptoms in patients with Sydenham's chorea. *American Journal of Psychiatry* 1989; **146**: 246–9.

98. Asbahr FR, Negrao AB, Gentil V *et al.* Obsessive-compulsive and related symptoms in children and adolescents with rheumatic fever with and without chorea: a prospective 6–month study. *American Journal of Psychiatry* 1998; **155**: 1122–4.

99. Baxter LR, Schwartz JM, Bergman KS. Caudate glucose metabolic rate changes with drug and behavior therapy for obsessive-compulsive disorder. *Archives of General Psychiatry* 1992; **49**: 681–9.

100. Berthier ML, Kulisevsky J, Gironell A, Heras JA. Obsessive-compulsive disorder associated with brain lesions. *Neurology* 1996; **47**: 353–61.

101. Zegart KN, Schwarz RH. Chorea gravidarum. *Obstetrics and Gynecology* 1968; **32**: 24–7.

102. Branch DW. Antiphospholipid antibodies and pregnancy: maternal implications. *Seminars in Perinatology* 1990; **14**: 139–46.

103. Lubbe WF, Butler WS, Palmer SS, Liggins GC. Lupus anticoagulant in pregnancy. *British Journal of Obstetrics and Gynecology* 1984; **91**: 357–63.

104. Omdal R, Roalso S. Chorea gravidarum and chorea associated with oral contraceptives – diseases due to antiphospholipid antibodies? *Acta Neurologica Scandinavica* 1992; **86**: 219–20.

105. Asherson RA, Derksen HWM, Harris EN *et al.* Chorea in systemic lupus erythematosus and 'lupus-like' disease association with antiphospholipid antibodies. *Journal of Rheumatology* 1988; **15**: 377–9.

106. Becker JB. Direct effect of 17β-estradiol on striatum: sex differences in dopamine release. *Synapse* 1996; **5**: 157–64.

107. Barber PV, Arnold AG, Evans G. Recurrent hormone dependent chorea: effects of oestrogens and progestogens. *Clinical Endocrinology* 1976; **5**: 291–3.

108. Fernando SJM. An attack of chorea complicating oral contraceptive therapy. *Practitioner* 1966; **197**: 210–11.

109. Solomon BL, Fein HG, Smallridge RC. Usefulness of antimicrosomal antibody titers in the diagnosis and treatment of postpartum thyroiditis. *Journal of Family Practitioner* 1993; **36**: 177–82.

9

Eating disorders and hyperemesis gravidarum

TANA A. GRADY-WELIKY

EATING DISORDERS

Many women maintain certain attitudes with regard to body weight during pregnancy, including over-concern about weight gain and body shape. These attitudes may reflect a cultural norm for women of childbearing age in Western societies. Alternatively, such concerns may represent 'disordered eating' patterns or a frank eating disorder. In one study of 100 otherwise healthy pregnant women, 59 women reported that they would have preferred a smaller or much smaller weight gain.[1] In addition, Abraham and colleagues[1] found that women who experienced 'disordered eating' during pregnancy were more likely to have difficulty gaining weight and more likely to have a preconception history of an eating disorder. The presence of eating disorder symptoms during pregnancy may have significant implications for the course and outcome of the pregnancy. Taken together, these findings highlight the importance of comprehensive assessment of eating behaviors, attitudes toward weight and history of past or current eating disorders during preconception and antenatal visits.

Changes in eating patterns, such as short-lived food cravings, are also frequently observed during pregnancy.[2,3] Of the women in the study by Abraham and colleagues, 53% reported having specific food cravings (e.g. fruit, cheese, chocolate, ice cream).[1] Pica is an eating disorder characterized by the ingestion of non-nutritive substances, which usually presents during childhood. A small number of pregnant women also experience these unusual cravings, and may ingest soap, clay or dirt.[2] In fact, 3% of the women in the study by Abraham and colleagues[1] reported non-nutritive substance craving. These unusual cravings generally remit after the pregnancy.

Anorexia nervosa and bulimia are more complex eating disorders which may complicate the course of pregnancy and have a negative effect on outcome. Anorexia nervosa is characterized by a refusal to maintain a minimally normal body weight, marked disturbance of body image, and a fear of gaining weight. Thus the requirement to gain 20 to 30 pounds during the course of a normal pregnancy is extremely difficult for women with anorexia nervosa. There are two types of anorexia nervosa according to the *Diagnostic and Statistical Manual of Mental Disorders*, Fourth Edition (DSM-IV).[4] These are the restricting type (in which the patient restricts her food intake and does not engage in any binge-eating or purging behaviors) and the binge-eating and purging type, in which the patient regularly engages in binge-eating and purging behaviors and remains 15% below her minimal expected weight.

Binge-eating and inappropriate compensatory methods of losing weight are the essential features of bulimia nervosa.[4] Patients with bulimia nervosa may engage in self-induced vomiting, laxative or diuretic abuse or excessive and compulsive exercise behavior in an attempt to prevent weight gain. Women with bulimia also have distorted body images and frequently measure their self-worth by their weight. Women with bulimia alone generally remain within their expected weight range. However, weight gain associated with pregnancy is also quite difficult for these patients, because of the association between weight and self-esteem. The connection between anorexia and bulimia and the usual symptoms of pregnancy such as weight gain, food cravings and nausea and vomiting has been the subject of only limited study.

Of particular interest is the role that hyperemesis gravidarum may play in the exacerbation or development of disordered eating behaviors. Hyperemesis gravidarum is characterized by severe and persistent nausea and vomiting during the first 20 weeks of pregnancy, which frequently results in marked dehydration, metabolic disturbances, weight loss (usually > 5% of body weight) and a need for hospitalization.[5-8] This is a relatively rare condition with incidence estimates of 0.03–1% of pregnancies.[7] Anorexia, bulimia and hyperemesis gravidarum are illnesses which are best understood from a biopsychosocial perspective. Each of these conditions has underlying biological, psychological and social factors which contribute to the etiology and treatment recommendations. There is some overlap of the biopsychosocial elements of these three conditions. This chapter will address the symptoms, proposed risk factors, biopsychosocial factors related to etiology and treatment, obstetrical complications and outcomes of hyperemesis gravidarum, anorexia nervosa and bulimia.

HYPEREMESIS GRAVIDARUM

Mild nausea and vomiting, commonly known as 'morning sickness,' is frequently one of the first diagnostic indicators of pregnancy. However, women with hyperemesis gravidarum will present with severe and persistent nausea and vomiting within the first half of the pregnancy. The onset of hyperemesis gravidarum is usually between 4 and 10 weeks, with spontaneous resolution of symptoms, usually by 20 weeks.[7] In addition to marked nausea and vomiting, patients with hyperemesis gravidarum will exhibit signs of dehydration, including tachycardia, hypotension and reduced skin elasticity.[6,7] A weight loss of more than 5% of the patient's body weight may also be present. Laboratory findings will include elevated hematocrit, elevated blood urea nitrogen, increased specific gravity of urine, ketonuria and chemistries consistent with metabolic alkalosis.[7] In addition, some patients show abnormalities of thyroid function tests consistent with hyperthyroidism, including elevation of free T_4 and decreased TSH levels.

Several risk factors have been identified for the development of hyperemesis gravidarum, including nulliparity, twin/other multiple pregnancy, increased body weight and a past history of unsuccessful pregnancy.[6,7] Hypertension, gastrointestinal disease (e.g. liver problems, gall-bladder disease, gastritis) and renal disease are medical comorbidities that may increase the risk of hyperemesis gravidarum during pregnancy.[7] A past history of an eating disorder has also been reported as a potential risk factor for the development of hyperemesis gravidarum.[9] No association has been found between hyperemesis gravidarum and race or socio-economic status.[6]

The exact etiology of hyperemesis gravidarum remains unknown. It is currently a diagnosis of exclusion. A number of biological factors have been studied and appear to play a role in the development of the condition. These include significantly elevated levels of human chorionic gonadotropin hormone (HCG), hyperthyroidism and alterations in gastric pH and motility.[6-8] A recent study investigated the potential role of serotonin in the etiology of hyperemesis gravidarum. Serotonergic mechanisms were examined because of the association of increased serotonin liberation with patients experiencing nausea and vomiting during cancer chemotherapies. Borgeat and colleagues[10] prospectively measured urinary excretion of 5–hydroxyindoleacetic acid (5–HIAA) in three groups – first, pregnant women with hyperemesis gravidarum, second, pregnant women without any nausea and vomiting, and third, non-pregnant women without nausea and vomiting. They observed no significant difference in serotonin excretion between the groups, which suggests that there is no direct association between serotonin and hyperemesis gravidarum. Borgeat and colleagues[10] have urged further systematic investigation of the potential connection of central serotonin release through stimulation of gastrointestinal afferents.

Several psychological mechanisms have also been proposed to be related to the development of hyperemesis gravidarum. An association between hyperemesis and hysteria has been noted in several clinical studies and case series.[5,11,12] Hyperemesis gravidarum as a symbolic rejection of pregnancy or femininity has been postulated as a psychoanalytic mechanism, which is similar to the psychoanalytic theory with regard to anorexia nervosa.[5,12] Finally, some authors have suggested that women who develop hyperemesis are immature and may demonstrate excessive dependence on their mothers or other significant figures.[5,12,13]

Katon and colleagues suggested that an increased vulnerability to stress and decreased social supports are social components of the etiology of hyperemesis.[12] The results of another study suggested that hyperemesis gravidarum is a physiologically based response to social difficulty.[14] Thus hyperemesis may be conceptualized as a biopsychosocial illness with etiologic factors in all three domains.

Several studies have suggested that the presence of nausea and vomiting during the first trimester is often predictive of a positive outcome.[5,15,16] However, there have been conflicting reports on the effect of hyperemesis on fetal outcome. Several studies have suggested an association with low-birth-weight infants in hyperemesis gravidarum patients who experience marked weight loss (> 5%).[17,18] Moreover, Gross and colleagues[18] noted an increased risk of fetal malformations among hyperemesis patients. However, more recent studies have demonstrated no difference in outcome (birth weight, congenital abnormalities or prematurity) between hyperemesis gravidarum patients and controls.[11,19,20]

Without adequate treatment, hyperemesis gravidarum can progress to confusion, coma and death secondary to metabolic disturbances and liver disease. Due to the potentially life-threatening nature of the illness, treatment of hyperemesis gravidarum is essential. Reflecting the biopsychosocial nature of its proposed etiology, the treatment of hyperemesis requires a multimodal approach. The initial treatment strategy is to correct dehydration and electrolyte imbalances. This is achieved by administering intravenous fluids for re-hydration and keeping the patient NPO in an attempt to rest her gut. Parenteral vitamins, specifically vitamins B_6, C and K, are also administered. These interventions are followed by a gradual reintroduction of a fat-restricted diet. Hospitalization may be required and is dependent on a number of factors, including the severity of the nausea and vomiting. The length of admission is also dependent upon the severity of the illness. Interestingly, the study by Stewart[9] noted that patients with an eating disorder history were less likely to respond to typical treatments and had longer durations of inpatient admission.

In addition to these medical interventions, brief psychotherapies may also be employed. In general, behavioral therapy paradigms have been found to be effective in the treatment of hyperemesis based on classical conditioning theory. Behavioral therapeutic approaches have included the use of relaxation training, coping strategies, stimulus deprivation and stimulus conditioning.[7,8] By means of these techniques the patient with hyperemesis learns to avoid conditioned stimuli associated with the nausea and vomiting. Through imagery, she may be taught to imagine the stimuli without feeling nausea.[13] Other forms of supportive psychotherapy may be effective, particularly if the patient is experiencing a high level of psychosocial stress in her relationships with significant others.

Lub-Moss and colleagues[21] have proposed the use of three subtypes of hyperemesis gravidarum in the prescription of the most appropriate form of psychotherapeutic treatment for patients with the disorder. The three subtypes of hyperemesis gravidarum are based on personality features, psychiatric symptoms and psychosocial stressors, respectively. Several examples of the semi-targeted treatment strategies proposed by Lub-Moss and colleagues[21] are given below. Patients in the personality feature subgroup may be best treated with specific forms of therapy based on the particular personality traits. For example, a patient with dependent personality traits would receive a targeted combination of supportive structuring and insight-giving therapy together with cognitive restructuring and assertiveness training. For patients with comorbid psychiatric conditions, such as eating disorders, a combination of cognitive restructuring and behavioral therapy related to their eating behaviors may be the best strategy. Finally, conjoint therapy with the patient's partner or significant others may be the best intervention for those individuals with extreme psychosocial stressors.

It is important to bear the biopsychosocial nature of hyperemesis gravidarum in mind when thinking about medication therapy. Anti-emetic medications should be viewed as adjunctive to nutritional and psychotherapeutic strategies. Antihistamines and sedative or tranquilizing agents may be useful for alleviating the nausea and vomiting associated with the condition. A recent study examined the combination of diphenhydramine and droperidol in patients with hyperemesis gravidarum. In that study, Nageotte and colleagues[22] found that this combination of medications resulted in a shorter length of hospital stay and a reduced number of readmissions for continued nausea and vomiting, compared to the control group which received other anti-emetic agents. There were no congenital anomalies or adverse maternal outcomes related to the medications used in the study. Anti-emetic therapy alone is inadequate treatment, but it is a useful adjunctive strategy, particularly if the patient is experiencing intractable nausea and vomiting. Due to its relative safety and lack of adverse effects, in combination with its utility in chemotherapy-related nausea and vomiting, ondansetron, a $5HT_3$ antagonist, has been examined in patients with hyperemesis gravidarum. A recent case report suggests that ondansetron may be an effective and safe alternative for patients with hyperemesis gravidarum.[23] However, a double-blind pilot study of ondansetron in hyperemesis gravidarum did not confirm the clinical finding. Sullivan and colleagues compared ondansetron with promethazine in a small group of women with hyperemesis gravidarum.[24] They reported no significant difference between women treated with ondansetron and with promethazine with regard to the reduction of nausea, weight gain, length of hospital stay or total doses of medication. Thus it is not clear what role, if any, ondansetron or other $5HT_3$-receptor antagonists may play in the treatment of hyperemesis gravidarum. When the previous data demonstrating a lack of increased serotonin liberation in patients with hyperemesis[10] are taken into consideration, the negative result obtained with ondansetron is not surprising.

In summary, hyperemesis gravidarum is an enigmatic disorder with biopsychosocial components. It has been associated with a number of negative outcomes, including low birth weight, congenital abnormalities and prematurity. The provision of multimodal treatment that incorporates rehydration, nutritional supplementation, psychotherapy and adjunctive pharmacologic therapy can effectively improve the course and outcome of pregnancy.

EATING DISORDERS AND PREGNANCY

The biopsychosocial nature of eating disorders is similar to that found for hyperemesis gravidarum. A wide range of biological factors has been implicated in the etiology of anorexia and bulimia. Serotonin dysregulation is one of these proposed biological factors contributing to the development of eating disorders.[25] Interestingly, serotonin has not been found to play a significant role in the etiology of hyperemesis gravidarum.[10] A full review of the biological factors involved in eating disorders is beyond the scope of this chapter. The psychological components of eating disorders include dependency, adult sexuality problems and enmeshed parental relationships. Several of these features are shared with women who develop hyperemesis gravidarum. The cultural drive for thinness in Western society, in combination with the proposed 'beauty ideal' represented by fashion models and beauty pageant contestants and winners, have been identified as the sociocultural factors contributing to the development of eating disorders. The multifactorial etiology of eating disorders contributes to their complexity. Eating disorders influence many aspects of the affected person's life and overall health. The following section will address the impact of eating disorders on reproductive function and pregnancy.

A variety of disorders of reproductive function, such as anovulation, amenorrhea, reduced libido and infertility, have been linked to eating disorders.[9] However, infertility rates among patients with eating disorders do not appear to be much lower than those of the general population.[9,26,27] However, for women with infertility and histories of eating disorders enhanced fertility methods are increasing the likelihood of conception. Bearing this in mind, it clearly becomes increasingly important to understand the relationship between eating disorders and pregnancy. This area has received more attention over the past few years through systematic investigation, but there are still conflicting data. There are two central questions with regard to the relationship between eating disorders and pregnancy. First, how does pregnancy affect the course of the underlying illness? Are eating disorder symptoms improved or worsened during and after pregnancy? A potential association between the presence of hyperemesis gravidarum and the development or worsening of eating disorders has been suggested.[8] This association has not been conclusively confirmed. However, Abraham[26] described an increased risk of postpartum depression and relationship difficulties in two women with bulimia nervosa who developed hyperemesis gravidarum. Second, how does a current or past history of an eating disorder influence the course and outcome of a pregnancy? Are there differences between women with an active eating disorder at conception and those who are asymptomatic at conception? What is the likelihood of a patient with an eating disorder maintaining the pregnancy to term, and what are the potential obstetrical and neonatal complications? In an attempt to answer these questions, a brief review of the research literature follows.

Whether pregnancy exacerbates or improves eating disorder symptomatology remains debatable. Stewart and colleagues[28] compared pregnant women ($n = 15$) with active eating disorders (anorexia alone or anorexia with bulimic symptoms) and women with an eating disorder in remission (controls). They found that the majority of women with an active eating disorder at conception ($n = 7$) remained ill or experienced an exacerbation of their symptoms during pregnancy. Six of the eight patients who were in remission at the time of conception remained well during and after pregnancy. Conversely, in a study of 20 patients with bulimia, Lacey and Smith[29] described a reduction in binge-eating and purging behaviors over the course of the pregnancy. However, they did report a return of preconception eating behaviors during the postpartum period. Lemberg and Phillips also observed an improvement in eating disorder symptoms during pregnancy in a group of 43 women with both bulimia and restrictive anorexia.[30] There was also a return of symptoms during the postpartum period in this cohort. Clinical improvement during pregnancy was noted to be greater among the patients with bulimia than in those with restrictive anorexia in a study by Conti and colleagues [31] of 88 women who give birth to low-birth-weight infants. In a larger and more recent study of 94 patients with bulimia, Morgan and colleagues replicated the finding of an improvement in aberrant eating behaviors during the course of pregnancy. In this study, 38% of the subjects reported that pregnancy 'improved' or 'cured' their bulimic symptoms. As with the earlier findings, 62% of the sample were unable to sustain their recovery and relapsed during the postpartum period. Morgan and colleagues described the following risk factors for postpartum relapse of bulimic symptoms: more severe symptoms prior to conception; a history of anorexia nervosa; gestational diabetes mellitus; an unplanned pregnancy and bulimic symptoms during the second trimester of the pregnancy.[32] Interestingly, Abraham[26] in her study of 43 bulimic patients, found no specific pattern of symptom improvement during pregnancy. Thus whether eating disorder symptoms are improved or exacerbated during pregnancy remains a somewhat open issue. However, the majority of data support the notion that there is an improvement in eating disorder symptoms during pregnancy. This improvement may be related to a number of factors, including the patient's desire to take care of herself because of the baby.[29–31] Lacey and Smith[29] also proposed the potential effect of the reduced physical space during pregnancy on binge-eating, which may result in a decline in the binge-purge-binge cycle and lead to symptomatic improvement during pregnancy.

The impact of eating disorders on the course and outcome of pregnancy has also been studied. Eating disorders have been associated with a number of complications during pregnancy and negative outcomes. A higher rate of miscarriages has been reported in women with eating disorders (anorexia and bulimia).[26,30] Stewart and colleagues[28] found that patients with eating disorders in remission gained more weight during pregnancy than did those with active eating disorder symptoms. Moreover, the patients in remission had higher-birth-weight babies with better 5 min Apgar scores. In a study of 50 women with anorexia, including 36 patients in remission, Brinch and colleagues[33] found that women with a history of anorexia had higher rates of premature births, perinatal mortality and low-birth-weight babies. In addition, Bulik and colleagues,[30] also noted that women with a lifetime history of anorexia nervosa were also more like to have a low-birth-weight infant compared to controls. As in the study by Brinch and colleagues, this finding was independent of whether the anorexia was active or in remission. In their study of women who gave birth to low-birth-weight infants, Conti and colleagues[31] found that 32% of women with small-for-gestational age (SGA) term infants had abnormal eating patterns, including behaviors consistent with anorexia nervosa, bulimia, and eating disorder not otherwise specified (NOS). Taken together, these findings support a connection between eating disorders and several adverse pregnancy outcomes, including miscarriage, prematurity, low-birth-weight infants, and higher perinatal mortality. Several of these negative events are also associated with hyperemesis gravidarum.

Specific pregnancy complications have also been noted in patients with eating disorders. Lacey and Smith[29] reported that 9 in 20 pregnant women with bulimia developed hypertension during pregnancy and experienced more complicated deliveries involving the use of forceps or Cesarean sections. Bulik and colleagues[27] also noted that women with anorexia were more likely to undergo Cesarean section compared to normal controls.

During the postpartum period most investigators have reported a return of eating disorder symptoms. Postpartum mood changes have also been described in women with eating disorders. Abraham[26] found that patients with bulimia were more likely to have a postpartum depression compared to controls. In the study by Stewart and colleagues,[28] patients with a past history of anorexia nervosa or active bulimic symptoms at the time of conception also demonstrated an increased likelihood of developing postpartum depression. The finding of an increased rate of postpartum depression among patients with bulimia nervosa has been replicated in the work by Morgan and colleagues.[32] These findings with regard to postpartum mood changes are not surprising, as there is a probable connection between eating disorders and affective illness.

In a recent study of the offspring of women with bulimia, Waugh and Bulik[34] noted lower birth weight and length, which was independent of whether the women were actively bulimic during the pregnancy. Interestingly, Waugh and Bulik[34] found that these differences did not persist beyond 6 weeks, and there was no evidence of any delay in developmental milestones or of differences in temperament between the children of bulimic mothers and those of non-eating-disordered mothers. However, feeding behaviors and interactions with their infants at mealtimes were problematic in the eating disorder cohort, which may contribute to an increased risk of offspring developing an eating disorder beyond the genetic factors. Further research in this area is warranted.

In summary, anorexia nervosa and bulimia are complex eating disorders which can have a significant impact on a woman's overall reproductive function and the overall course and outcome of pregnancy. Whether pregnancy is helpful in reducing eating disorder symptoms remains a controversial issue. Further research involving larger patient samples needs to be completed in order to improve the understanding of the impact of eating disorders on the course of pregnancy, including any potential association with hyperemesis gravidarum or other complications of pregnancy. With regard to the outcome of pregnancy, it appears that eating disorder patients, like those with hyperemesis, are more at risk for miscarriage, prematurity and small-for-gestational-age infants. The underlying fear of gaining weight and an inability to maintain adequate nutrition in the pregnant patient with a history of a current or past eating disorder may contribute to the higher rates of miscarriages and lower-birth-weight babies. Taking all of these factors into consideration it is clearly important for clinicians to perform comprehensive preconception and antenatal assessments with regard to the patient's attitudes towards weight, eating habits and behaviors and any personal history of eating disorder. By passing increased attention during the preconception and early antenatal stages, it is possible that some of the aberrant eating behaviors may be modified through the use of multimodal treatments, which should help to increase weight gain during pregnancy and ultimately improve outcome.

REFERENCES

1. Abraham S, King W, Llewellyn-Jones D. Attitudes to body weight, weight gain and eating behavior in pregnancy. *Journal of Psychosomatic Obstetrics and Gynecology* 1994; **15**: 189–95.
2. Fahy TA, O'Donoghue. Eating disorders in pregnancy. *Psychological Medicine* 1991; **21**: 577–580.
3. Fairburn CG, Stein A, Jones R. Eating habits and eating disorders during pregnancy. *Psychosomatic Medicine* 1992; **54**: 665–72.
4. American Psychiatric Association. *Diagnostic and statistical manual of mental disorders*, 4th edn (DSM-IV). Washington, DC: American Psychiatric Association Press, 1994.
5. Fairweather DVI. Nausea and vomiting in pregnancy. *American Journal of Obstetrics and Gynecology* 1968; **102**: 135–75.

6. Hod M, Orvieto R, Kaplan B, Friedman S, Ovadia J. Hyperemesis gravidarum: a review. *Journal of Reproductive Medicine* 1994; **39**: 605–12.
7. Abell TL, Reily CA. Hyperemesis gravidarum. *Gastroenterology Clinics of North America* 1992; **21**: 835–49.
8. Lingham R, McCluskey S. Eating disorders associated with hyperemesis gravidarum. *Journal of Psychosomatic Research* 1996; **40**: 231–4.
9. Stewart DE. Reproductive functions in eating disorders. *Annals of Medicine* 1992; **24**: 287–91.
10. Borgeat A, Fathi M, Valiton A. Hyperemesis gravidarum: is serotonin implicated? *American Journal of Obstetrics and Gynecology* 1997; **176**: 476–7.
11. Guze SB, Allen DH, Grollmus JJ. The prevalence of hyperemesis gravidarum: a study of 162 psychiatric patients and 98 medical patients. *American Journal of Obstetrics and Gynecology* 1962; **84**: 1859–64.
12. Katon WJ, Ries RK, Bokan JA, Kleinman A. Hyperemesis gravidarum: a biopsychosocial approach. *International Journal of Psychiatry in Medicine* 1980–81; **10**: 151–62.
13. Iancu I, Kotler M, Spivak B, Radwan M, Weizman A. Psychiatric aspects of hyperemesis gravidarum. *Psychotherapy and Psychosomatics* 1994; **61**: 143–9.
14. Tylden E. Hyperemesis and physiological vomiting. *Journal of Psychosomatic Research* 1968; **12**: 85.
15. Brandes JM. First-trimester nausea and vomiting as related to outcome of pregnancy. *Obstetrics and Gynecology* 1967; **30**: 427–31.
16. Hallak M, Tsalamandris K, Dombrowski MP, Isada NB, Pryde PG, Evans MI. Hyperemesis gravidarum: effects on fetal outcome. *Journal of Reproductive Medicine* 1996; **41**: 871–6.
17. Chin RKH, Lao TT. Low birth weight and hyperemesis gravidarum. *European Journal of Obstetrics, Gynecology and Reproductive Biology* 1988; **28**: 179–83.
18. Gross S, Librach C, Cecutti A. Maternal weight loss associated with hyperemesis gravidarum: a predictor of fetal outcome. *American Journal of Obstetrics and Gynecology* 1989; **160**: 906–9.
19. Tsang IS, Katz VL, Wells SD. Maternal and fetal outcomes in hyperemesis gravidarum. *International Journal of Obstetrics and Gynecology* 1996; **55**: 231–5.
20. Bashiri A, Neumann L, Maymon E, Katz M. Hyperemesis gravidarum: epidemiologic features, complications and outcome. *European Journal of Obstetrics, Gynecology, and Reproductive Biology* 1995; **63**: 135–8.
21. Lub-Moss MMH, Eurelings-Bontekoe EHM. Clinical experiences with patients suffering from hyperemesis gravidarum (severe nausea and vomiting during pregnancy): thoughts about subtyping of patients, treatment and counseling methods. *Patient Education and Counseling* 1997; **31**: 65–75.
22. Nageotte MP, Briggs GG, Towers CV, Asrat T. Droperidol and diphenhydramine in the management of hyperemesis gravidarum. *American Journal of Obstetrics and Gynecology* 1996; **174**: 1801–6.
23. Tincello DG, Johnstone MJ. Treatment of hyperemesis gravidarum with the 5–HT$_3$ antagonist ondansetron. *Postgraduate Medical Journal* 1996; **72**: 688–9.
24. Sullivan CA, Johnson CA, Roach H, Martin RW, Stewart DK, Morrison JC. A pilot study of intravenous ondansetron for hyperemesis gravidarum. *American Journal of Obstetrics and Gynecology* 1996; **174**: 1565–8.
25. Jimerson DC, Wolfe BE, Metzger ED, Finkelstein DM, Cooper TB, Levine JM. Decreased serotonin function in bulimia nervosa. *Archives of General Psychiatry* 1997; **54**: 529–34.
26. Abraham S. Sexuality and reproduction in bulimia nervosa patients over 10 years. *Journal of Psychosomatic Research* 1998; **44**: 491–502.
27. Bulik C, Sullivan PF, Fear JL, Pickering A, Dawn A, McCullin M. Fertility and reproduction in women with anorexia nervosa: a controlled study. *Journal of Clinical Psychiatry* 1999; **60**: 130–5.

28. Stewart DE, Raskin J, Garfinkel PE, MacDonald OL, Robinson GE. Anorexia nervosa, bulimia and pregnancy. *American Journal of Obstetrics and Gynecology* 1987; **157**: 1194–8.
29. Lacey JH, Smith G. Bulimia nervosa: the impact of pregnancy on mother and baby. *British Journal of Psychiatry* 1987; **150**: 777–81.
30. Lemberg R, Phillips J. The impact of pregnancy on anorexia nervosa and bulimia. *International Journal of Eating Disorders* 1989; **8**: 285–95.
31. Conti J, Abraham S, Taylor A. Eating behavior and pregnancy outcome. *Journal of Psychosomatic Research* 1998; **44**: 465–77.
32. Morgan JF, Lacey JH, Sedgwick PM. Impact of pregnancy on bulimia nervosa. *British Journal of Psychiatry* 1999; **174**: 135–40.
33. Brinch M, Isager T, Tolstrup K. Anorexia nervosa and motherhood: Reproduction pattern and mothering behavior of 50 women. *Acta Psychiatrica Scandinavica* 1988; **77**: 611–17.
34. Waugh E, Bulik C. Offspring of women with eating disorders. *International Journal of Eating Disorders* 1999; **25**: 123–33.

10

Phenomenology, fertility and sexual issues in women with schizophrenia

JANET L. TEKELL

INTRODUCTION

Schizophrenia is a heterogeneous, chronic and typically debilitating illness that has the potential to negatively affect a patient's judgement and reasoning. Thus, the medical management of the pregnant schizophrenic woman presents a unique challenge for the obstetrician, psychiatrist and family physician. Medical decisions, like the illness itself, are multifactorial, involving medication issues, competency issues, educational issues and social issues.

To provide a theoretical background for understanding clinical management issues, this chapter will begin with a review of clinical syndrome characteristics, general diagnostic and treatment issues, and gender-specific epidemiologic, clinical and pathophysiologic findings. This will include a brief discussion of the role of estrogen in brain development and the subsequent phenotypic expression of the disease, as well as the impact of antipsychotic treatment and illness characteristics on fertility.

SYNDROMAL CHARACTERISTICS/DIAGNOSTIC CRITERIA

Schizophrenia is a chronic mental illness first described by Kraeplin in 1919 and initially labeled 'dementia praecox.'[1] Unlike most physical illnesses which are diagnosed on the basis of etiology, schizophrenia is defined by specific clinical characteristics (see Box 10.1) as outlined in the *Diagnostic and Statistical Manual of Mental Disorders*, 4th Edition (DSM-IV).[2] Whether this clinical syndrome is caused by one or multiple etiologies is a matter of ongoing research. Heterogeneity of clinical symptoms is a hallmark of the illness. In particular,

---

Box 10.1 *Diagnostic criteria for schizophrenia*

A Characteristic symptoms – two or more
  1 Delusions
  2 Hallucinations
  3 Disorganized speech
  4 Grossly disorganized or catatonic behavior
  5 Negative symptoms
    Note: Only one symptom is required if:
    • Delusions bizarre
    • Hallucinations
        Voice keeps up a running commentary of the person's behavior/thoughts
        Two or more voices converse with each other
B Social/occupational dysfunction
C Duration – continuous signs for at least 6 months
D Schizoaffective and mood disorder exclusion
E Substance/general medical condition exclusion
Subtypes
  • Paranoid
  • Disorganized
  • Catatonic
  • Undifferentiated
  • Residual

Source: American Psychiatric Association.[2]

---

patients who meet diagnostic criteria must have at least two of the following symptoms: delusions, hallucinations, disorganized speech, grossly disorganized or catatonic behavior or negative symptoms (alogia, affective flattening, avolition) for at least 1 month. In addition, they must exhibit social and occupational dysfunction. Medical problems and substance abuse must be excluded as causes for the syndrome. Clinical subtypes include the paranoid, disorganized, catatonic, undifferentiated and residual types.

Despite these specific phenomenologic criteria, schizophrenia is quite variable in its clinical presentation. Some patients may exhibit a predominance of negative symptoms, possibly displaying isolative behavior and minimal speech with poor initiation of normal activities of daily living, while other patients may demonstrate more positive symptoms with a dominant paranoia, constant auditory hallucinations and/or agitation. As might be expected, regardless of which symptoms predominate, patients with schizophrenia have problems with social interaction. Those who are paranoid have difficulty in trusting anyone sufficiently to relate well, and those with severe negative symptoms have no desire to interact with others. These patients tend to be difficult to engage in relationships and productive activity, and tend to be downwardly socially mobile.

GENDER-RELATED DIFFERENCES IN SCHIZOPHRENIA

Age of onset and premorbid history

The heterogeneity of schizophrenia also extends to gender-related differences in the epidemiology, phenomenology and clinical course of the illness. Earlier age of onset and earlier age at first hospitalization for men compared to women has been consistently reported regardless of diagnostic system, culture and historical time periods.[3–5] Goldstein,[6] in a study of schizophrenic patients with onset during adolescence, found the male-to-female ratio to be 2:1, while in a study of patients with onset at age 50 years or above,[5] the female-to-male ratio was 2:1. This reported variability in age of onset might account for the predominance of males in some samples of young patients, and it explains the overall equal incidence of the illness in men and women. In general, men tend to have onset of illness between the ages of 18 and 25 years, while the onset in women is typically at 25–35 years of age.[7,8] In addition to this initial peak of onset in women, there is another smaller peak of onset around age 40–50 years.[8,9] Faraone and colleagues have reported that 3–10% of women with schizophrenia are diagnosed when they are over 45 years of age.[10]

Box 10.2 *Peak ages of onset in schizophrenia*

Men   18–25 years[7,8]
Women   25–35 years[7,8]/40–50 years[8,9]

This later age of onset probably accounts at least in part for reports of a better premorbid history in women with schizophrenia. They have a longer period in which they can function before illness onset than men, so they are more likely to display better school performance, social achievement and occupational performance.[9–11] Women are also more likely than men to have been married. The longer time allowed for brain maturation and social functioning with later age of onset may account for this gender-related difference in the expression of schizophrenic illness.

Illness severity

The issues of differential clinical characteristics between men and women are not clearly proven. Findings in this area have been more variable than research on the age of onset. Some reports indicate that men tend to exhibit more negative symptoms than women.[12] The severity of positive symptoms seems to be the same in both sexes, but some specific types of positive symptoms may cluster in specific genders. For example, women have been reported to exhibit more persecutory delusions[13] and auditory hallucinations.[14]

Despite the equivalent severity of positive symptoms, women are generally thought to have a less severe clinical course than men. Women with schizophrenia appear to be more responsive to medication, less frequently hospitalized, and to have a less severe clinical course.[15] These findings were initially identified in chronic populations, but a 1-year study of first-episode schizophrenics found a similar pattern of treatment response. Szymanski and colleagues found an initial full response rate to medication of 87% in women and 55% in men.[16] Similarly, in a German study of first-admitted patients with schizophrenia, Angermeyer and colleagues found that women had shorter hospital stays, showed more improvement during hospitalization, and survived longer in the community after their first hospital admission.[7] Flor-Henry suggests that these gender differences in symptoms may not be specific to schizophrenia, but rather an exaggeration of normal gender differences in brain maturation.[17] The variation in findings across studies has been attributed to lack of diagnostic precision, variable follow-up times, sample selection and differential definition of outcome.[18] Several investigators[19] have suggested that the longer the observation time, the less marked the gender differences in treatment outcome become.

> **Box 10.3** *Hospital course in new-onset schizophrenic women*
>
> - Better response to treatment (full response: women, 87%; men, 55%)[16]
> - Shorter hospital stay[7]
> - Longer survival in the community after discharge[7]

Some explanations for the treatment response are linked to differences in pharmacokinetics and pharmacodynamics between men and women. Several researchers have found higher blood levels of neuroleptic medication in female subjects at similar dose levels.[20–23] This could possibly be attributed to differences in absorption (which could affect the bioavailability of drugs) and differences in distribution (women have a lower ratio of lean body mass to adipose tissue),[20] as well as possible differences in drug metabolism due to hepatic enzyme variation and menstrual cycle or exogenous ovarian hormone effects.[24]

Brain development

The phenotypic expression of schizophrenia may also vary as a function of the normal dimorphic development of the brain. In normal brain development, sex hormones exert organizational and activation influences.[25,26] Organizational influences refer to prenatal development, which affects the permanent structural development of the brain. For example, sexually dimorphic brain nuclei in primates are present in the central amygdala, preoptic area and hypothalamus. These areas exert substantial influence on neurotransmitter secretion, certain types of learning, feeding and other important life functions.[27] It is not clear whether these sexually dimorphic nuclei differ with regard to numbers of receptors. However, a difference in receptor affinities and receptor site has been postulated.[28] Estrogen receptors appear to be present both cortically and subcortically.[27,29]

One of the known gender differences in normal brain development involves the pace at which the brain matures. The brains of women have earlier neuronal myelinization and cerebral lateralization, and earlier neuronal connections. Therefore the female brain is relatively more mature at birth and thus less vulnerable to the potential trauma of the birth process.[27,30] This could account for the higher prevalence of birth trauma in male schizophrenic patients. It might also explain the earlier age of onset in males who are genetically predisposed to schizophrenia. With this earlier age of onset, the male schizophrenic is exposed to an earlier interruption in cognitive and social development, resulting in the more impoverished premorbid personality associated with male schizophrenic patients. In one study of 184 patients with functional psychoses,[31] obstetric complications did not affect the age of onset in patients with affective psychoses. However, there was a subgroup of male schizophrenic patients with a history of obstetric complications in which the age of onset was on average 3.5 years earlier. Another gender variation in brain development occurs with aging. Dopamine receptors deteriorate more rapidly in men as they get older.[32] This could explain why short-term outcomes favor women, but long-term outcomes are indistinguishable between men and women, due to a greater female:male ratio of neuroleptic need in older age.[33]

THE ROLE OF ESTROGEN – POTENTIAL ANTIDOPAMINERGIC EFFECTS

These gender differences in neuroleptic requirement and age of onset may also be related to estrogen effects on symptom expression in schizophrenia. Some studies suggest that an increase in psychosis is related to a decline in estrogen. This view is supported by the higher incidence of illness onset in postmenopausal women. The second peak in illness onset at approximately the time of the menopause was replicated transnationally by Hambrecht and colleagues in 1992.[3] In one study of schizophrenic patients with age of onset over 60 years, very-late-onset patients were mostly women with good premorbid histories who displayed positive symptoms (hallucinations and persecutory delusions). This group was less likely than patients with an earlier onset to have a family history of schizophrenia, an association with obstetric complications, or to exhibit alogia, anergia or other negative symptoms.[8] This late-onset peak may also be related to the differential decrease in the number of dopamine receptors with age.

This putative antidopaminergic effect of estrogen is demonstrated by studies which indicate that a lower neuroleptic dosage is required in premenopausal women for control of psychotic symptoms. Although the data on this topic are conflicting,[34] some research suggests that ovarian hormones may alter and increase the efficacy of antipsychotic treatment in women.[20] This indirect clinical evidence of the antidopaminergic activity of estrogen has been more directly studied in preclinical studies, the result of which are also inconsistent. However, evidence suggests that estrogen may act similarly to neuroleptics on dopamine-associated behaviors.[35–37] Biochemical studies have shown that estrogen can alter dopamine-receptor density and affinity, although the effect is dependent on the time-course of administration.[38] In general, these reports indirectly suggest that estradiol down-regulates dopamine receptors.

Further support for these ideas can be found in various case reports and clinical studies which have commented on the relationship between clinical symptoms and estrogen levels over the course of the menstrual cycle and life cycle. Several reports have noted that in some schizophrenic women, psychotic symptoms became worse premenstrually (when estrogen levels drop).[39,40] Other epidemiologic studies have noted an exacerbation of psychiatric symptoms in the luteal phase,[41] or an increase in psychiatric admissions in the late luteal phase.[42] Hallonquist and colleagues[43] found a decrease in psychotic symptoms during the mid-luteal phase, as compared to the early follicular phase of the menstrual cycle. Gattaz and colleagues[44] found a non-significant excess of admissions among schizophrenic women in the luteal phase of the menstrual cycle (62%), compared to the high-estrogen phase (38%; $P <$ 0.11). In 1994, Riecher-Rossler and colleagues studied 32 acutely admitted female schizophrenic patients with regular menstrual cycles. They monitored their patients' clinical symptoms and serum estradiol levels. There was a significant negative correlation between symptoms and estradiol levels on all subscores of the Brief Psychiatric Rating Scale (BPRS), with the exception of the anxiety/depression scale. Negative correlations with estradiol levels included thought disturbance ($P < 0.01$), activation ($P < 0.01$) anergia ($P < 0.10$) and hostile–suspiciousness ($P < 0.10$). The strong association with the thought disturbance subscale (which primarily measures psychotic symptoms) suggests more specificity for psychosis as opposed to depressive symptoms.[45] In another study, Riecher-Rossler and colleagues studied 32 acutely admitted schizophrenic women and compared them to 29 women with mental illnesses other than schizophrenia (primarily depressive illness).[19] Correlations were evaluated between serum estradiol levels and clinical psychopathology. With the exception of the depressive subscale, almost all measures of psychopathology decreased with increasing estrogen levels. In the age-matched control group, symptoms were not correlated with estradiol levels. These researchers concluded that the clinical effect of estrogen resembles that of neuroleptics. Estrogen appears to alleviate psychotic symptoms and possibly some other behaviors, but not depressive symptoms.[19]

A few case reports support the view that estrogen influences symptom expression. One case report described a woman with schizoaffective disorder whose symptoms improved with 3 mg of estradiol/day.[46] Another report by Kulkarni and colleagues,[47] published in the same year, indicated a decrease in positive symptoms with 0.02 mg of estradiol during the first 30 days of treatment, but subsequent worsening of symptoms in the next 30 days. This case was part of a study of 11 premenopausal schizophrenic women with acute psychotic symptoms who were treated with 0.02 mg of estradiol in combination with standard neuroleptic treatment. These women were compared with a control group of 7 women who received neuroleptics alone. The study group showed rapid improvement in psychotic symptoms compared to control group in the early part of the study, but both groups reached similar symptom levels at the end of the study in 8 weeks.[47] Another case report from research on postmenopausal schizophrenic women was reported by Lindamer and colleagues in 1997.[38] In this instance, a 49–year-old woman showed a decrease in positive symptoms (but unchanged negative symptoms and global pathology) after 4 months on 0.05 mg transdermal β-estradiol in conjunction with a low-dose neuroleptic. Two weeks after discontinuation of the transdermal β-estradiol she required an increase in her neuroleptic dose. Six weeks after discontinuation of estrogen, her positive symptoms had returned to her pre-estrogen rating. These few treatment cases and other previously described reports of changes in symptom severity based on estrogen level provide more indirect evidence of the possible role that estrogen plays in delaying illness onset and attenuating the strength of psychotic symptoms associated with schizophrenia.

The possible protective role of estrogen in alleviating positive symptoms is further demonstrated by symptom manifestation during pregnancy and postpartum. According to Lindamer and colleagues,[38] during the high-estrogen state of pregnancy, schizophrenic patients tended to have a stable course and occasionally showed improved positive symptoms. However, a subset of schizophrenic women appeared to be vulnerable to decompensation postpartum. Kendall and colleagues reported an increase in acute hospitalization in postpartum schizophrenic women.[48] McNeil found a relapse rate of 23.5% for schizophrenic women postpartum, compared to a relapse rate of 46.7% among mothers with affective psychosis.[49] These reports suggest that lower estrogen states do not put all schizophrenic women at risk for decompensation,[38] but rather only a subset of patients.

Box 10.4 *Relationship of estrogen to age of onset and symptom expression*

- Second peak of illness onset at age of menopause[8,9]
- Decreased psychiatric symptoms with estrogen supplementation in some case reports[38,46,47]
- Exacerbation of symptoms and increased psychiatric admissions in luteal phase[39–42,44]
- Association between lower estradiol levels and thought disturbance subscale of the Brief Psychiatric Rating Scale (BPRS)[45]
- Postpartum worsening of symptoms in a subset of schizophrenic women[38,48,49]
- Possible increased efficacy of antipsychotic therapy in women[20]

SEXUAL BEHAVIOR AND BELIEFS

Compatible with the multiple manifestations of schizophrenic illness, the sexual attitudes and practices of schizophrenic women are varied and complex. Most of the sparse literature on this topic has focused on chronic psychiatric populations in general, as opposed to schizophrenic patients. A few early inpatient studies of hospitalized schizophrenic patients suggest that these patients have a high incidence of sexual dysfunction and decreased sexual activity.[50–53] One of the first studies of schizophrenic sexual behavior by Verhulst and Schneidman[53] reported less sexual activity in male patients but not in female schizophrenic patients. However, this study did not have a normal control group for comparison. The data reported by Lukianowicz[54] do not support the hypothesis of decreased sexual activity. A number of other reports also argue against the concept of decreased sexual interest and activity in schizophrenia, particularly in women.[53,55,56]

In general, earlier reports of sexual attitudes and habits focused on pathology rather than providing general review of sexual behaviors and beliefs. In a later study, Friedman and Harrison[57] collected data on 20 schizophrenic women and 15 normal volunteers. In these inpatients from a predominantly African-American population, schizophrenic patients were found to have an increased incidence of sexual abuse both premorbidly and after onset, earlier menstruation, more negative feelings about menstruation, and increased sexual dysfunction. Specifically, 60% of the schizophrenic group had never had an orgasm, compared to 13.4% of the normal group. In fact, in this group, 40% of the schizophrenic group did not know the meaning of the word 'orgasm.'[57] Rozensky and Berman studied 61 outpatients and discovered a conflict between patients' actual sexual practices and their emotional ease with sexual acts and feelings, resulting in a negative perception of sexuality.[58] Lukoff's work confirmed these previous studies with reports of sexual dysfunction in 63% of his population of recent-onset male outpatients.[59] In this study, all 16 participants were sexually active, with autoerotic sexual activity predominating.

Box 10.5 *Sexual experiences and attitudes of schizophrenic women*

- Increased incidence of sexual abuse[57]
- Earlier onset of menstruation[7]
- More negative feelings and emotional conflict about sexual activity[58]
- Increased problems with sexual dysfunction[57,59]
- Impaired understanding of sexual activities and procreation[57]

One further report by McEvoy and colleagues in 1983,[60] describes a study of 23 chronically institutionalized refractory schizophrenic women. In this severely ill population, the majority were interested in and continued to engage in sexual activity. While the majority of these patients reported that they understood the reasons for and methods of birth control, their practical knowledge was limited. For example, 10 of the 23 women did not understand that birth control methods could be used to avoid pregnancy if they were unable to afford another child or if they were incapable for caring for another baby.[60] Three women did not understand how sex was related to pregnancy, and 11 women said that birth control was immoral and used by 'loose women'. These women were also inaccurate about their own sexual histories, giving inaccurate responses regarding their ability to procreate, the number of children they had produced, and their chosen method of birth control.[60]

SEXUAL EDUCATION

As described above, the need for disease-informed sex education programs for schizophrenic patients is evident. Major obstacles to the institution of such programs have included: professional misconception of and unease about patient needs and sexual behavior, professional fears that such information could cause patients to decompensate, patients' refractory delusions and disorganization, and patients' cognitive deficits and difficulty with abstraction.[59] Lukoff and colleagues have outlined the important needs for sexual education in schizophrenic patients as related to quality of life, a high incidence of sexual dysfunction which could lead to decompensation, medication non-compliance, the need for intimacy skills training, inappropriate sexual behavior and an increasing pregnancy rate (many unwanted and unplanned pregnancies).[59]

Box 10.6 *Obstacles to sexual education*

Professional contribution:
• Discomfort with sexual issues
• Misconception about patients assuming parental role
• Fears that information may cause decompensation
Patient contribution:
• Disorganized thoughts and delusions
• Cognitive deficits and difficulty with abstraction

Source: Lukoff *et al.*[59]

Although these studies support the need for sexual education in the chronic schizophrenic patient,[61–63] little research has been conducted to assess the subgroups that would benefit, and the characteristics of useful programs. One of the first articles on patient sex education in 1980 reviewed the course content and staff training of a group program attended by patients in transitional housing at a Washington state hospital.[64] While no formal program evaluation was conducted, the authors report that group members were attentive, and no verbal or behavioral signs of distress or unease were noted. Sadow and Corman reported positive results from an educational approach to sex education in a Veterans' Administration (VA) day program in 1983.[65] The first controlled research on the effects of sex education on the chronic psychiatric population was reported by Berman and Rozensky in 1984.[66] In this study of 26 psychiatric patients (16 schizophrenic patients) in a day-treatment center, subjects were randomized to a life skills group or a sexual issues group. The objective of the latter group was to provide information, help members to identify feelings about their sexuality, expose members to alternative perspectives, and help members to choose appropriate means of expressing their own sexuality. Thus it was geared to providing both knowledge and values clarification. The results indicate that the group improved in its awareness of birth control, social skills and sexual hygiene. Attitudinal changes compared to the control group included a greater awareness of the spectrum of sexual behavior, and an increased perception of sexuality as a positive aspect of life.

Lukoff and colleagues reported on another VA-sponsored group sex education program in an outpatient clinic population, the aim of which was to provide information, clarify values,

---

Box 10.7 *Goals of sexual education*

• Improve quality of life
• Decrease sexual dysfunction
• Increase capacity for sexual/emotional intimacy
• Decrease inappropriate sexual behavior
• Decrease unwanted/unplanned pregnancies

Sources: Lukoff *et al.*,[59] Miller and Finnerty.[68]

address sexual dysfunction and enhance intimacy skills.[59] In 1988, Edith Pepper reported on a sexual education program in the Boston area which confirmed previous findings of a positive patient response to group education.[67] Based on these cited studies, the most experience in teaching sexual topics to schizophrenic patients has been gained through the use of group education in stable outpatients. These groups are geared not only to provide information about contraception and the effect of medication on sexual behavior, but also to help patients to clarify their own values, increase their sexual vocabulary and knowledge, and improve their capacity to relate at a more intimate level.

Box 10.8 *Potential focus of sexual education groups*

Information:
- About their bodies and sexual behavior/hygiene
- About contraception
- About sexually transmitted diseases
- About medication effects on sexual function

Value clarification:
- About sexual practices and personal choices
- About relationships and comfortable ways to express intimacy

Source: Lukoff *et al.*,[59] Miller and Finnerty.[68]

Treatment education groups have also been used to prevent the occurrence of AIDS in the chronically mentally ill. Research has indicated that people with serious mental illness are at increased risk of infection with the HIV virus[68–70] through high-risk sexual behavior as well as comorbid drug use. Schizophrenic women frequently suffer from increased impulsivity and cognitive impairment which may result in unwanted pregnancies, repeated abortions, and increased risk for sexually transmitted diseases, including AIDS.[71] In one group of 352 psychiatric inpatients, 0.6% of those with low-risk sexual behavior were seropositive, while 14.4% of patients with high-risk sexual behavior were positive for the HIV virus. Another study of 147 female psychiatric outpatients (50% schizophrenic patients) showed that patients scored less well on 5 out of 10 questions about AIDS, compared to a matched control group.[72] In another study of outpatients, 19% of women reported multiple sexual partners and infrequent use of condoms during intercourse.[73] A 6-week, HIV-risk reduction group was held in New York, with subsequent data indicating enhanced HIV-related knowledge as well as increased practical skill in condom use.[74] Other reviews suggest that patients who require psychiatric hospitalization may benefit from education groups about AIDS and HIV[69,75–77] to augment ongoing programs sponsored by chronic care outpatient programs.[78] Problems which are characteristic of schizophrenic patients (e.g. difficulty with abstraction, decreased executive functioning) should be used as foci to modify general programs in order to address the barriers to treatment specific to this population. McDermott and colleagues[79] identified different types of risk behaviors that varied according to psychiatric diagnosis. In particular, schizophrenic patients displayed poor knowledge of AIDS and HIV infection compared to controls or other psychiatric patients. The only consistent factor associated with risk control in schizophrenic patients was whether they believed that their behavior affected their chances of becoming infected. On the basis of this information, McDermott and colleagues recommend that programs for schizophrenic patients should be geared to provide them with concrete, cause–effect information as well as a sense of control over their own behavior.[79]

In addition to the use of groups to provide education about HIV, Carmen and colleagues have also described a prevention program which combines an individual assessment and outreach effort with an outpatient drop-in group.[71] Group content varies according to the specific membership of that group, and ranges from being primarily educational (using films, role-playing activity, etc.) to being a more spontaneous group that addresses varied topics. Condom distribution and use of an anatomical model are a routine part of this group, and are considered to be an essential part of AIDS education.[71,76,80] Resistance to change in this population can be partially attributed to compromised cognition and reality perception. In addition, if patients have been chronically abused and thus have adopted a social role as a sexual object, change could threaten their sense of self.[71]

Box 10.9 *Sexually transmitted diseases in schizophrenic women*

Disease-related problems:
- Increased impulsivity
- Cognitive impairment
- Poor insight

Potential effects of disease-related problems on sexual behavior:
- Multiple sexual partners
- Infrequent use of condoms during intercourse
- Impaired capacity to understand and decrease sexual risk behaviors

Source: Aruffo *et al*.,[72] Weinhardt *et al*.[74]

FERTILITY ISSUES IN SCHIZOPHRENIA

As might be expected, the findings of early studies of marital and reproductive behavior in these patients are characterized by generally low rates of fertility and marriage.[81–83] In the 1950s, prior to the use of neuroleptic medication, most studies of fertility in schizophrenic patients involved examination of census data. Low birth rates among patients were thought to be secondary to social and cultural factors, such as low marriage rates, high divorce rates and institutionalization during the most fertile years.[84] Early studies using census data did not control for ethnicity, socio-economic status, age and other variables associated with measures of fertility.[85,86]

With the advent of traditional neuroleptics and the deinstitutionalization of patient treatment, initial surveys of reproductive capacity of schizophrenic patients indicated increased fertility rates.[81,87] Nimgaonkar and colleagues attributed this phenomena partially to decreased hospital stays and a change in social attitudes.[86] Again, these studies were poorly controlled and had multiple potential confounding variables. More recent studies of procreation in the schizophrenic population have been conducted as controlled studies in the community setting.[68,85,86,88–91] These studies, with only a few exceptions,[91] indicate reduced rates of reproduction in the schizophrenic population compared to normal control subjects. In a study of 79 female schizophrenic women, 124 screened female controls and 86 schizophrenic men, no significant differences in fertility between female patients and controls were detected, but reduced fecundity was noted among female patients past the reproductive period. Male patients showed a significant reduction in both fertility and fecundity compared to female patients.[86] This gender-related effect was independent of age of onset and clinical course.

In all of these studies, the effect of psychotropic medications on fertility was not factored into the evaluation of fertility and fecundity. All medications for schizophrenia, with the exception of the newer atypical antipsychotics that have been developed since 1980, have treated psychosis by the same mechanism, namely non-selective blocking of dopaminergic (D_2) pathways. This non-selective blockade is responsible for most of the side-effects of these medications (i.e. extrapyramidal symptoms secondary to D_2-receptor antagonism in the nigrostriatal areas). Elevated prolactin levels, sometimes up to 8–10 times normal values,[92] are caused by acute non-specific blockade of dopamine receptors in the tuberoinfundibular system, while direct neuroleptic action on the hypothalamic–pituitary axis (HPA) modulates pituitary response independent of the activity of prolactin. By these two mechanisms neuroleptic medications can interrupt ovulation.[84,93,94] Sustained neuroleptic usage has been variably noted to cause persistent prolactin elevation[95] or a gradual return of prolactin to baseline levels.[96] Increased prolactin levels can cause various side-effects, including galactorrhea and amenorrhea. In a study by Ghadirian and colleagues, 91% of 29 female patients who were treated with thioridazine reported alterations in menstruation.[50] Of those women, 50% had reversible amenorrhea. Thus some infertility in the schizophrenic population can probably be attributed to the secondary hyperprolactinemia or direct action on the HPA axis caused by traditional neuroleptic medication.

Some of the newer atypical antipsychotics, which work by mechanisms other than non-specific D_2-receptor antagonism, cause minimal or no elevation of prolactin levels. The current FDA-approved atypical medications which do not elevate prolactin levels (or do so only minimally) include olanzapine, clozapine and quetiapine. Consequently, these new drugs should not cause secondary amenorrhea and may serve to increase fertility in a subgroup of this population.[97,98] Although risperidone is a newer antipsychotic, it still exhibits significant D_2-receptor blockade and elicits an equal (and sometimes higher) elevation of prolactin levels compared to traditional neuroleptic medication. Thus when switching from a traditional neuroleptic to an atypical medication, it is important to be aware of these potential changes in endocrine side-effects, to inform the patient of the potential for increased fertility, and to facilitate decision-making regarding birth control.

REFERENCES

1. Kraeplin E. *Dementia Praecox and Paraphrenia*, New York, Robert E. Krieger; 1971.
2. American Psychiatric Association. *Diagnostic and statistical manual of mental disorders*, 4th edn, Washington, DC: American Psychiatric Association, 1994.
3. Hambrecht M, Maurer K, Sartorious N. Transnational stability of gender differences in schizophrenia? *European Archives of Psychiatry and Clinical Neuroscience* 1992; **242**: 6–12.
4. Sartorius N, Jablensky A, Korten A et al. Early manifestations and first-contact incidence of schizophrenia in different cultures. *Psychology Medicine* 1986; **16**: 909–28.
5. Häfner J, Maurer K, Loffler W, Riecher-Rössler A. The influence of age and sex on the onset and early course of schizophrenia. *British Journal of Psychiatry* 1994; **164**: 625–9.
6. Goldstein JM, Tsuang MT, Faraone SV. Gender and schizophrenia: implications for understanding the nature of the disorder. *Psychiatry Research* 1989; **28**: 243–53.
7. Angermeyer MC, Kuhn L, Goldstein JM. Gender and the course of schizophrenia: differences in treated outcomes. *Schizophrenia Bulletin* 1990; **16**: 293–9.
8. Castle DJ, Wessely S, Howard R, Murray RM. Schizophrenia with onset at the extremes of adult life. *International Journal of Geriatric Psychiatry* 1997; **12**: 712–17.
9. Salokangas RKR. Prognostic implications of the sex of schizophrenic patients. *British Journal of Psychiatry* 1983; **142**: 145–51.

10. Faraone SV, Chen WJ, Goldstein JM *et al*. Gender differences in age at onset in schizophrenia. *British Journal of Psychiatry* 1988; **22**: 141–55.
11. Seeman MV. Gender differences in schizophrenia. *Canadian Journal of Psychiatry* 1998; **27**: 108–11.
12. Cheek FE. A serendipitous finding: Sex roles and schizophrenia. *Journal of Abnormal Social Psychology* 1984; **69**: 392–400.
13. Goldstein JM, Link BG. Gender and the expression of schizophrenia. *Journal of Psychiatric Research* 1988; **22**: 141–55.
14. Rector N, Seeman MV. Auditory hallucinations in women and men. *Schizophrenia Research* 1992; **7**: 233–6.
15. Tamminga C. Gender differences in schizophrenia. Abstract from Symposium on Gender Differences in Psychiatric Disorders at 149th Annual Meeting of the American Psychiatric Association, New York, 1996.
16. Szymanski S, Lieberman JA, Alvir JM *et al*. Gender differences in onset of illness, treatment response, course, and biologic indexes in first-episode schizophrenic patients. *American Journal of Psychiatry* 1995; **152**: 698–703.
17. Flor-Henry P. The influence of gender on psychopathology: Animal experiments. In Flor-Henry P. *Cerebral basis of psychopathology*. Boston: John Wright PSG; 1983: 97–116.
18. Goldstein JM. The impact of gender on understanding the epidemiology of schizophrenia. In: Seeman MV (ed) *Gender and psychopathology*. Washington DC: American Psychiatric Association Press, Inc.; 1995: 159–200.
19. Reicher-Rössler A, Häfner H, Stumbaum M, Maurer K, Schmidt R: Can estradiol modulate schizophrenic symptomatology? *Schizophrenia Bulletin* 1994; **20**: 203–14.
20. Seeman MV. Neuroleptic prescriptions for men and women. *Social Pharmacology* 1989; **3**: 219–36.
21. Simpson GM, Yadalam KG, Levinson DF, Stephanos MJ, Lo ES, Cooper TB. Single-dose pharmacokinetics of fluphenazine after fluphenazine decanoate administration. *Journal of Clinical Psychopharmacology* 1990; **10**: 417–21.
22. Chouinard G, Annable L, Collu R. Plasma prolactin levels: A psychiatric tool. In Collu R, Ducharme JR, Tolis G, Barbeau A. *Brain peptides and hormones*. New York: Raven Press; 1982: 333–41.
23. Ereshefsky L, Saklad SR, Watanabe MD, Davis CM, Jann MW. Thiothixene pharmacokinetic interactions: a study of hepatic enzyme inducers, clearance inhibitors, and demographic variables. *Journal of Clinical Psychopharmacology* 1991; **11**: 296–301.
24. Yonkers KA, Kando JC, Cole JO, Blumenthal S. Gender differences in pharmacokinetics and pharmacodynamics of psychotropic medication. *American Journal of Psychiatry* 1992; **149**: 587–95.
25. Seeman MV. Prenatal gonadal steroids and schizophrenia. *Psychiatric Journal of University of Ottawa* 1989; **14**: 473–5.
26. McEwen BS. Actions of sex hormones on the brain: 'Organization' and 'activation' in relation to functional teratology. *Progress in Brain Research* 1988; **73**: 121–34.
27. Seeman MV, Lang M. The role of estrogens in schizophrenia gender differences. *Schizophrenia Bulletin* 1990; **16**: 185–94.
28. Seeman MV, Seeman P. Molecular psychiatry, receptor density, and receptor sensitivity states. *Integrative Psychiatry* 1986; **4**: 41–43.
29. MacLusky NJ, Naftolin F. Sexual differentiation of the central nervous system. *Science* 1981; **211**: 1294–303.
30. McMillan MM: Differential mortality by sex in fetal and neonatal deaths. *Science* 1979; **204**: 89–91.
31. Kirov G, Jones PB, Harvey I *et al*. Do obstetric complications cause the earlier age at onset in male than female schizophrenics? *Schizophrenia Research* 1996; **20**: 117–24.

32. Wong DF, Wagner HN Jr, Dannals RF, Links JM *et al*. Effects of age on dopamine and serotonin receptors measured by positron tomography in the living human brain. *Science* 1984; **226**: 1393–6.
33. D'Mello DA, McNeil JA. Sex differences in bipolar affective disorder: neuroleptic dosage variance. *Comprehensive Psychiatry* 1990; **31**: 80–3.
34. Jeste DV, Harris MJ, Krull A, Kuck J, McAdams LA, Heaton R. Clinical and neuropsychological characteristics of patients with late-onset schizophrenia. *American Journal of Psychiatry* 1995; **152**: 722–30.
35. Hafner H, Behrens S, De Vry J, Gattaz WF. An animal model for the effects of estradiol on dopaine-mediated behavior: Implications for sex differences in schizophrenia. *Psychiatric Research* 1991; **38**: 125–34.
36. Gordon JH. Modulation of apomorphine-induced stereotypy by estrogen: time course and dose response. *Brain Research Bulletin* 1980; **5**: 679–82.
37. Hruska RE, Ludmer LM, Silbergold EK. Hypophysectomy prevents the striatal dopamine receptor supersensitivity produced by chronic haloperidol treatment. *European Journal of Pharmacology* 1980; **65**: 445–56.
38. Lindamer LA, Lohr JB, Harris MJ, Jeste DV. Gender, estrogen and schizophrenia. *Psychopharmacology Bulletin* 1997; **33**: 221–8.
39. Endo M, Asano Y, Yamashita I, Daiguji M, Takahashi S. Periodic psychosis recurring in association with menstrual cycle. *Journal of Clinical Psychiatry* 1978; **39**: 456–61.
40. Glick J, Steward D. A new drug treatment for premenstrual exacerbation of schizophrenia. *Comprehensive Psychiatry* 1980; **21**: 281–7.
41. Dalton K. Menstruation and acute psychiatric illness. *British Medical Journal* 1959; **1**: 148–9.
42. Janowsky DS, Gorney R, Castelnuovo-Tedesco P, Stone CB. Premenstrual-menstrual increases in psychiatric admission rates. *American Journal of Obstetrics and Gynecology* 1969; **103**: 189–91.
43. Hallonquist JD, Seeman MV, Lang M, Rector NA. Variation in symptom severity over the menstrual cycle in schizophrenics. *Biological Psychiatry* 1993; **33**: 207–9.
44. Gattaz WF, Vogel P, Riecher-Rossler A, Soddu G. Influence of the menstrual cycle phase on the therapeutic response in schizophrenia. *Biological Psychiatry* 1994; **36**: 137–9.
45. Riecher-Rössler A, Häfner H, Dutsch-Ströbel A *et al*. Further evidence for a specific role of estradiol in schizophrenia. *Biological Psychiatry* 1994; **36**: 492–5.
46. Korhonen S, Saarijarvi S, Arto M. Successful estradiol treatment of psychotic symptoms in the premenstrual phase: A case report. *Acta Psychiatrica Scandinavica* 1995; **92**: 237–8.
47. Kulkarni J, de Castella A, Smith D. Adjunctive estrogen treatment in women with schizophrenia. *Schizophrenia Research* 1995; **15**: 157.
48. Kendell RE, Chalmers JC, Platz C. Epidemiology of puerperal psychoses. *British Journal of Psychiatry* 1987; **150**: 662–73.
49. McNeil TF. A prospective study of postpartum psychoses in a high-risk group. *Acta Psychiatrica Scandinavica* 1986; **74**: 205–16.
50. Ghadirian AM, Chouinard G, Annable L. Sexual dysfunction and plasma prolactin levels in neuroleptic-treated schizophrenic outpatients. *Journal of Nervous Mental Disorder* 1982; **170**: 463–7.
51. Rozan G, Tuchin T, Kurland M. Some implications of sexual activity for mental illness. *Mental Hygiene* 1971; **55**: 318–23.
52. Akhtar S, Thomson J. Schizophrenia and sexuality: a review and a report of twelve unusual cases-Part II. *Journal of Clinical Psychiatry* 1980; **41**: 166–74.
53. Verhulst J, Schneidman B. Schizophrenic and sexual functioning. *Hospital and Community Psychiatry* 1981; **4**: 259–62.
54. Lukianowicz N. Sexual drive and its gratification in schizophrenia. *International Journal of Social Psychiatry* 1963; **9**: 250–58.

55. Shearer ML, Davidson RT, Finch SM. The sex ratio of offspring born to state hospitalized schizophrenic women. *Journal of Psychiatric Research* 1967; **5**: 349–50.
56. Erlenmeyer-Kimling L, Ranier JD, Kallmann FJ. Current reproductive trends in schizophrenia. In: Proceedings of the Annual Meeting of the American Psychopathological Association 1966; **54**: 252–76.
57. Friedman S, Harrison G. Sexual histories, attitudes, and behavior of schizophrenic and 'normal' women. *Archives of Sexual Behavior* 1984; **13**: 555–67.
58. Rozensky RH, Berman C. Sexual knowledge, attitudes, and experiences of chronic psychiatric patients. *Psychosocial Rehabilitation Journal* 1984; **8**: 21–7.
59. Lukoff D, Gioia-Hasick D, Sullivan G, Golden JS, Nuechterlein KH. Sex education and rehabilitation with schizophrenic male outpatients. *Schizophrenia Bulletin* 1986; **12**: 669–76.
60. McEvoy JP, Hatcher A, Appelbaum PS, Abernathy V. Chronic schizophrenic women's attitudes toward sex, pregnancy, birth control, and childrearing. *Hospital Community Psychiatry* 1983; **34**: 536–9.
61. Dincin J, Wise S. Sexual attitude reassessment for psychiatric patients. *Rehabilitation Literature* 1979; **40**: 222–9.
62. Wolfe SD, Menninger WW. Fostering open communications about sexual concerns in a mental hospital. *Hospital and Community Psychiatry* 1973; **24**: 147–50.
63. Grunebaum H, Abernathy V, Rofman ES, Weiss JL. The family planning attitudes, practices, and motivations of mental patients. *American Journal of Psychiatry* 1971; **128**: 740–4.
64. Shaul S, Morrey L. Sexuality education in a state mental hospital. *Hospital and Community Psychiatry* 1980; **31**: 175–9.
65. Sadow D, Corman AG. Teaching a human sexuality course to psychiatric patients: the process, pitfalls and rewards. *Sexuality and Disability* 1983; **6**: 47–63.
66. Berman C, Rozensky RH. Sex education for the chronic psychiatric patient: the effects of a sexual-issues group on knowledge and attitudes. *Psychosocial Rehabilitation Journal* 1984; **8**: 28–34.
67. Pepper E. Sexual awareness groups in a psychiatric day treatment program. *Psychosocial Rehabilitation Journal* 1988; **11**: 45–52.
68. Miller LJ, Finnerty M. Sexuality, pregnancy, and childrearing among women with schizophrenia-spectrum disorders. *Psychiatric Service* 1996; **47**: 502–6.
69. Abernathy VD, Grunebaum H. Toward a family planning program in psychiatric hospitals. *American Journal of Public Health* 1972; **62**: 1638–46.
70. Thompson SC, Checkley GE, Hocking JS, Crofts N *et al*. HIV risk behaviour and HIV testing of psychiatric patients in Melbourne. *Australian and New Zealand Journal of Psychiatry* 1997; **31**: 566–76.
71. Carmen E, Brady SM. AIDS risk and prevention for the chronic mentally ill. *Hospital and Community Psychiatry* 1990; **41**: 652–7.
72. Aruffo JF, Coverdale JH, Chacko RC, Dworkin RJ. Knowledge about AIDS among women psychiatric outpatients. *Hospital and Community Psychiatry* 1990; **41**: 326–8.
73. Kelly JA, Murphy DA, Bahr GR *et al*. AIDS/HIV risk behavior among the chronic mentally ill. *American Journal of Psychiatry* 1992; **149**: 886–9.
74. Weinhardt LS, Carey MP, Carey KB. HIV risk reduction for the seriously mentally ill: pilot investigation and call for research. *Journal of Behavior Therapy in Experimental Psychiatry* 1997; **28**: 87–95.
75. Hoffman B, Arthurs K, Lunn S *et al*. AIDS: clinical and ethical issues on a psychiatric unit. *Canadian Journal of Psychiatry* 1989; **34**: 847–52.
76. Baer JW, Dwyer PC, Koehler-Lewitter S. Knowledge about AIDS among psychiatric patients. *Hospital and Community Psychiatry* 1988; **39**: 986–8.
77. Sacks MH, Silberstein C, Weiler P *et al*. HIV- related risk factors in acute psychiatric inpatients. *Hospital and Community Psychiatry* 1990; **41**: 449–51.

78. Seeman MV, Lang M, Rector N. Chronic schizophrenia: A risk factor for HIV? *Canadian Journal of Psychiatry* 1990; **35**: 765–8.

79. McDermott BE, Sautter FJ, Winstead DK, Quirk T. Diagnosis, health beliefs, and risk of HIV infection in psychiatric patients. *Hospital and Community Psychiatry* 1994; **45**: 580–5.

80. Solomon MZ, DeJong W. Preventing AIDS and other STDs through condom promotion: a patient education intervention. *American Journal of Public Health* 1989; **79**: 453–8.

81. Erlenmeyer-Kimling L, Rainer JD, Nicol S, Deming WE. Changes in fertility rates of schizophrenic patients in New York State. *American Journal of Psychiatry* 1969; **125**: 916–27.

82. Slater E, Hare EH, Price JS. Marriage and fertility of psychiatric patients compared with the national data. Fertility and reproduction in physically and mentally disordered individuals. *Social Biology* 1971; (Supplement 18): S60–S73.

83. Odegard O. Fertility of psychiatric first admissions in Norway. *Acta Psychiatrica Scandinavica* 1980; **62**: 212–20.

84. Currier GW, Simpson GM. Antipsychotic medications and fertility. *Psychiatric Service* 1998; **49**: 175–6.

85. Lane A, Byrne M, Mulvany F *et al*. Reproductive behavior in schizophrenia relative to other mental disorders: evidence for increased fertility in men despite decreased marital rate. *Acta Psychiatrica Scandinavica* 1995; **91**: 222–8.

86. Nimgaonkar VL, Ward SE, Agarde H, Weston N, Ganguli R. Fertility in schizophrenia: results from a contemporary US cohort. *Acta Psychiatrica Scandinavica* 1997; **95**: 364–9.

87. Goldfarb C, Erlenmeyer-Kimling L. Mating and fertility trends in schizophrenia. In: Kallman FJ, Erlenmeyer-Kimling L, Granville EV, Rainer JD. *Expanding goals of genetics in psychiatry*. New York, Grune & Stratton; 1962: 42–51.

88. Hilger T, Propping P, Haverkamp F. Is there an increase of reproductive rates in schizophrenics? *Archives Psychiatrie Nervenkrankenheiten* 1993; **233**: 177–86.

89. Burr WA, Falek A, Strauss LT, Brown SB. Fertility in psychiatric outpatients. *Hospital and Community Psychiatry* 1979; **30**: 527–31.

90. Fanasas L, Bertranpelt J. Reproductive rates in families of schizophrenic patients in a case control study. *Acta Psychiatrica Scandinavica* 1995; **91**: 202–4.

91. Bassett AS, McAlduff J, Bury A, Bindseil K, Hodgkinson KA, Honer WG. Reproductive fitness in familial schizophrenia. *Schizophrenia Research* 1995; **15**: 35–6.

92. Wetzel H, Wiesner J, Hiemke C, Bbenhart O. Acute antagonism of dopamine D_2–like receptors by amisulpride: Effects on hormone secretion in healthy volunteers. *Journal of Psychiatric Research* 1994; **28**: 461–73.

93. Gunnett JW, Moore KF. Neuroleptics and endocrine function. *Annual Review of Pharmacology and Toxicology* 1988; **28**: 347–66.

94. Kreig JR, Cassidy JR. Counteraction of the haloperidol blockade of ovulation by bromocriptine, and the effect of bromocriptine on LH and prolactin secretion. *Neuroendicrinology* 1984; **38**: 371–5.

95. Zelaschi NM, Delucchi GA, Rodriguez JL. High plasma prolactin levels after long-term neuroleptic treatment. *Biological Psychiatry* 1996; **39**: 900–1.

96. Green AI, Brown WA. Prolactin and neuroleptic drugs. *Endocrinology Metabolic Clinics of North America* 1988; **17**: 223–30.

97. Kaplan B, Modai I, Stoler M, Kitai E, Valevski A, Weizman A. Clozapine treatment and risk of unplanned pregnancy. *Journal of the American Board Family Practice* 1995; **8**: 239–41.

98. Canuso CM, Hanau M, Jhamb KK, Green AI. Olanzapine use in women with antipsychotic-induced hyperprolactinemia. *American Journal of Psychiatry* 1998; **155**: 1458.

11

Management of pregnancy in the schizophrenic woman

JANET L. TEKELL

INTRODUCTION

Prevention and management of the previously described problems of inadequate reproductive knowledge, lack of family planning, poor prenatal care and exposure to pregnancy risks need to be addressed by physicians caring for women with schizophrenia. In this chapter, disease-specific issues in family planning and education will be discussed. The impact of pregnancy on the clinical course of schizophrenia will be reviewed, as well as the specific problems that the schizophrenic illness imposes on the normal course of pregnancy and delivery. Finally, pharmacologic issues during pregnancy, delivery and lactation will be outlined prior to discussing parenting and custody issues.

FAMILY PLANNING

Despite the high incidence of unwanted pregnancies in the schizophrenic population, the literature includes few studies that address the contraceptive and family planning needs of this group. Coverdale and others focus on the need for a complete sexual history and integration of family planning services with mental health services in the treatment of schizophrenic patients.[1,2]

They also discuss the assessment of competency to participate in an informed-consent process. In particular, Coverdale notes that:

patients must first be able to attend to, absorb, retain and recall information disclosed. . . The patient should understand that the decision has consequences for the future (cognitive understanding) and should be helped to evaluate those consequences on the basis of her beliefs (evaluative understanding). . . The psychiatrist should help the patient achieve cognitive and evaluative understanding and to communicate a decision based on these types of understanding.[3]

In schizophrenia, patients who have the capacity to perform these activities may become variably impaired at different times in their lives.[4] Therefore ongoing assessment for capacity to consent is necessary. Rather than advocate a paternal approach to patients, the authors emphasize the need to treat the reversible barriers to decision-making by focusing on adequate symptom treatment and education.[1,4]

Box 11.1 *Informed consent*

(Capacity may be variably present over the course of the illness)
- Attend to information
- Understand, retain and recall information
- Comprehend that decisions have consequences for the future
- Evaluate potential consequences based on values
- Communicate evaluative and cognitive understanding
- Express decision based on that understanding

Sources: Coverdale *et al*.,[3] McCullogh *et al*.[4]

Coverdale and colleagues emphasized the urgent need for family planning in this population based on the pregnancy outcomes of schizophrenic women. In their 1989 study of 80 female chronic schizophrenic outpatients, 31% reported a history of at least one abortion. Of all the live births ($n = 75$), 60% were raised by individuals other than the mother. Of those sexually active patients who stated that they did not want to become pregnant, 33% had not used contraception at the time of last intercourse.[5] Other studies document system inadequacies in the provision of access to family planning services and education.[5–8]

Box 11.2 *Characteristics of 80 pregnant schizophrenic women*

- History of at least one abortion – 31%
- Children raised by someone other than mother – 60%
- Unwanted pregnancy, but no attempt at contraception – 33%

Source: Coverdale and Aruffo.[5]

Due to the compliance problems with most medications in this population, Coverdale and Aruffo recommend the use of an intrauterine device (IUD) or medroxyprogesterone (Depo-Provera) for schizophrenic women who request birth control.[5] An additional option could be any extended-release birth control method, such as levonorgestrel (Norplant).[4,5] The possibility of tubal ligation is also a consideration if the woman is competent and does not wish to bear any more children. If there is a spouse or a stable sexual partner who wishes to be involved in family planning, and the couple does not desire to have children, discussion might also include the possibility of a vasectomy. Although condoms protect against sexually transmitted diseases, research suggests that schizophrenic patients frequently fail to use condoms.[4,6] Although education about the prevention of sexually transmitted diseases and condom use is important, effective birth control in this population may realistically require long-acting or permanent methods.[5]

Box 11.3 *Most effective birth control options for schizophrenic outpatients*

Long-acting temporary methods
- Intrauterine device (IUD)
- Medroxyprogesterone (Depo-Provera)
- Levonorgestrel (Norplant)

Permanent method
- Tubal ligation

Source: Coverdale and Aruffo.[5]

Family planning education targeted at schizophrenic patients can be achieved either individually or in a group. The topic can also be combined with HIV/AIDS awareness. Education must be specifically tailored to the patient's capacity to understand and consent. In this population, a practical approach using behavior skills training may be most effective. Systematic training in fitting condoms, refusing unwanted advances and other social skills can all be useful for helping schizophrenic patients to adhere to their wishes with regard to family planning.[7,8]

Another way to provide optimal contraception services is to address the difficulty that mentally ill women experience in accessing consumer services. In addition, mental health professionals may feel uncomfortable addressing sexual, family planning or pregnancy issues. Yet, several studies of the effect of group treatment and education demonstrate increased knowledge, enhanced ease with sexual issues and increased contraceptive use in this population.[7,9,10] In her 1996 review, Miller describes the multiple problems in identifying access to care and delineates the specific services needed to provide comprehensive care to schizophrenic women.[11]

Like sexual education and HIV awareness, family planning for the schizophrenic woman must be tailored to her individual needs and disease-specific problems. Genetic counseling is most commonly presented in a non-directive manner geared to educate the patient to make autonomous decisions.[12,13] Due to the complex mode of inheritance of schizophrenia, it is impossible to calculate the exact risk of illness for any particular person. Using information from family, adoption and twin studies, Moldin estimated the risk of schizophrenia to be 9% for all first-degree relatives.[14] Asherman and colleagues report that a couple with one schizophrenic parent would have an approximately 3% risk of having a child affected by schizophrenia.[15] This approximate range of risk would be increased considerably in a family with many affected members.[16] Moldin[14] and Faraone and colleagues[17] have written comprehensive reviews of the stages and methodology of psychiatric genetic counseling.

IMPACT OF PREGNANCY ON MENTALLY ILL MOTHERS

Whether a pregnancy is planned or unplanned, the events of gestation and childbirth have an impact on the clinical course of schizophrenic illness. Bleuler first noted the impact of pregnancy on mentally ill mothers in 1911. He observed that 'too many' women with psychosis had an exacerbation of their symptoms in the puerperium.[18] In 1969, Yarden and Suranyi [19] noted an insignificant trend towards more frequent hospitalization in postpartum schizophrenic patients compared to other schizophrenic women. Their case–control study matched pregnant schizophrenic women with non-pregnant schizophrenic women, and the 67 subjects were followed for 5 years postpartum. In Trixler's 1995 study of 919 schizophrenic women, 109 women (11.9%) decompensated within 6 months after parturition, while only 3 women (0.32%) decompensated during pregnancy.[20] Curran suggested in his 1961 paper that for a schizophrenic mother the stress of child care may be more damaging than the biological effects of pregnancy or childbirth.[21]

Psychotic patients are known to have more social problems and to have a more negative experience of pregnancy than non-psychotic patients.[22] This negative experience appears to be correlated with the degree of psychotic symptoms and the social stressors experienced during the pregnancy.[23] Miller and Finnerty[24] utilized a semi-structured interview to assess the sexuality, reproductive and child-rearing characteristics of 46 women who fulfilled ICD-10 criteria for schizophrenia or schizoaffective disorder, compared to 50 control subjects without major mental illness. The groups were matched for age, race, education, employment status and religion. They were also comparable with regard to numbers of pregnancies and rates of infertility, miscarriage, Cesarean section, premature birth and other obstetric complications. Both groups reported high rates of substance abuse during unprotected intercourse and pregnancy. The two groups differed in that the subjects with schizophrenia spectrum disorders were less likely to have planned pregnancies and less likely to have received prenatal care. Those subjects were also more likely to have been physically abused during the pregnancy and to have had an abortion in the past.[24] Rejection of obstetrical and psychiatric care, irrational behavior, denial of pregnancy and potentially dangerous behavior in pregnant schizophrenic women have been noted in the literature.[23–27]

Referring back to Miller and Finnerty's study, other significant demographic characteristics of the schizophrenic spectrum group included more lifetime sex partners, a higher probability of having been raped or having engaged in prostitution, and less likelihood of having a current partner. This group was less likely to have been tested for HIV, even though they were at higher risk of being HIV-positive. With regard to child-rearing, the schizophrenic spectrum group had less social support, less confidence in their ability to meet their children's needs, and were more likely to lose custody of their children than the control group.[24] Rudolph's 1990 study of 35 severely mentally ill pregnant women (66% schizophrenic women, 8% bipolar patients and 26% atypical psychosis) demonstrated similar demographic characteristics. In total, 22 of the 35 women were separated or divorced, and social support from families was frequently lacking; 22 women were receiving disability payments and 5 women were homeless.[22] The literature regarding pregnancy issues indicates that some of the most important factors concerning adjustment to pregnancy and childbirth are quality support from a significant other, financial support and social support in the community.[22,23,27] The studies cited previously, as well as the schizophrenia literature in general, indicate that these resources are not usually available to the schizophrenic mother, leaving her with severe social stressors in addition to whatever biological factors predispose to decompensation in the postpartum period.

Inconsistently reported rates of decompensation in the puerperium can possibly be attributed to variable diagnostic criteria. Recent studies that utilize narrow definitions of schizophrenia are identifying higher rates of decompensation in affective disorders and lower rates in schizophrenia.[28] McNeil's 6-month postpartum study of schizophrenic and affective disorder patients showed that schizophrenic subjects decompensated slightly later postpartum than the affective disorder patients. He also noted that subjects who met the criteria for a more restrictive definition of schizophrenia had a lower rate of relapse than those patients who only met the broader diagnostic criteria.[29] Following up on this information, Davies and colleagues[28] used a retrospective case-note design to assess the 5-year postpartum progress of 45 schizophrenic mothers. Using ICD-10 criteria, a 'broad' diagnostic group of 21 was identified, while a 'narrow' diagnostic group of 16 was identified using more restrictive Feighner criteria. All of the subjects met DSM-III-R criteria for schizophrenia. Demographically, the more narrowly defined group was significantly younger, unemployed, more likely to be African-Caribbean in origin, more likely to be living in a 'supported hostel', and with an earlier age of onset. There was no difference between the groups with regard to medical treatment with neuroleptics, psychotic symptoms, mode of delivery or postnatal complications. The mode of delivery and incidence of postnatal complications were similar to those in the general population. Analysis of the clinical course postpartum of these two groups reveals a relapse rate acutely postpartum of 43% in the 'broadly' defined group of subjects compared to no decompensation in the patients who met 'narrow' diagnostic criteria. Thus the variation in the diagnostic criteria used to diagnose patients in the different studies in the literature could account for some of the conflicting reports.[28]

IMPACT OF SCHIZOPHRENIC ILLNESS ON PREGNANCY AND DELIVERY

Pregnancy

There are also conflicting reports on the impact of schizophrenia on pregnancy and delivery in the literature.[30] Some studies of childbearing women with histories of mental illness reveal an insignificantly altered course in chronic schizophrenia.[31,32] The patient may nonetheless deal with the pregnancy while hindered by residual psychotic symptoms and reduced psychosocial support. With reduced social and financial resources, it is difficult to create a nurturing environment for both the mother and the baby. Impaired reality, lack of insight and motivation and cognitive deficits can also impact on compliance with medical recommendations and treatment. As mentioned previously, many of these women have unwanted pregnancies, are physically abused when pregnant, and have limited resources to meet their own needs.[33,34] The literature contains various case reports referring to decompensated schizophrenic women who have acted in a self-harming manner during their pregnancies (e.g. induced their own abortions, performed their own Cesarean sections).[35] Other potential risks include fetal abuse,[36] neonaticide[37,38] and sudden unassisted delivery.[39]

Spielvogel and Wile[39] reviewed the clinical course of 22 pregnant psychiatric inpatients in an attempt to determine which psychiatric diagnoses were more frequently associated with problems during pregnancy and childbirth. In this small population, that included 10 schizophrenic women, those women who had delusions about the pregnancy or psychotic denial were significantly less likely to detect labor than non-delusional women. Substance abuse patients, personality-disordered patients and bipolar patients were more likely to detect signs of labor and co-operate with instructions than women with schizophrenia.[39] In Miller's review of 26 consecutive admissions to a specialized inpatient unit for women with mental illness who decompensated during pregnancy, 12 women exhibited psychotic denial of pregnancy.[40] In three of these women, denial was related more to belief about the viability of the pregnancy than to denial of the pregnancy. In total, 11 of these 12 women had a principal diagnosis of chronic schizophrenia. The groups were comparable with regard to age, race, marital status and employment status. The women who exhibited psychotic denial of pregnancy significantly more often lost custody of their children and were significantly more likely to face the possibility of separation due to loss of custody during the current pregnancy.

Most women with this delusion were chronically homeless and impoverished, with no social support, impaired capacity to access health care, and little ability to manage frustration.[40]

Medical management of psychotic denial of pregnancy consisted of treatment with antipsychotic medication and supportive psychotherapy to identify stressors and deal with anticipated loss. After evaluation of their parenting skills and social network, some mothers were referred to parenting classes and other community resources so that they could safely retain custody of their babies.[40] Although the clinical course of schizophrenia may be cited as being 'stable' during pregnancy, the pregnancy can nonetheless be complicated by residual psychotic symptoms, severe psychosocial stressors or persistent cognitive and executive deficits which threaten the woman's capacity to bear her child safely or maintain custody after birth.

Box 11.4 *Psychotic denial of pregnancy*

- Increased incidence of loss of custody
- Less social support
- Fewer internal resources to manage frustration/crises
- Increased likelihood of precipitous delivery
- Less capacity to follow labor instructions

Source: Miller.[40]

Birth complications

The incidence of pregnancy and birth complications in children of schizophrenic mothers is also variably reported in the literature. In 1975, Reider and colleagues noted an increase in the rate of fetal and neonatal deaths among offspring of schizophrenic parents.[41] This was also reported by Modrzewska in 1980.[42] McNeil and Kaij's review of the literature found mixed results, but some studies indicated that there were no differences between schizophrenic and control subjects.[20,43] Cohler and colleagues[44] found no significant increase in the rate of pregnancy and birth complications in schizophrenic women, while Zax's study[45] suggested lower birth weights, more premature births and lower Apgar scores in severely ill (although not necessarily schizophrenic) mothers.

Another study in 1980 by Wrede and colleagues[46] reviewed the history of all children born to schizophrenic women between 1960 and 1964 in Helskinki. A total of 212 deliveries were found for 192 women (5 twin births). In this socialized country, no correlation was found between socio-economic status and pregnancy and birth complications. In the schizophrenic group, as compared to the matched non-mentally ill group, there were more stillbirths and neonatal deaths. More perinatal and pregnancy complications occurred in the chronic group (higher number of admissions prior to pregnancy) than in the mild group (1–3 psychiatric hospitalizations prior to pregnancy).[46]

A 1996 meta-analysis of the literature on obstetric complications examined studies that met the following three criteria: schizophrenic parents included both father and mother; control groups were normal controls; and non-schizophrenic psychotic parents were excluded. A total of 14 studies that met these criteria were analyzed and, although the effect sizes were small, parents with schizophrenia had an increased risk of pregnancy and birth complications, low birth weight and compromised neonatal outcome. The risk appeared to be greatest for offspring of schizophrenic mothers as opposed to schizophrenic fathers. This implies that the increase in obstetric complications may be an epiphenomenon due to environmental contributions rather than genetic factors.[47]

More recently, Bennedsen[48] conducted an extensive review of the literature which focuses on the incidence of low birth weight, preterm births and perinatal death in the infants of schizophrenic mothers. Her paper carefully outlines general obstetric risk factors and their incidence in women with schizophrenia. Since the incidence of poverty, smoking, substance abuse and many other general risk factors for obstetric complications is increased in many women with schizophrenia, a higher frequency of complications in these babies could be expected on the basis of environmental factors alone. Bennedsen concludes that evidence for a solely genetic increase in premature births, low birth weight and perinatal death in schizophrenic women is still lacking. She emphasizes the importance of future work focusing on the relationship between environmental conditions and genetic influences in order to clarify issues that are specific to schizophrenia and to identify general risk factors which should be addressed in pregnant schizophrenic women in order to prevent complications.

Box 11.5 *Birth complications in children of schizophrenic patients*

1 Variably reported, and not well controlled for general risk factors such as:
   - Smoking
   - Lower socio-economic status
   - Substance use
   - Age
2 Recent meta-analysis suggests:
   - Risks are greatest in offspring of schizophrenic mother – suggesting epiphenomena
   - Problems include more pregnancy/birth complications, low birth weight and compromised neonatal outcome

Source: Sacker *et al.*[47] Bennedsen *et al.*[48]

Perinatal complications

Perinatal complications in the offspring of schizophrenic parents may include low muscle tone, poor motor maturity, variations in alertness, abnormally low activity level and decreased capacity to cuddle.[49] While earlier reviews[50,51] reported various perinatal abnormalities in the children of schizophrenic patients, Fish and colleagues reviewed 12 studies of high-risk infants conducted in the 1980s and concluded that a subset of schizophrenic offspring had more delayed gross motor and visual motor development.[52] Fish coined the term 'pandysmaturation' as an index of an inherited neurointegrative defect in infancy which might be a marker to detect those children of schizophrenic parents who were genetically vulnerable to later schizophrenia.[53] A replication analysis using Jerusalem data showed a diagnosis of pandysmaturation to be significantly related to a parental diagnosis of schizophrenia and to cognitive and motor deficits at 10 years of age. Although motor problems seemed to result from obstetric and birth complications, only perceptual cognitive signs were correlated with parental diagnosis and infant problems.[49]

In a later report of 108 children with various risk factors (schizophrenia, non-schizophrenic mothers, parental maltreatment), Bergman and colleagues noted a specific relationship between neuromotor dysfunction and behavior which varies as a function of parental diagnosis.[54] Other studies also indicate a heightened rate of motor abnormalities in some offspring of schizophrenic parents.[55] Although it is beyond the scope of this chapter to review the high-risk literature, the New York High-Risk Project has reported diverse behaviors,[56] cognitive patterns[57] and attentional deficits[58–60] in some children with a schizophrenic parent.

In the perinatal period, infants of schizophrenic parents should be observed for neuro-motor and visual motor delays, variations in alertness, and the possible side-effects of maternal medication, which will be discussed in the next section.

RISK/BENEFIT ASSESSMENT OF MEDICAL TREATMENT

While many issues related to schizophrenia and pregnancy are complicated and unclear, the decisions related to medication treatment vs. non-treatment are less ambiguous due to the typical morbidity of untreated schizophrenic illness. As in all medical decisions, the physician treating a pregnant schizophrenic patient must assess the risk/benefit ratio prior to prescribing medication. In the pregnant patient this involves assessment of the medical effects on the fetus as well as the mother. In addition, the physician must consider the risk posed by untreated mental illness to the mother and baby.[61] The latter risk is especially high in the schizophrenic patient.[62,63]

Pharmacodynamics and pharmacokinetics in the mother and fetus

When assessing risk, as well as deciding on medication dosage, the physician must consider the pharmacodynamics and pharmacokinetics related to pregnancy in order to determine the drug effectiveness and side-effects. Although there are only limited clinical data to define these issues, some theoretical gender differences that have been explored by Yonkers and colleagues[64] include decreased gastric absorption (due to less gastric acid), decreased transit time through the gastrointestinal tract for both solids and liquids,[65] and less lean body mass[66] (which may cause a prolonged half-life in patients who are taking highly lipophilic medications).

Applying this information to antipsychotic medication, the decreased gastrointestinal transit time may account for better absorption of medication, and the increased adipose/lean tissue ratio may lead to greater retention of the highly lipophilic antipsychotic medications. Several studies indicate that women generally have higher blood levels of antipsychotic medications at comparable dosing, age and weight.[67–69] In a study by Ereschefsky and colleagues[70] thiothixene was needed in higher dosages in men, due to higher oral clearance rates that were not related to body weight. Clearance was also noted to be reduced in subjects over the age of 50 years, but smoking and concurrent drug usage were not factored into the analysis. As previously discussed, another possible factor contributing to this decreased dose requirement in women could be explained by the proposed antidopaminergic effect of estrogen.[71,72] Confirmation of these varied ideas awaits studies which control for age, other medications, menstrual status, menstrual cycle phase, weight and exogenous hormone administration in the study subjects.[64]

The alterations in antipsychotic pharmacodynamics and pharmacokinetics that occur during pregnancy are due to the multiple physiologic changes of the puerperium. In his review of psychopharmacology during pregnancy and lactation, Zachary Stowe identified five changes which may occur during pregnancy and which could effect psychotropic drug concentrations. These were delayed gastric emptying, further decreased gastrointestinal mobility (thought to be mediated by progesterone), increased volume of distribution diluting the concentration of medication), decreased-drug binding capacity (leading to higher free drug concentrations) and increased hepatic metabolism.[73] Thus it is important to closely monitor side-effects or any change in medication efficacy.

With regard to the impact of antipsychotic drugs on the fetus, all psychotropic medications are known to cross the placenta, which has its own metabolism.[74] The placenta allows medication to enter by simple diffusion. Although the mother and baby are at equilibrium, the fetus is known to have decreased plasma protein binding, increased cardiac output, decreased hepatic functioning and increased permeability of the blood–brain barrier.[73] This creates an increased risk for CNS exposure to medication in the fetus.

Box 11.6 *Variables that affect psychotropic drug concentrations during pregnancy*

In mother:
- Delayed gastric emptying
- Decreased gastrointestinal motility
- Increased volume of distribution
- Decreased drug-binding capacity
- Increased hepatic metabolism

In fetus:
- Decreased plasma protein-binding
- Increased cardiac output
- Decreased hepatic functioning
- Increased permeability of the blood brain barrier

Sources: Dworkin *et al.*,[59] Erlenmeyer-Kimling and Cornblatt,[60] Miller,[61] Seeman.[68]

Antipsychotic medication

The impact of neuroleptic medication on the fetus has been discussed many times in the literature, although primarily in case reports and small studies that cannot adequately establish a causal relationship. The only large controlled outcome studies of low-potency and high-potency antipsychotics have been conducted on pregnant women suffering from hyperemesis gravidarum. Lower doses of medication are used for hyperemesis gravidarum than for schizophrenia, so this must be considered when drawing conclusions with regard to risk to the infant.

With regard to the high-potency antipsychotics, case reports include a limb reduction abnormality[75] as well as a case of limb deformity[76] in the offspring of two mothers who were treated with haloperidol. Two prospective controlled studies of neuroleptics for emesis[77,78] indicated that there were no significant increases in neonatal deaths or severe abnormalities. The results were similar in two retrospective studies of trifluoperazine when used for repeated abortions and emesis.[79,80] In a French study of 199 children of schizophrenic mothers, a minimal increase compared to normal values was noted, with 2.5% of children having malformations.[81] All of the traditional neuroleptics are considered to be drugs for which risk cannot be ruled out, and the risk/benefit ratio should be carefully considered before prescribing them during pregnancy.

Other large studies of neuroleptics have been retrospective chart reviews. The French National Institute of Health reviewed 12 764 births. Congenital malformations occurred at an overall rate of 1.6% in this population, and of 315 babies exposed to phenothiazines, 3.5% had malformations. Although this is a significant difference, this study did not control for maternal age, so the difference may not reflect an actual drug effect.[82] The California Child Health Development Project (1959–1966) studied more than 19 000 births and found no significant increase in congenital malformations in babies exposed to neuroleptics.[83] One study[82] suggests that the aliphatic phenothiazines may be especially problematic for the fetus. The many potential confounding variables in these studies that were not controlled include maternal age, other medication, alcohol, stress, dose and timing of dose, nutritional status, gravidity, environmental toxins, previous pregnancy loss, effects of illness and genetic influences. In Ananth's comprehensive review, the authors concluded that controlled studies had not adequately implicated the phenothiazines as factors in congenital malformations, and that the additional isolated case reports were not sufficient evidence to classify the phenothiazines as teratogens.[84]

Conflicting reports about neuroleptic use during pregnancy can be attributed in part to multiple confounding variables that have been inadequately considered in some studies.[77-79,82,83] Despite these problems and inconsistent findings, animal studies and reviews of human pregnancy have failed to clearly demonstrate any specific organ malformation with the use of chlorpromazine, haloperidol or perphenazine.[77,80-89]

A 1996 meta-analysis of the existing literature analyzed only those reports that included first-trimester exposure to phenothiazines. Altshuler and colleagues found that first trimester exposure to low-potency antipsychotics for non-psychotic women was associated with a 2.4% incidence of anomalies. With a baseline incidence of 2%, the antipsychotics conferred an additional risk of 4 in 1000 (0.4%).[90] The authors concluded that psychosis alone probably confers the greatest risk to fetal outcome. However, phenothiazines may contribute slightly to the possibility of a bad outcome.[90]

The potential for teratogenicity of the newer atypical antipsychotics is not known. A few case reports and case studies in the literature[91-93] have noted no obstetric or perinatal complications in the patients who became pregnant while being treated with clozapine. In one study, Waldman and Safferman[92] reported on 12 women who became pregnant while taking clozapine. No adverse sequelae had been noted. In a review of clozapine treatment in 59 pregnant women, Dev and Krupp reported that 51 of 61 births produced healthy babies. Of the 10 problematic births, 5 infants had perinatal symptoms and 5 infants had congenital malformations. However, the adverse effects of other medications used during the pregnancy could not be ruled out.[94] Further experience with atypical medications is needed before the risks and benefits of these medications to the mother and baby can be clarified.

With regard to the effects of neuroleptics on labor and delivery, Harer[95] noted that the short-term use of chlorpromazine does not increase the duration of labor or the number of deliveries. One case report notes an uncomplicated delivery after treatment of hyponatremia in a patient with psychogenic polydipsia.[96]

Neuroleptic effects on the neonate have been noted, partly due to the highly lipid-soluble and protein-bound nature of the drugs. In addition, the fetus has variably immature liver enzymes, resulting in decreased drug metabolism, decreased plasma protein concentrations causing increased levels of free drug, and an undeveloped central nervous system making the baby more sensitive to drug effects.[73] One specific effect noted in neonates whose mothers are treated with high-potency neuroleptics is extrapyramidal symptoms (EPS), that have been noted to continue up to 6–10 months postpartum.[20,45,97-99] Typically, this condition is not noted at birth, but starts 1–3 days postpartum if the mother was treated with oral medication, and 3–4 weeks after birth if she was treated with long-acting neuroleptic injections.[61] It has been reported that EPS in the neonate reflect a familial predisposition or drug dosage.[61] Brazelton[100] noted some effects on weight and neurosensory early learning tasks in babies who had been exposed to neuroleptics *in utero*, but problems were thought to be limited to the immediate postnatal period. There is one report of neonatal jaundice and hyperbilirubinemia in a premature infant,[101] and another report of functional bowel obstruction.[102,103] A previous study by Kris and Carmichael[104] found no first-week abnormalities in bilirubin levels in babies who had been exposed to chlorpromazine.

Other potential neuroleptic effects on the neonate include increased crying and sucking, sluggish primitive reflexes, vasomotor instability, weakness, hypertonicity and increased

---

Box 11.7 *Effect of fetal metabolism on drug concentration*

1 Increased levels of free drug due to:
   • Decreased metabolism of immature liver enzymes
   • Decreased plasma protein concentration
2 Increased fetal sensitivity to drug effects due to underdeveloped central nervous system

Source: Seeman.[68]

---

crying.[105,106] Desmond and colleagues[105] described the abnormal behavior as biphasic – decreased movement, crying and feeding difficulties characterized days 1–5, and from day 6 to month 7, behavior was noted to be agitated with excessive sucking, tremors and hyper-reflexia. Another fetal side-effect, namely respiratory depression, has been noted immediately postpartum in neonates whose mothers were treated with 500–600 mg/day of chlorpromazine in the third trimester.[89] This was not noted with lower doses or other neuroleptics. In another case report involving a mother who received 1800 mg of chlorpromazine daily, the infant was noted to show extreme apathy for several days after birth.[107]

Box 11.8 *Potential neuroleptic effects on neonate*

• Increased crying or sucking
• Sluggish primitive reflexes
• Vasomotor instability
• Weakness
• Hypertonicity

Sources: Brazelton,[100] Scokel and Jones.[101]

In addition to these immediate postpartum effects on the baby, a few studies have looked at long-term sequelae of neuroleptic exposure during pregnancy. Kris and Carmichael[104] followed babies for 4–5 years after birth who were exposed to 50–100 mg of chlorpromazine. These 52 babies were assessed as healthy with no behavioral or mental abnormalities, but the mode of assessment was not described. It should also be noted that the protocol was used on babies of mothers who had been treated with low doses of medication. Slone[108] prospectively followed 151 babies exposed to unspecified phenothiazines up to age 4 years and found that their IQs were equal to those of controls as well as of infants who were irregularly exposed to phenothiazines. Another study[109] reports significantly increased height and/or weight in children who were exposed to antipsychotic drugs *in utero*. These differences were noted at different points in development between 4 months and 7 years of age, and the size of the effect was positively correlated with the duration of exposure. The etiology was postulated to be related to eating behavior, growth hormone and/or motor activity.[61] Finally, in a case–control study of children exposed to antipsychotics *in utero* during the second half of pregnancy, the exposed children were found to show no difference in school behavior compared to the matched controls.[110] Due to the limited number of controlled studies and problems with controlling for confounding variables, the issue of behavioral teratogenicity due to neuroleptics is not clearly established in humans. In animal studies, neuroleptics have been noted to cause persistent learning and memory abnormalities,[111–114] although there is at least one conflicting study.[115] To date, there have been no reports of animal teratogenicity with clozapine.[61]

Anticholinergic medication

A review of the medication effects of neuroleptics on the fetus would not be complete without including the anticholinergic medications that are frequently used to control antipsychotic side-effects. Again, the existing literature is limited. Diphenhydramine has not been found to be a teratogen in animal studies. In a review of the safety of anti-emetics for hyperemesis gravidarum, Leathem suggests that benadryl has a low risk.[116] However, some reports of congenital anomalies exist.[117,118] In addition, there has been one report of a possible neonatal withdrawal syndrome associated with third-trimester diphenhydramine use, characterized by diarrhea and tremulousness.[119] The combination of diphenhydramine and benzodiazepines near term has also been associated with stillbirth in one report.[120]

Amantadine, another medication used to control extrapyramidal symptoms, has been noted to cause congenital anomalies in animals, and it poses a high risk for organ dysgenesis.[121–123] However in humans, only one case report has documented a possible association with amantadine and a cardiovascular malformation.[124] Finally, a possible association between the use of trihexyphenidyl and benztropine and congenital malformation has been reported in one study.[123] Thus antiparkinsonian agents should be avoided in pregnancy. In patients with extrapyramidal side-effects, the use of lower-potency antipsychotic medication or calcium supplementation should be considered.[122]

Beta-blockers

Beta-blockers constitute an additional class of medication that is used to treat neuroleptic side-effects. They are most frequently used to manage akathisia. Propanolol and atenolol are most commonly used, and it is important to maintain adequate blood pressure and pulse while patients are on these medications. Beta-blockers have been reported to cause intrauterine growth retardation when used as antihypertensive treatment in non-psychiatric pregnant patients.[125] However, the findings of this retrospective analysis were not well supported by subsequent prospective studies.[126] Rubin, in his extensive review of the topic,[127] cites no evidence of teratogenesis reported for beta-blockers in 94 subjects. He does note two cases of neonatal bradycardia and hypoglycemia with no apparent lasting sequelae. Despite a few case series and retrospective analyses which suggest the possibility of adverse events, Rubin reviews the confounders in these studies and concludes that beta-blocker treatment of hypertension in pregnancy 'appears to improve the likelihood that the fetus will be normal, although it is still not clear whether such therapy specifically improves the outcome in patients with hypertension induced by pregnancy.'[127]

Breastfeeding

In addition to issues during pregnancy and delivery, medication management issues continue postpartum if the mother wishes to breastfeed her infant. Antipsychotics, like all psychotropic medications, are secreted into breast-milk.[128] Drug concentrations in breast-milk vary considerably. The effects of these agents on the neonate depend on the specific medication bioavailability and the maturity of the infant's brain, central nervous system and metabolism.[129] Breast-milk concentrations have been measured during lactation for several specific neuroleptic drugs, including thiothixenes,[130] haloperidol,[131,132] trifluoperazine and perphenazine[133] and clozapine.[134] In the case of clozapine, the level in breast-milk was more than twice the mother's blood level. This was attributed to higher lipid concentrations in breast-milk. A case study of four infants who were breastfed by mothers who were being treated with clozapine noted that two infants had no problems, while one infant became sedated and another developed agranulocytosis. The agranulocytosis resolved with discontinuation of breastfeeding.[94]

In a study by Whalley and colleagues,[135] breast-milk contained two-thirds the levels of haloperidol that were found in maternal serum. Infants of mothers taking 30 mg/day fed normally, were not sedated, and achieved the expected developmental milestones at 6 months and 1 year. No behavioral abnormalities were noted. However, Trixler and Tenyi note that haloperidol concentrations in milk appear to be higher than the concentrations of lower-potency antipsychotics.[136] Because there are no data clarifying the effects of these drugs on the developing brain, patients who require antipsychotic medication should be advised about the risks and benefits and consider deferring breastfeeding until the possible risks to the fetus are better understood.[129] If a mother still elects to breastfeed, the infant should be closely watched for symptoms of toxicity. Drug concentrations both in breast-milk and in the baby should be rigorously monitored.[137]

ASSESSMENT OF PARENTING SKILLS AND EDUCATION

The mother with schizophrenia typically has few internal or external resources to help her deal with the challenges of motherhood. In a study of 100 consecutive admissions to a mother and baby unit in England, the main problem hindering competent parenthood was maternal lack of insight or inability to concentrate and sustain consistently safe behavior. In total, 50% of schizophrenic mothers were separated from their infants at discharge. In some cases, voluntary fostering arrangements were made with relatives. Even in these cases, only one mother was able to regain custody of her child.[30] This poor outcome may have been influenced by the fact that only 30% of schizophrenic mothers were returning to a home and partner, and only 35% were being discharged to a non-supervisory setting (compared to 70% of affective disorder patients returning home with a partner). The data from another study of a mother and baby unit were consistent with Kumar's work, showing that approximately 50% of schizophrenic mothers lost custody of their babies.[40] Both reports were generated from inpatient settings, so those schizophrenic mothers who do not require hospitalization during the puerperium may have had higher rates of maintaining custody. Further research on outcome in more stable schizophrenic outpatients is needed.

Despite the high percentage of inpatient schizophrenic mothers who do not retain custody of their babies, the assessment of parental competency and the provision of rehabilitation of parenting skills in the mentally ill mother are rarely addressed in the psychiatric, obstetric and pediatric literature. The legal definition of parental competency has historically been restricted to capacity to provide for a child's minimal needs for physical sustenance, such as food, shelter and clothing.[138] If the mother has a planned pregnancy and receives prenatal care, her capacity to care for her infant can be assessed longitudinally throughout the pregnancy. In this situation, the patient can be referred for parenting education if this is indicated. An interdisciplinary team should perform ongoing assessments and make recommendations for custody prior to delivery.

Stewart and Gangbar have commented on the useful, although longitudinally incomplete, assessment of the schizophrenic mother and her baby while hospitalized postpartum. They suggest that there should be a focus on more measurable issues, such as housing, ability to obtain and prepare food, ability to access social resources and capacity to maintain hygiene and cleanliness.[139] More specifically, observation of the mother's current mental state, capacity to learn, ability to respond to her baby's non-verbal cues and capacity to function within her social system may help to predict the environment of the baby after discharge. Observation of the maternal–infant interaction postpartum can also be useful when making such an assessment.[140] Rudolph suggests the use of the Nursing Child Assessment Feeding Scale (NCAST) as one objective measure of child-care ability.[22]

In addition, an assessment of social support and parenting history is useful when determining the mother's capacity to care for her child.[139] A check-list of parenting history could include the number of pregnancies, the number of children and their ages, and the number of abortions, as well as the legal custodian of the children. Other factors to be considered would include history of dangerous behavior, and history of child neglect or abuse, or substance use.[22]

Box 11.9 *Hospital assessment of parental competency*

History:
- Parental history
- Social support
- Housing
- Capacity to obtain/prepare food
- Ability to access social resources

Observation:
  Ability to respond to non-verbal cues from infant
- Ability to maintain hygiene/cleanliness
- Ability to learn and carry out functions necessary to provide for infant's needs

Source: Stewart *et al.*[139]

Although useful initially, hospital evaluation is longitudinally limited, and the need for ongoing support, evaluation and rehabilitation for the schizophrenic mother is a critical although rarely addressed issue. The need for increased resources in parental rehabilitation is reflected in a report on a 1990 national survey of state mental health authorities. The authors found that only 69 programs in 19 states addressed parenting skills, despite one report that 45% of mentally ill women under the age of 35 years have children under the age of 18 years. Only nine of these programs focused specifically on the mentally ill mother's evaluation and needs (as opposed to those of the child) and addressed training in parenting skills.[141] Nicholson and Blanch have described the need for rehabilitation for mentally ill parents. They delineate a comprehensive program which should include parental assessment (caregiving skills/relationship skills/cognitive capacity), skills development (parenting, medication compliance, social interaction) and support development (peer, parental, professional).[138] Because mentally ill adults have the normal desires for intimacy and procreation, the successful accomplishment of this life role would be facilitated by the development of such programs.

Box 11.10 *Comprehensive rehabilitation for mentally ill parents*

- Parental assessment (caregiving and relationship skills, cognitive capacity)
- Skills development (parenting, medication compliance, social interaction)
- Support development (peer, parental, professional)

Source: Nicholson *et al.*[138]

Although a comprehensive approach is a goal, the implementation of programs is limited by funding and social service structures. One program described by Waldo and colleagues in 1987 outlines a supplemental program called the Denver Mothers and Childrens Project.[142] This program makes extensive use of volunteer mothers to run a program that focuses on schizophrenic mothers and their infants. Groups that use directed play and role-modeling as well as developmental education have been noted to improve mother–infant interaction as well as maternal symptoms. Although they did not define the methodology for assessing the interaction, they did report a decrease in the number of children in foster care. Maternal improvement is defined by a marked decrease in hospitalization in 83% of participating mothers. Several other programs have been reported in the literature,[143–146] but in general this is an area which needs development if schizophrenic women who wish to have children are to optimize their potential for success in the parental role.

GENERAL SUMMARY AND GUIDELINES

This chapter ends with a final summary of education and treatment of the pregnant schizophrenic woman. Treatment begins with the primary intervention provided by education and family planning. An initial evaluation of all patients should include a complete sexual history and physical examination in order to assess the woman's problems and needs. Contraception, if desired, will probably be most successful if the method selected is easy to use and has extended effects, thus requiring minimal attention and executive functioning (which is often impaired in these patients). Suitable examples would include an intrauterine device, medroxyprogesterone, or other long-acting hormonal methods (e.g. levonorgestrel). If a patient is switched from a traditional neuroleptic to an atypical antipsychotic, she should be advised of the possibility of an increased likelihood of becoming pregnant if she is not currently using any form of birth control. If the woman chooses an oral contraceptive, it should be noted that external estrogens have been associated with an increase in parkinsonian symptoms. Estrogens may also potentiate some neuroleptics.[147]

In addition, the risks of sexually transmitted diseases (STDs) and education regarding the reduction of this risk should be assessed and discussed with all patients. If the need is indicated, the patient should receive education about STD risks and the means of avoiding such risks. Periodic screening for pregnancy and HIV status may be indicated in some patients who show high-risk behavior. In addition, due to the high incidence of rape and physical abuse in these patients, there should be ongoing assessment for evidence of abuse. Individual educational efforts can be augmented by group education which should emphasize a concrete behavior-oriented approach to educating patients about condoms and other methods of avoiding STDs. All of these decisions require evaluation of a patient's competence to make decisions at the time of the interview, as well as ongoing evaluation over the course of the illness. Attention to and compliance with this aspect of treatment could be enhanced by the availability of a consultation service in the mental health clinic to improve access to reproductive services.

If a pregnancy is planned, with adequate time for consultation, the potential heritability of the mental illness, as well as the potential risks of medication effects on the fetus and the impact of pregnancy on maternal mental health, can be discussed in detail with the patient. Planning can allow for a trial of minimizing medication as well as consideration of the least potentially toxic medication before pregnancy ensues. Periodic pregnancy tests may be required based on the patient's sexual and abuse history, menstrual history and medication compliance history. A serum beta-subunit human chorionic gonadotropin assay (β-HCG), physical examination and detailed history should be obtained to confirm any positive urine tests.[61]

Once pregnancy is confirmed, the patient's thoughts and concerns about the pregnancy should be clarified. Her obstetric history, parenting history and social support should all be assessed in order to facilitate decision-making. If the patient wishes, and if there is a partici-pating spouse/partner involved, he should also be included in this process. If the patient wishes to continue the pregnancy, prenatal care should include a risk–benefit assessment of continued treatment with antipsychotic medication. Based on a solely pharmacologic perspective of safety for the fetus, it is best to withhold treatment in the first 4–10 weeks, during organogenesis.[61] However, due to the usual extreme morbidity of untreated illness in this population (which could include severe decompensation that could potentially endanger the lives of both the mother and the fetus), the mother will probably need continued medica-tion treatment during the pregnancy. Nurnberg and colleagues have identified several situa-tions which would indicate the need for psychotropic medication during pregnancy in the schizophrenic woman. These include, but are not limited to, 'inability to care for herself or to provide proper prenatal care; impaired reality testing to the extent that she may be danger-ous to herself or others; manifests disorganized thoughts or behavior; and perception is unresponsive to supportive interventions up to and including hospitalization.'[88] If the mother has a history of instability when she is not taking medication, continuing treatment is proba-bly the best course of action. The lowest possible dose of medication (especially in the first 4–10 weeks post-conception) is recommended. Due to the risk of neonatal extrapyramidal symptoms, some authors suggest discontinuing the antipsychotic for up to 2 weeks before the estimated date of confinement.[128,129] Again, the risks and benefits of treatment must be continually evaluated due to the high risk of decompensation in this population.

Box 11.11 *Indications for medication during pregnancy in the schizophrenic woman*

- Inability to provide self-care
- Inability to comply with prenatal care
- Impaired reality causing potential danger to self or others
- Disorganized thoughts or behavior
- Problems that are unresponsive to supportive interventions

Source: Nurnberg *et al.*[88]

The medication treatment should probably be a higher-potency, non-aliphatic neurolep-tic. If ongoing review of the atypical antipsychotic literature begins to indicate safety during pregnancy, the use of atypical antipsychotics during gestation may eventually be recom-mended. The potential risk of agranulocytosis and seizures in both baby and mother associ-ated with clozapine use, as well as its association with orthostasis and hypotension, restrict the potential of this drug for use during pregnancy. If the mother requires medication and is stable at the time of conception, it may be best to maintain her on the current antipsychotic, since no single drug (with the possible exception of the aliphatic neuroleptics) appears to confer any disadvantage over others. Due to their prolonged side-effects, some authors have discouraged the use of depot neuroleptics, preferring the use of other measures to ensure compliance.[56] However, it would be wise to review the literature on the specific drug at the time when pregnancy is diagnosed, in order to inform the mother, and any invited family members in as much detail as possible. Prophylactic antiparkinsonian agents are not recommended. Miller advocates the use of calcium supplementation as an alternative method of preventing extrapyramidal symptoms.[148,122]

Apart from pharmacologic issues, the pregnant schizophrenic woman should undergo an early assessment of her capacity to meet the nutritional, parenting and housing needs of her unborn child. Contact with social services should be initiated as soon as possible, so that any resources that are available for the mother and baby can be mobilized by the time of the birth. Parenting skills classes that utilize a behavioral skills approach should be useful not only for educating the mother, but also for assessing her capacity to learn the skills necessary to feed, bathe and nurture her baby.

If the pregnant woman is under- or unmedicated at the time of presentation, an assessment of her competency and need for inpatient treatment will need to be made. If she is decompensated and unable to participate voluntarily in adequate prenatal care, thus putting the fetus at risk, the need for legal intervention will also need to be ascertained. Medication treatment, combined with a supportive alliance, may facilitate her co-operation with medical monitoring during pregnancy. In some cases, involuntary hospitalization with court-mandated medical and prenatal care may be necessary. Worsening of psychiatric symptoms during pregnancy requires a thorough evaluation to rule out infection, electrolyte abnormalities, toxic substances and other organic causes.[129] Collaboration between the psychiatrist and the obstetrician and/or gynecologist will be necessary in order to identify potential problems. In women who display psychotic denial of the pregnancy, Miller suggests hospitalization for acute crises. Due to the risk of precipitous birth in these patients, she also recommends hospitalization at the end of the third trimester. Indications for hospitalization for all pregnant schizophrenic women would include, but are not limited to, inability to meet nutritional needs during pregnancy or prenatal care, the possibility of precipitous delivery, any threat of violence towards the fetus, and any attempt to self-harm or perform premature self-delivery.[61]

Box 11.12 *Indications for hospitalization of the pregnant woman*

- Inability to meet nutritional needs, or poor prenatal care
- Possibility of precipitous delivery
- Threat of violence towards fetus
- Any attempt to self-harm or precipitate premature self-delivery

Source: Miller.[61]

Obstetric care of the schizophrenic woman during pregnancy may need to include more frequent monitoring, depending on the mother's previous pregnancy history, social support, current and baseline mental state, and any specific problems associated with this particular pregnancy. One program utilizes a psychiatric/obstetric nursing team for weekly home visits.[149] Techniques that are useful with these patients during examinations include the use of a concrete educational approach and specific directed questions about important symptoms (e.g. vaginal secretions, bleeding, etc.). Such methods should improve compliance and communication of important information, since schizophrenic patients may have impaired cognitive and executive functioning which could hinder their capacity to volunteer information. Plans for other children and options for birth control after delivery can be discussed at this time. If the pregnant woman is competent and wishes to have a tubal ligation after delivery, discussion during the early phase of the pregnancy allows her adequate time for decision-making.

When the patient is close to the estimated delivery date, closer monitoring may be necessary. Some reports suggest that pregnant schizophrenic women have a higher pain threshold and may have difficulty in recognizing and communicating the signs of labor onset.[61] The use of a psychiatric clinical nurse specialist during labor and delivery may help labor and delivery staff in their interactions with the patient.[149] Because each patient varies in her expression of illness, an adequate history should be taken and an ongoing analysis of symptoms should be made throughout all phases of the pregnancy and delivery. After delivery, the mother's psychotic symptoms should be optimally treated, especially in view of the increased risk of decompensation postpartum. Prior to discharge, future birth control (if it was not decided during pregnancy) can be discussed and initiated if the mother so wishes. Breastfeeding the baby is typically discouraged, since antipsychotic medication is present in maternal breast-milk and the effect of medication on the developing brain is unknown. The mother should be closely monitored for social stressors and signs of decompensation after delivery. Continued parenting skills classes and group support have been found to be useful in other populations of schizophrenic women after delivery.[138,150]

After birth, the neonate should receive a regular examination with extra attention being paid to the presence of any EPS and problems with respiration or elimination. If EPS are diagnosed in the neonate, they can be treated with diphenhydramine elixir.[61,97,99] If the baby fails to pass meconium or develops abdominal distension, a gastrograffin enema has been suggested by Miller[122] to differentiate between antipsychotic side-effects and gastrointestinal atresia and Hirschsprung's disease.[102,122]

If the issues of custody and parenting skills were not addressed prior to delivery, the baby and mother should both be observed in the hospital. Maternal parenting history, physical resources, social support and maternal interaction with the baby can all be evaluated prior to discharge from the hospital. However, it may be difficult to mobilize any necessary social services support at short notice. In addition, this cross-sectional evaluation should be further augmented by ongoing support and assessment after discharge. If the mother is not thought to be capable of caring for her baby, social services must be contacted. Alternatives to maternal custody may include placement of the baby with a close relative until the mother stabilizes and/or is trained in necessary parenting skills.

In conclusion, treatment of the schizophrenic patient during pregnancy involves multiple medical and social decisions. Optimal management will most probably be achieved by systems integration and the inclusion of sexual education, family planning and parenting skills programs in a single facility.[11] Each patient varies in her expression of the illness and must be individually assessed with a risk/benefit evaluation in order to determine appropriate treatment management. Attention to ongoing communication and education in this population can facilitate the capacity of the schizophrenic woman to successfully carry out an important life role.

REFERENCES

1. Coverdale J, Aruffo J, Grunebaum H. Developing family planning services for female chronic mentally ill outpatients. *Hospital and Community Psychiatry* 1992; **43**: 475–8.
2. Coverdale JH, Turbott SH, Roberts H. Family planning needs and STD risk behaviours of female psychiatric out-patients. *British Journal of Psychiatry* 1997; **171**: 69–72.
3. Coverdale JH, Bayer TL, McCullough LB, Chervenak FA. Respecting the autonomy of chronic mentally ill women in decisions about contraception. *Hospital and Community Psychiatry* 1993; **44**: 672.

4. McCullough LB, Coverdale J, Bayer T, Chervenak FA. Ethically justified guidelines for family planning interventions to prevent pregnancy in female patients with chronic mental illness. *American Journal of Obstetrics and Gynecology* 1992; **167**: 19–25.

5. Coverdale JH, Aruffo JA. Family planning needs of female chronic psychiatric outpatients. *American Journal of Psychiatry* 1989; **146**: 1489–91.

6. Coverdale JH, McCullough LB, Chervenak FA. Sexually transmitted diseases and unwanted pregnancies in chronically ill psychiatric patients. *Medical Journal of Australia* 1997; **166**: 231–2.

7. Carmen E, Brady SM. AIDS risk and prevention for the chronic mentally ill. *Hospital and Community Psychiatry* 1990; **41**: 652–7.

8. Lukoff D, Gioia-Hasick D, Sullivan G, Golden JS, Nuechterlein KH. Sex education and rehabilitation with schizophrenic male outpatients. *Schizophrenia Bulletin* 1986; **12**: 669–76.

9. Solomon MZ, DeJong W. Preventing AIDS and other STDs through condom promotion: a patient education intervention. *American Journal of Public Health* 1989; **79**: 453–8.

10. Berman C, Rozensky RH. Sex education for the chronic psychiatric patient: the effects of a sexual-issues group on knowledge and attitudes. *Psychosocial Rehabilitation Journal* 1984; **8**: 28–34.

11. Miller LJ. Comprehensive care of pregnant mentally ill women. *Journal of Mental Health Administration* 1992; **19**: 170–6.

12. Harper PS. *Practical genetic counseling*. Bristol: Wright and Sims, 1988.

13. McGuffin P, Owen M, O'Donovan M, Thapar A, Gottesman II. *Genetic Counseling and Ethical Issues. Seminars in Psychiatric Genetics*, London: Galkell Press, 1994.

14. Moldin SO. Psychiatric genetic counseling. In: Guze SB (ed.) *Washington University Adult Psychiatry*. St Louis, MO: Mosby, 1996: 365–81.

15. Asherman P, Mant R, McGuffin P. Genetics and schizophrenia. In: Hirsch SR, Weinberger DR (eds) *Schizophrenia*. Oxford: Blackwell Science Ltd, 1995: 253–74.

16. Gottesman II. *Schizophrenia genesis. Origins of madness*. San Francisco, CA: WH Freeman, 1991.

17. Faraone SV, Tsuang MT, Tsuang DW. Clinical applications of psychiatric genetics. *Genetics of mental disorders*. New York: Guilford Press, 1997: 159–95.

18. Bleuler E. *Dementia praecox of the group of schizophrenias*. New York: J. Zinkin, 1950.

19. Yarden PE, Suranyi I. The early development of institutionalized children of schizophrenic mothers. *Diseases of the Nervous System* 1968; **29**: 380–4.

20. Trixler M, Gati A, Tenyi T. Risks associated with childbearing in schizophrenia. *Acta Psychiatrica Scandinavica* 1995; **95**: 159–62.

21. Curran D. Psychiatric indications for the termination of pregnancy. *New Zealand Medical Journal* 1961; **60**: 467–9.

22. Rudolph B, Larson GL, Sweeney S, Hough EH, Arorian K. Hospitalized pregnant psychotic women: characteristics and treatment issues. *Hospital and Community Psychiatry* 1990; **41**: 159–63.

23. Spielvogel A, Wile J. Treatment of the psychotic pregnant patient. *Psychosomatics* 1986; **27**: 487–92.

24. Miller LJ, Finnerty M. Sexuality, pregnancy, and childrearing among women with schizophrenia-spectrum disorders. *Psychiatric Services* 1996; **47**: 502–6.

25. Carmack BJ, Corwin TA. Nursing care of the schizophrenic maternity patient during labor. *American Journal of Maternal Child Nursing* 1980; **5**: 107–13.

26. Targum SD. Dealing with psychosis during pregnancy. *American Pharmacy* 1979; **19**: 18–21.

27. Burgess HA. Schizophrenia in pregnancy. *Issues in Health Care of Women* 1980; **2**: 61–9.

28. Davies A, McIvor RJ, Kumar RC. Impact of childbirth on a series of schizophrenic mothers: a comment on the possible influence of oestrogen on schizophrenia. *Schizophrenia Research* 1995; **16**: 25–31.

29. McNeil TF. A prospective study of postpartum psychoses in a high-risk group. *Acta Psychiatrica Scandinavica* 1986; **74**: 205–16.
30. Kumar R, Marks M, Platz C, Yoshida K. Clinical survey of a psychiatric mother and baby unit: characteristics of 100 consecutive admissions. *Journal of Affective Disorders* 1995; **33**: 11–22.
31. McNeil TF, Kaij L, Malmquist-Larsson A. Women with nonorganic psychosis: pregnancy's effect on mental health during pregnancy. *Acta Psychiatrica Scandinavica* 1984; **70**: 140–8.
32. Yarden PE, Max DM, Eisenbach Z. The effect of childbirth on the prognosis of married schizophrenic women. *British Journal of Psychiatry* 1966; **112**: 491–9.
33. Winfield I, George LK, Swartz M, Blazer DG. Sexual assault and psychiatric disorders among a community sample of women. *American Journal of Psychiatry* 1990; **147**: 335–41.
34. McEvoy JP, Hatcher A, Appelbaum PS, Abernathy V. Chronic schizophrenic women's attitudes toward sex, pregnancy, birth control and childrearing. *Hospital and Community Psychiatry* 1983; **34**: 536–9.
35. Zynep Y, Akin I, Tahir Y, Levent E, Cemalettin A. A woman who did her own cesarean section. *Lancet* 1996; **348**: 135.
36. Condon JT. The spectrum of fetal abuse in pregnant women. *Journal of Nervous and Mental Diseases* 1986; **174**: 509–16.
37. Resnick PJ. Murder of the newborn: a psychiatric review of neonaticide. *American Journal of Psychiatry* 1970; **126**: 1414–20.
38. Brozovsky M, Falit H. Neonaticide: clinical and psychodynamic considerations. *Journal of the American Academy of Child and Adolescent Psychiatry* 1971; **10**: 673–83.
39. Spielvogel A, Wile J. Treatment and outcomes of psychotic patients during pregnancy and childbirth. *Birth* 1992; **19**: 131–7.
40. Miller LJ. Psychotic denial of pregnancy: phenomenology and clinical management. *Hospital and Community Psychiatry* 1990; **41**: 1233–7.
41. Reider RO, Rosenthal D, Wender P *et al*. The offspring of schizophrenics. Fetal and neonatal deaths. *Archives of General Psychiatry* 1975; **32**: 200–11.
42. Modrzewska K. The offspring of schizophrenic parents in a North Swedish isolate. *Clinical Genetics* 1980; **17**: 191–201.
43. McNeil TF, Kaij L, Malmquist-Larsson A. Women with nonorganic psychosis: factors associated with pregnancy's effect on mental health. *Acta Psychiatrica Scandinavica* 1984; **70**: 209–19.
44. Cohler BJ, Gallant DH, Grunebaum HU, Weiss JL, Gamer E. Pregnancy and birth complications among mentally ill and well mothers and their children. *Social Biology* 1975; **22**: 269–78.
45. Zax M, Sameroff AJ, Babigian HM. Birth outcomes in the offspring of mentally disordered women. *American Journal of Orthopsychiatry* 1977; **47**: 218–30.
46. Wrede G, Mednick SA, Huttunen MO, Nielsson CG. Pregnancy and delivery complications in the births of an unselected series of Finnish children with schizophrenic mothers. *Acta Psychiatrica Scandinavica* 1980; **62**: 369–81.
47. Sacker A, Done DJ, Crow TJ. Obstetric complications in children born to parents with schizophrenia: a meta-analysis of case–control studies. *Psychological Medicine* 1996; **26**. 279–87.
48. Bennedsen BE. Adverse pregnancy outcome in schizophrenic women: occurrence and risk factors. *Schizophrenia Research* 1998; **33**: 1–26.
49. Marcus J, Hans SL, Auerbach JG, Auerbach AG. Children at risk for schizophrenia: the Jerusalem infant development study. *Archives of General Psychiatry* 1993; **50**: 797–809.
50. Erlenmeyer-Kimling L, Cornblatt B. Biobehavioral risk factors in children of schizophrenic parents. *Journal of Autism and Development Disorder* 1984; **14**: 357–74.
51. Walker E, Emory E. Infants at risk for psychopathology: offspring of schizophrenic parents. *Child Development* 1983; **54**: 1269–85.
52. Fish B, Marcus J, Hans SL, Auerbach JG, Perdue S. Infants at risk for schizophrenia: sequelae of a genetic neurointegrative defect. *Infants and Schizophrenia* 1992; **49**: 221–35.

53. Fish B. Neurobiological antecedents of schizophrenia in children: evidence for an inherited, congenital neurointegrative defect. *Archives of General Psychiatry* 1977; **34**: 1297–313.
54. Bergman AJ, Wolfson MA, Walker EF. Neuromotor functioning and behavior problems in children at risk for psychopathology. *Journal of Abnormal Child Psychology* 1997; **25**: 229–37.
55. McNeil TJ, Harty B, Blennow G, Cantor-Graae E. Neuromotor deviation in offspring of psychotic mothers: a selective developmental deficiency in two groups of children at heightened psychiatric risk? *Journal of Psychiatric Research* 1993; **27**: 39–54.
56. Amminger GP, Pape S, Rock D *et al*. Relationship between childhood behavioral disturbance and later schizophrenia in the New York High-Risk Project. *Amercian Journal of Psychiatry* 1999; **156**: 525–30.
57. Ott SL, Spinelli S, Rock D *et al*. The New York High-Risk Project: social and general intelligence in children at risk for schizophrenia. *Schizophrenia Research* 1998; **31**: 1–11.
58. Erlenmeyer-Kimling L, Cornblatt BA, Rock D *et al*. The New York High-Risk Project: anhedonia, attentional deviance, and psychopathology. *Schizophrenia Bulletin* 1993; **19**: 141–53.
59. Dworkin RH, Cornblatt BA, Friedman R *et al*. Childhood precursors of affective vs. social deficits in adolescents at risk for schizophrenia. *Schizophrenia Bulletin* 1993; **19**: 563–77.
60. Erlenmeyer-Kimling L, Cornblatt BA. A summary of attentional findings in the New York High-Risk Project. *Journal of Psychiatric Research* 1992; **26**: 405–26.
61. Miller LJ. Clinical strategies for the use of psychotropic drugs during pregnancy. *Psychiatric Medicine* 1991; **9**: 275–298.
62. Abernathy VD, Grunebaum H. Toward a family planning program in psychiatric hospitals. *American Journal of Public Health* 1972; **62**: 1638–46.
63. Carpenter Jr WT, Hanlon TE, Heinrichs DW *et al*. Continuous versus targeted medication in schizophrenic outpatients: outcome results. *American Journal of Psychiatry* 1990; **147**: 1138–48.
64. Yonkers KA, Kando JC, Cole JO, Blumenthal S. Gender differences in pharmacokinetics and pharmacodynamics of psychotropic medication. *American Journal of Psychiatry* 1992; **149**: 587–95.
65. Datz FL, Christian PE, Moore J. Gender-related differences in gastric emptying. *Journal of Nuclear Medicine* 1987; **28**: 1204–7.
66. Seeman MV. Neuroleptic prescriptions for men and women. *Social Pharmacology* 1989; **3**: 219–36.
67. Simpson GM, Yadalam KG, Levinson DF, Stephanos MJ, Lo ES, Cooper TB. Single-dose pharmacokinetics of fluphenazine after fluphenazine decanoate administration. *Journal of Clinical Psychopharmacology* 1990; **10**: 417–21.
68. Seeman MV. Interaction of sex, age and neuroleptic dose. *Comprehensive Psychiatry* 1983; **24**: 125–8.
69. Dawkins K, Potter WZ. Gender differences in pharmacokinetics and pharmacodynamics of psychotropics: focus on women. *Psychopharmacology Bulletin* 1991; **27**: 417–21.
70. Ereshefsky L, Saklad SR, Watanabe MD, Davis CM, Jann MW. Thiothixene pharmacokinetic interactions: a study of hepatic enzyme inducers, clearance inhibitors and demographic variables. *Journal of Clinical Psychopharmacology* 1991; **11**: 296–301.
71. Seeman MV, Lang M, Rector N. Chronic schizophrenia: a risk factor for HIV? *Canadian Journal of Psychiatry* 1990; **35**: 765–8.
72. Chouinard G, Annable L, Collu R. Plasma prolactin levels: a psychiatric tool. In Collu R, Ducharme JR, Tolis G, Barbeau A (eds) *Brain peptides and hormones*. New York: Raven Press, 1982: 333–41.
73. Stowe ZN, Nemeroff CB. Psychopharmacology during pregnancy and lactation. In: Schatzberg AF, Nemeroff CB (eds) *American psychiatric press textbook of psychopharmacology*. Washington, DC; American Psychiatric Press, 1998: 823–37.

74. Moya F, Thorndyde V. Passage of drugs across the placenta. *American Journal of Obstetrics and Gynecology* 1962; **84**: 1778–98.

75. Hanson JW, Oakley GP Jr. Haldol and limb deformity. *Journal of the American Medical Association* 1975; **231**: 26.

76. Kopelman AE, McCullar FW, Heggeness L. Limb malformations following maternal use of haloperidol. *Journal of the American Medical Association* 1975; **231**: 62–4.

77. Van Waes A, Van De Velde E. Safety evaluation of haloperidol in the treatment of hyperemesis gravidarum. *Journal of Clinical Pharmacology* 1969; **9**: 224–7.

78. Milkovich L, van den Berg BJ. An evaluation of the teratogenicity of certain anti-nausea drugs. *American Journal of Obstetrics and Gynecology* 1976; **125**: 244–8.

79. Moriarty AJ, Nance NR. Trifluoperazine and pregnancy. *Canadian Medical Association Journal* 1963; **88**: 375–6.

80. Rawlings WJ, Ferguson R, Maddison TG. Phenmertazine and trifluoperazine. *Medical Journal of Australia* 1963; **1**: 370.

81. Rumeau-Rouquette C, Goujard J, Huel G. Possible teratogenic effect of phenothiazines in human beings. *Teratology* 1977; **15**: 57–64.

82. Godet PF, Marie-Cardine M. Neuroleptiques, schizophrenie et grossesse: étude epidemiologique et teratologique. *Encephale* 1991; **17**: 543–7.

83. Slone D, Siskind V, Heinonen RP, Monson RR, Kaufman D, Shapiro S. Antenatal exposure to the phenothiazines in relation to congenital malformations, perinatal mortality rate, birth weight, and intelligence quotient score. *American Journal of Obstetrics and Gynecology* 1977; **128**: 486–8.

84. Ananth J. Congenital malformations with psychopharmacologic agents. *Comprehensive Psychiatry* 1975; **16**: 437–45.

85. Coyle I, Wagner MJ, Singer G. Behavioral teratogenesis: a critical evaluation. *Pharmacology, Biochemistry and Behavior* 1976; **4**: 191–200.

86. Ayd FJ. Children born to mothers treated with chlorpromazine during pregnancy. *Clinical Medicine* 1964; **71**: 1758–63.

87. Kris EB. Children of mothers maintained on pharmacotherapy during pregnancy and postpartum. *Current Therapeutic Reearch* 1965; **7**: 785–9.

88. Nurnberg HG, Prudic J. Guidelines for treatment of psychosis during pregnancy. *Hospital and Community Psychiatry* 1984; **35**: 67–71.

89. Sobel DE. Fetal damage due to ECT, insulin coma and chlorpromazine. *Archives of General Psychiatry* 1960; **2**: 606–11.

90. Altshuler LL, Cohen L, Szuba MP, Burt VK, Gitlin M, Mintz J. Pharmacologic management of psychiatric illness during pregnancy: dilemmas and guidelines. *American Journal of Psychiatry* 1996; **153**: 592–606.

91. Dickson RA, Edwards A. Clozapine and fertility. *American Journal of Psychiatry* 1997; **154**: 582–3.

92. Waldman MD, Safferman AZ. Pregnancy and clozapine. *American Journal of Psychiatry* 1993; **150**: 168–9.

93. Lieberman J, Safferman AZ. Clinical profile of clozapine: adverse reactions and agranulocytosis. *Psychiatric Quarterly* 1992; **63**: 51–70.

94. Dev V, Krupp P. The side-effects and safety of clozapine. *Reviews of Contemporary Pharmacotherapy* 1995; **6**: 197–208.

95. Harer WB. Chlorpromazine in normal labour. *Obstetrics and Gynecology* 1956; **8**: 1–9.

96. Goodner DM, Arnas GM, Andros GJ, Waterhouse RB. Psychogenic polydipsia causing acute water intoxication in pregnancy at term. *Obstetrics and Gynecology* 1971; **37**: 873–6.

97. O'Connor MO, Johnson GH, James DI. Intrauterine effect of phenothiazines. *Medical Journal of Australia* 1981; **1**: 416–17.

98. Tamer A, McKey R, Arias D, Worley L, Fogel BJ. Phenothiazine-induced extrapyramidal dysfunction in the neonate. *Journal of Pediatrics* 1969; **75**: 479–80.

99. Cleary MF. Fluphenazine decanoate during pregnancy. *American Journal of Psychiatry* 1977; **134**: 815–16.

100. Brazelton TB. Effect of prenatal drugs on the behaviour of the neonate. *American Journal of Psychiatry* 1970; **126**: 1261–6.

101. Scokel PW, Jones WN. Infant jaundice after phenothiazine drugs for labor: an enigma. *Obstetrics and Gynecology* 1962; **20**: 124–7.

102. Falterman CG, Richardson CJ. Small left colon syndrome associated with maternal ingestion of psychotropic drugs. *Journal of Pediatrics* 1980; **97**: 308–10.

103. Margulies AI, Berris B. Jaundice associated with the administration of trifluoperazine. *Canadian Medical Association Journal* 1968; **98**: 1063–4.

104. Kris E, Carmichael D. Chlorpromazine maintenance therapy during pregnancy and confinement. *Psychiatric Quarterly* 1957; **31**: 690–5.

105. Desmond MM, Rudolph AJ, Hill RM *et al.* Behavioral alterations in infants born to mothers on psychoactive medication during pregnancy. In; Farrell G (ed.) *Congenital mental retardation.* Austin, TX: University of Texas Press, 1969: 235–44.

106. Hauser LA. Pregnancy and psychiatric drugs. *Hospital and Community Psychiatry* 1985; **36**: 817–18.

107. Hammond JE, Toseland PA. Placental transfer of chlorpromazine. *Archives of Diseases in Childhood* 1970; **45**: 139–40.

108. Slone BR. The unwanted pregnancy. *New England Journal of Medicine* 1969; **280**: 1206–13.

109. Platt JE, Friedhoff AJ, Broman SH *et al.* Effects of prenatal exposure to neuroleptic drugs on children's growth. *Neuropsychopharmacology* 1988; **1**: 205–12.

110. Stika L, Elisova K, Honzakova L *et al.* Effects of drug administration in pregnancy on children's school behavior. *Pharmaceutish Weekblad (Scientific Edition)* 1990; **12**: 252–5.

111. Vorhees CV, Brunner RL, Butcher RE. Psychotropic drugs as behavioral teratogens. *Science* 1979; **205**: 1220–5.

112. Hoffeld DR, McNew J, Webster RL. Effect of tranquilizing drugs during pregnancy on activity of offspring. *Nature* 1968; **218**: 357–8.

113. Ordy JM, Samorajski T, Collins RL. Prenatal chlorpromazine effects on liver survival and behavior of mice offspring. *Journal of Pharmacology and Experimental Therapeutics* 1966; **151**: 110–25.

114. Robertson RT, Majka JA, Peter CP, *et al.* Effects of prenatal exposure to chlorpromazine on postnatal development and behavior of rats. *Toxicology and Applied Pharmacology* 1980; **53**: 541–9.

115. Dallemagne G, Weiss B. Altered behavior of mice following postnatal treatment with haloperidol. *Pharmacology, Biochemistry and Behavior* 1982; **16**: 761–7.

116. Leathem AM. Safety and effiacy of antiemetics used to treat nausea and vomiting in pregnancy. *Clinical Pharmacokinetics* 1986; **5**: 660–8.

117. Saxen I. Cleft palate and maternal diphenhydramine intake. *Lancet* 1974; **1**: 407–8.

118. Wisner KL, Perel JM. Psychopharmacologic agents and electroconvulsive therapy during pregnancy and the puerperium. In: Cohen RL (ed.) *Psychiatric consultation in childbirth settings: parent- and child-oriented approaches.* New York: Plenum, 1988: 165–206.

119. Parkin DE, Bliss RW. Probable benadryl withdrawal manifestations in a newborn infant. *Journal of Pediatrics* 1974; **85**: 580–1.

120. Kargas GA, Kargas SA, Bruyere J Jr, *et al.* Perinatal mortality due to interaction of diphenhydramine and temazepam. *New England Journal of Medicine* 1985; **313**: 14–17.

121. Hirsh MS, Swartz MN. Antiviral agents. *New England Journal of Medicine* 1980; **302**: 903–7.

122. Miller L, Martis B. Treating pregnant patients with psychotropic drugs. *Psychiatric Times* 1997; **14**: 31–2.

123. Heinonen OP, Slone D, Shapiro S. *Birth defects and drugs in pregnancy*. Littleton, MA: Publishing Services Group, 1977.
124. Nora JJ, Nora AH, Way GL. Cardiovascular maldevelopment associated with maternal exposure to amantadine. *Lancet* 1975; **2**: 607.
125. Pruyn SC, Phelan JP, Buchanan GC. Long-term propanolol therapy in pregnancy: maternal and fetal outcome. *American Journal of Obstetrics and Gynecology* 1979; **135**: 485–9.
126. Gallery EDM, Saunders DM, Hunyor SN, Gyory AZ. Randomized comparison of methyldopa and oxprenolol for treatment of hypertension in pregnancy. *British Medical Journal* 1979; **1**: 1591–4.
127. Rubin PC. Beta-blockers in pregnancy. *New England Journal of Medicine* 1981; **305**: 1325.
128. Calabrese JR, Gulledge AD. Psychotropics during pregnancy and lactation: a review. *Psychosomatics* 1985; **26**: 413–26.
129. Cohen LS, Heller VL, Rosenbaum JF. Treatment guidelines for psychotropic drug use in pregnancy. *Psychosomatics* 1989; **30**: 25–33.
130. Matheson I, Skjaeraasen J. Milk concentrations of flupenthixol, nortriptyline and zuclopenthixol and between-breast differences in two patients. *European Journal of Clinical Pharmacology* 1988; **35**: 217–20.
131. Woerner MG, Pollack M, Klein DF. Pregnancy and birth complications in psychiatric patients: a comparison of schizophrenic and personality disorder patients with their siblings. *Acta Psychiatrica Scandinavica* 1973; **49**: 712–21.
132. Grunebaum H, Cohler B, Kauffman C *et al.* Children of depressed and schizophrenic mothers. *Child Psychiatry and Human Development* 1978; **8**: 219–28.
133. Wilson JT, Brown RD, Cherek DR *et al.* Drug excretion in human breast milk: principles, pharmacokinetics and projected consequences. *Clinical Pharmacokinetics* 1980; **5**: 1–66.
134. Barnas C, Bergant A, Hummer M, Saria A, Fleischhacker WW. Clozapine concentrations in maternal and fetal plasma, amniotic fluid and breast milk. *American Journal of Psychiatry* 1994; **151**: 945.
135. Whalley IJ, Blain PG, Prim JK. Haloperidol secreted in breast milk. *British Medical Journal* 1981; **282**: 1746–7.
136. Trixler M, Tenyi T. Antipsychotic use in pregnancy. *Drug Safety* 1997; **16**: 403–10.
137. Goldberg HL, Nissem R. Psychotropic drugs in pregnancy and lactation. *International Journal of Psychiatry in Medicine* 1994; **24**: 129–49.
138. Nicholson J, Blanch A. Rehabilitation for parenting roles for people with serious mental illness. *Psychosocial Rehabilitation Journal* 1994; **18**: 109–19.
139. Stewart D, Gangbar R. Psychiatric assessment of competency to care for a new born. *Canadian Journal of Psychiatry* 1984; **29**: 583–9.
140. Persson-Blennow I, Naslund B, McNeil TF, Kaij L, Malmquist-Larsson A. Offspring of women with nonorganic psychosis: mother–infant interaction at three days of age. *Acta Psychiatrica Scandinavica* 1984; **70**: 149–59.
141. Nicholson J, Geller JL, Fisher WH, Dion CL. State policies and programs that address the needs of mentally ill mothers in the public sector. *Hospital and Community Psychiatry* 1993; **44**: 484–9.
142. Waldo MC, Roath M, Levine W, Freedman R. A model program to teach parenting skills to schizophrenic mothers. *Hospital and Community Psychiatry* 1987; **38**: 1110–12.
143. Goodman SH. Children of emotionally disturbed mothers: problems and alternatives. *Child Today* 1984; March-April: **13**: 6–9.
144. Cohler BJ, Musick J. *Intervention among psychiatrically impaired parents and their young children*. No. 24. Washington, DC: Jossey Bass, Inc., New Directions for Mental Health, 1984.
145. Grunbaum L, Gammeltoff M. Young children of schizophrenic mothers: difficulties of intervention. *American Journal of Orthopsychiatry* 1993; **63**: 16–27.
146. Liberman RP, Massel HK, Moch MD, Wong SE. Social skills training for chronic mental patients. *Hospital and Community Psychiatry* 1985; **36**: 396–403.

147. Jensvold MF. Non-pregnant reproductive-age women. Part II. Exogenous sex steroid hormones and psychopharmacology. In Jensvold MF, Halbreich U, Hamilton JA (eds) *Psychopharmacology and women: sex, gender, and hormones.* Washington, DC: American Psychiatric Press, 1996: 171–90.

148. Kuny S, Binswanger U. Neuroleptic-induced extrapyramidal symptoms and serum calcium levels. *Neuropsychobiology* 1989; **21**: 60–67.

149. Forcier KI. Management and care of pregnant psychiatric patients. *Journal of Psychosocial Nursing* 1990; **28**: 11–16.

150. Blanch AK, Nicholson J, Purcell J. Parents with severe mental illness and their children: the need for human services integration. *Journal of Mental Health Administration* 1994; **21**: 388–96.

12

The treatment and consequences of alcohol abuse and dependence during pregnancy

SHELLY F. GREENFIELD AND DAWN E. SUGARMAN

INTRODUCTION

Although no universally safe level of alcohol consumption has been identified, approximately 20% of all pregnant women will consume some alcohol during pregnancy.[1] Alcohol use during pregnancy can have adverse consequences for the pregnancy itself,[2] as well as a spectrum of harmful effects on the exposed offspring.[3] This chapter will review the epidemiology of alcohol use during pregnancy, the *in utero*, neonatal and long-term postnatal effects of alcohol exposure during pregnancy, and the role of prevention (including education and screening), as well as possible treatment for pregnant women who consume alcohol.

SCOPE OF THE PROBLEM

It is estimated that 2.6 million infants are born in the USA each year following significant intrauterine alcohol exposure, resulting in a wide range of abnormalities.[4] The total annual cost of fetal alcohol syndrome (FAS) alone is estimated to be 74.6 million dollars. About 75% of this cost is associated with the treatment and care of FAS-related mental retardation and

16% with the care of infants with low birth weight.[5,6] Costs of other alcohol-related abnor-malities are not included in this expenditure figure.

Approximately 60% of adult women in the USA have a drink containing alcohol at least occasionally. Most of these women consume small or moderate amounts of alcohol. However, it is significant that the rates of drinking and heavy drinking are highest among young women and decline with age.[1] According to the 1991–1993 and 1994–1995 National Household Surveys on Drug Abuse, an estimated 21.2% of pregnant women reported alcohol use in the past month.[7] The results of several other studies are consistent with this finding. For example, the 1989 National Longitudinal Survey of Youth, the 1991 Centers for Disease Control (CDC) Behavioral Risk Factors Surveillance Survey and the 1994 National Institute on Drug Abuse Pregnancy and Health Survey[1] all found that less than 25% of pregnant women reported any use of alcohol. Among pregnant women who drink alcohol, approximately 6–8% have serious alcohol-related problems.[8]

A number of sociodemographic characteristics have been associated with any alcohol use as well as heavy alcohol use during pregnancy.[9–11] One study compared 1712 pregnant women with 36 057 non-pregnant women and found that pregnant women consumed a lower median number of drinks per month (4.2) than non-pregnant women (8.7).[10] In the first year of the study, consumption was found to be more common among pregnant women who were smokers, unmarried, college graduates and between the ages of 35–45 years. However, alcohol use among the older and more educated pregnant women declined as the study continued, while levels of alcohol use remained high among the smokers and the unmarried subjects. This study also found that among the pregnant women, those who were smokers, unmarried and black reported drinking the highest number of drinks per month.[10] An earlier study reported that alcohol consumption during pregnancy was associated with having a male partner who drank.[11] Heavy drinking during pregnancy has also been found to be associated with older maternal age, high parity, low level of education, and unemployment of the father or present partner.[9]

Alcohol use during pregnancy can be associated with a number of serious health conse-quences for the pregnant woman, the fetus, and the newborn infant. We shall explore these consequences, as well as prevention and treatment in this chapter.

DRINKING DURING PREGNANCY – HEALTH CONSEQUENCES FOR THE MOTHER

Excessive alcohol consumption during pregnancy is associated with the possible development of many of the same medical complications as occur in the non-pregnant woman. These include nutritional deficiencies, gastritis, ulcer disease, pancreatitis, alcoholic hepatitis, alcoholic ketoacidosis, and cirrhosis of the liver.[12,13] Of course, any of these alcohol-induced medical problems can adversely affect the pregnancy and its outcome. It is important to note that women are generally more vulnerable to the negative consequences of alcohol consump-tion than are men because of gender differences in the way in which alcohol is metabo-lized.[13,14] For example, women have less alcohol dehydrogenase in the gastric mucosa than do men, thereby decreasing the amount of so-called 'first-pass metabolism' in women. Compared to men, women absorb a higher proportion of unmetabolized ethanol directly from the gastric mucosa. Because of this and other metabolic and physiologic factors, women experience a more rapid transition to both the medically and socially adverse consequences of drinking than do their male counterparts. This so-called 'telescoping effect' of alcohol problems among women has been well documented.[13,15] In addition to these more general effects on women's health status, excessive alcohol consumption may precipitate preterm labor,[12] and may contribute to deficient lactation in the postpartum period.[12]

IN UTERO EXPOSURE – EFFECTS ON THE DEVELOPING FETUS

Alcohol crosses the placenta. Therefore, when a pregnant woman drinks, the alcohol levels in the mother and the fetus equilibrate approximately 15 min after alcohol consumption.[2,16] In addition, the fetus has only a limited ability to metabolize alcohol because of a deficiency of the hepatic enzyme alcohol dehydrogenase, which is the primary pathway for alcohol metabolism. The fetus must therefore rely on passive diffusion across the placenta and maternal elimination of alcohol. Alcohol elimination from the amniotic fluid is approximately twice as slow as that from the maternal bloodstream. Thus the fetus is exposed to higher levels of alcohol for longer periods of time than the mother.[16] In addition, cigarette smoking may exacerbate the teratogenic effect of prenatal drinking.[2,17] This is of particular concern since findings from the 1997 National Household Survey on Drug Abuse indicate that around 40% of all current alcohol users have also smoked cigarettes in the past month.[18]

The risk of fetal abnormalities increases with the amount of alcohol consumed daily, and there appears to be no clear risk of abnormalities with less than 1 ounce of pure alcohol a day. However, the risk increases to 10% with 1 or 2 ounces, to 50% with 5 ounces, and to 75% with over 5 ounces.[2] The exact threshold is difficult to determine because there is a wide range of defects associated with prenatal alcohol exposure, and subtle effects often go unnoticed.[4,19]

The effects of alcohol may also vary with genetic susceptibility, gestational stage and dosage schedule.[20] Exposure to alcohol in the first trimester is associated with organ and musculoskeletal anomalies, while exposure in the second and third trimesters is associated with growth and intellectual and behavioral deficits.[16] In addition, the risk of adverse effects increases with maternal age.[21] It has been found that binge-drinking results in more severe deficits than continuous exposure to the same overall dose of alcohol.[1,16] Therefore the only safe drinking level that has been established is abstinence. In addition to alcohol consumption, other related factors influence the effects of *in utero* exposure to alcohol on the neonate, including maternal health and nutritional status, parity, timing of exposure to alcohol, and the use of other substances.[16]

EFFECTS OF ALCOHOL ON THE COURSE OF PREGNANCY AND ON THE NEONATE

Drinking during pregnancy has been associated with an increased risk of stillbirth and spontaneous abortion.[2] In one study, women who were heavy drinkers reported at least one clinically recognized spontaneous abortion at a rate 2 to 3 times higher than the general population.[22] While several other studies have reported an increase in spontaneous abortion[23,24] and low birth weight,[25] other studies have found weak[26] or no associations,[27,28] between alcohol consumption and these outcomes.[13] If the neonate survives past birth, it is at significant risk of demonstrating a wide range of abnormalities that range from severe disabilities to no apparent abnormalities.

One study found that 3–day-old infants that had been exposed prenatally to alcohol were more likely to have abnormal reflexes, heightened arousal, immature motor function, higher activity levels and an increased incidence of hypertonia and tremors. This study grouped the infants as follows according to the duration of maternal alcohol use during pregnancy: 'never', 'stopped' or 'continued'. The infants in the 'continued' group were more severely affected than those in the 'stopped' group. The authors did not specify during which trimesters of gestation the neonates were exposed.[22] Lower mental and motor development indices as measured by the Bayley's Scales of Infant Mental and Motor Development[29] have also been found in infants exposed to alcohol prenatally.[22,30] These infants may also exhibit irritability, tremulousness, poor sucking, inconsolable crying and hypertonia.[4]

LONG-TERM EFFECTS OF PRENATAL EXPOSURE TO ALCOHOL

The most severe abnormalities that result from prenatal exposure to alcohol are characterized as fetal alcohol syndrome (FAS). The less severe effects of fetal alcohol exposure are often categorized as fetal alcohol effects (FAE) and alcohol-related birth defects (ARBD). The distinction between these two terms is imprecise and confusing. The term 'fetal alcohol effects' is often used when alcohol is being considered as one of the possible causes of a child's birth defects.[19] Children with FAE usually have a less severe set of the symptoms associated with FAS.[31] In 1987 it was estimated that 36 000 infants per year were born with FAE, which was 10 times the number of those diagnosed with FAS.[11] A 1996 estimate indicated that 50 000 children showed symptoms of FAE, while 5000 children were born with FAS.[31] The term 'alcohol-related birth defects' commonly refers to anatomic or functional abnormalities attributed to prenatal alcohol exposure, including malformations (which can be cardiac, skeletal, renal, ocular or auditory).[1,19] Since FAE and ARBD are very broad and varied categories, this chapter will focus mainly on FAS.

It is estimated that FAS occurs in between 1 in 300 and 1 in 1000 births.[4] The Centers for Disease Control (CDC) report the incidence of FAS to be between 0.3 and 0.9 per 10 000 births, excluding Native Americans. The ethnic breakdown of FAS per 10 000 births is as follows: Asians, 0.3; Hispanics, 0.8; Whites, 0.9; Blacks, 6.0; Native Americans, 29.9. A higher prevalence was found in Southwest Plains Indians than in Navajo and Pueblo Indians. Suggested factors that may contribute to this difference include cultural influences, patterns of alcohol consumption and population differences in the baseline prevalence of alcohol use disorders, maternal nutrition and metabolic differences.[19]

The diagnostic criteria for FAS consists of three categories, namely growth retardation (below the tenth percentile in weight and/or length or height), central nervous system dysfunction and characteristic facial dysmorphology.[9,22,32,33]

More than 80% of children with a diagnosis of FAS show prenatal or postnatal growth deficiency.[34] The diagnostic criteria for FAS require at least one of the following for evidence of growth retardation: low birth weight for gestational age; decelerating weight over time not due to nutrition; and disproportionally low weight to height.[1] Low birth weight is defined as less than 2500 g and is prevalent in 77% of children with FAS.[22] Most children with FAS have growth deficiencies that persist throughout adolescence.[16,22] The median birth weight for children with FAS is 37% lower than the normal median birth weight.[22]

The central nervous system impairments that are characteristic of FAS include borderline intelligence or mental retardation, delayed attainment of motor skills, speech and language disorders, balance difficulties and attention deficit hyperactivity disorder behaviors.[35] The diagnostic criteria for FAS require at least one of the following for evidence of central nervous system neurodevelopmental abnormalities: decreased cranial size at birth, structural brain abnormalities (microcephaly, partial or complete agenesis of the corpus callosum, cerebellar hypoplasia); or neurological hard or soft signs (e.g. impaired fine motor skills, neurosensory hearing loss, poor tandem gait, or poor eye-hand coordination).[1]

Microcephaly, which is defined as less than 2.5 standard deviation units below the mean for head circumference, occurs in more than 80% of FAS infants and becomes more evident as the child grows older.[2,22] Around 50% of FAS children qualify as borderline mentally retarded,[2] and FAS is the leading known cause of mental retardation in the USA with 85% of children with FAS having some degree of mental retardation.[4] The IQ of a person with FAS can range from normal to severely mentally retarded.[1] Osborn and colleagues summarized several studies that examined the IQ ranges for people diagnosed with FAS or FAE.[16] One of these studies reported that the average IQ of 82 people with FAS who were tested as adolescents and adults was 70, which falls within the borderline to mildly retarded range. Another study of 20 children with FAS found a mean IQ of 65, with a range of 16–105.[16] A follow-up study of 24 children of alcoholic mothers found that six of the children attended a school for the mentally retarded and 11 children received some form of special education.[36]

Facial dysmorphology is the most unique identifier of FAS. The characteristic facial features associated with FAS are small palpebral fissure, flat maxillary area, poorly developed philtrum, epicanthal folds and a thin upper lip.[1,8,16] In one study, the medical records of 60 FAS patients revealed that the commonest facial features were long and flat philtrum (60%), low nasal bridge (52%), short palpebral fissures (42%), thin upper lip (30%) and midface hypoplasia (28%).[37]

The effects of prenatal alcohol exposure persist over time. Children with FAS may display a range of behavioral and emotional disorders, including hyperactivity, poor toilet training skills, a higher incidence of eating and sleeping problems, stereotypic behaviors and social immaturity.[2] As toddlers, children with FAS may exhibit clumsy and impulsive behavior, emotional lability, short attention span and easy distractibility.[6] Larroque and Kaminski found that children who had been exposed to a moderate amount of alcohol prenatally displayed developmental deficits at preschool age.[9] Compared to non-exposed children, these children showed an increased prevalence of the other features of FAS, such as minor neurological anomalies, facial dysmorphologies and shorter stature.

Another study examined 24 preadolescent children who had been exposed prenatally to abusive levels of alcohol consumption. Abusive levels were defined as the equivalent of a daily intake of 200 mL of hard liquor or more. It was found that the majority of these children had attention deficits and motor control problems. Learning disorders were also prevalent. The most severe problems were detected in children whose mothers abused alcohol throughout their pregnancy.[36] Other studies have also reported the association of attention deficit disorder (ADHD) in children and adolescents with prenatal alcohol exposure.[22] Steinhausen and Spohr assessed children with FAS at preschool, early school and late school age.[38] They found some persistent psychiatric disorders, including hyperkinetic disorders, emotional disorders, sleep disorders, and abnormal habits and stereotypes. One or more psychiatric disorders were present in 63% of the children.[38]

Research clearly shows that the effects of prenatal alcohol exposure can be serious, persistent, and irreversible. It is therefore important to educate women about the risks associated with alcohol use during pregnancy in order to prevent FAS and other associated syndromes.

PREVENTION

Fetal alcohol syndrome and other abnormalities associated with *in utero* exposure to alcohol are 100% preventable through elimination of the use of alcohol during pregnancy. Since some women consume alcohol before realizing that they are pregnant, it is important to educate a wide range of women, as well as their partners, about the risks of drinking alcohol during pregnancy. Educational programs on the risks of drinking alcohol, including the risks incurred by pregnant women, could be integrated into mandatory health curricula for elementary, junior-high and high-school students, as well as in colleges and adult centers of learning.

Within the health-care sector, obstetricians and gynecologists, general internists, family physicians, psychiatrists and other mental health clinicians, as well as clinical nurse practitioners and other health professionals who care for women, should increase their awareness of alcohol and its effects on women, pregnancy, the developing fetus and the infant and child after birth.[39] Since women with alcohol problems are more likely to be seen in non-alcohol-treatment settings than in alcohol-treatment facilities,[40] it is important for physical and mental health caregivers who see such women to take a careful alcohol history from all of their patients, and to be prepared to refer these patients to appropriate treatment settings if necessary.

In reviewing the health behaviors of all women of childbearing age, in addition to discussion of the other health risks posed by alcohol (e.g. liver disease, possible increased risk of breast cancer, etc.), clinicians should educate women about the risk to the fetus should a woman become pregnant. It is most helpful if women receive such education prior to considering or planning a pregnancy, so that they are aware of the risks and have the opportunity to discontinue alcohol use before becoming pregnant. In the case of an unwanted or unplanned pregnancy, women may be unaware that they are pregnant for at least part of the first trimester. In this case, it is appropriate to review the use of any medications or substances, including alcohol, that they have used during the initial part of the pregnancy, and they should receive counseling about the possible effects on the developing fetus. Clearly, at any time that a pregnancy is recognized and brought to the attention of a clinician, access to prenatal care is a high priority.

Women of childbearing age who abuse alcohol or are alcohol dependent should receive as part of any intervention education about the possible risk to a pregnancy and a developing fetus should they become pregnant. In some instances, women who are considering starting a family can use this as a powerful motivator to discontinue their alcohol use or to enter treatment. In addition, women of childbearing age with alcohol use disorders should be offered birth control information, referral, and access to community and treatment services.[1]

With regard to pregnant women who are using alcohol, early recognition of prenatal drinking and cessation of alcohol consumption can help to reduce the risk the severity of FAS.[22,33] Therefore, it is important for all pregnant women to be screened for alcohol use, abuse or dependence. Clinicians can achieve this by first taking a complete history. Women may fear the consequences of admitting to the use of alcohol during pregnancy, and for this reason the attitude of the clinician is important.[22] It is most helpful if the clinician taking the history adopts an attitude that is sincere, non-judgemental and accepting in order to encourage the woman to be open and honest. A woman's past medical and psychiatric history, family history, psychosocial history, and previous obstetric history may provide signs of risk.[8] It is useful to ask whether there is a family history of alcohol abuse or dependence, especially in biological parents, because this increases the individual risk for alcohol use disorders and should prompt further history-taking regarding drinking behavior. In addition, the drinking habits of the pregnant woman may be similar to those of her partner.[6,11] It is often less threatening to begin with questions about the family history as well as the drinking habits of other household members, and then to explore the woman's own drinking pattern.[6] It is also important to ask about the use of other substances, such as caffeine and nicotine, as well as marijuana and other illicit drugs.

A number of screening questionnaires can be used to determine maternal alcohol consumption. The TWEAK,[41] T-ACE,[42] CAGE,[43] and Michigan Alcoholism Screening Test

Table 12.1 *Summary of screening tool questions and cut-off scores*[*]

CAGE	**C** Have you ever felt you ought to **c**ut down on your drinking?
	A Have people ever **a**nnoyed you by criticizing your drinking?
	G Have you ever felt bad or **g**uilty about your drinking?
	E Have you ever had a drink early in the morning (**e**ye opener) to steady your nerves or get rid of a hangover?
	Scoring: 1 point for a positive response
	Cut-off score: 2 or more
TWEAK	**T** How many drinks does it take for you to feel high or how many drinks can you hold (tolerance)?
	W Do friends or relatives **w**orry about your drinking?
	E '**E**ye opener' from CAGE
	A Has a friend or family member ever told you things you said or did while you were drinking that you cannot remember (**a**mnesia)?
	K '**K**/cut down' from CAGE
	Scoring: 2 points for the tolerance question, 1 point for the other questions
	Cut-off score: 3 or more
T-ACE	**T** 'Tolerance' question from TWEAK
	A 'Annoyed' question from CAGE
	C 'Cut down' question from CAGE
	E 'Eye opener' question from CAGE
	Scoring: 2 points for the tolerance question, 1 point for the other questions
	Cut-off score: 2 or more
MAST	(**M**ichigan **A**lcoholism **S**creening **T**est)
	25 questions
	Scoring: each question weighted 0, 1, 2 or 5; score range: 0–53
	Cut-off score: 4 or more

[*] Table derived from Bradley *et al.*,[50] Smart *et al.*,[49] Chan *et al.*,[41] Russell *et al.*,[47] Selzer.[44]

(MAST)[44] are all screening instruments that have been shown to be effective in detecting prenatal drinking (see Table 12.1).[6,33,41,45–47]

The CAGE is an acronym for the following four questions. Have you ever felt you ought to *Cut down* on your drinking? Have people ever *Annoyed* you by criticizing your drinking? Have you ever felt bad or *Guilty* about your drinking? Have you ever had a drink first thing in the morning to steady your nerves or to get rid of a hangover (*Eye-opener*)? Each item is given a score of 1 point for a positive response.[47] A score of 1 or above is an indication that there is a problem with alcohol, and a further alcohol history should be obtained. The advantages of the CAGE are its brevity and high clinical validity.[48,49] In a number of studies, a score of ≥ 2 positively identified individuals on surgical and alcoholic rehabilitative services with alcohol dependence.[48,49] The disadvantages of the CAGE are its reported low sensitivity in a number of populations, as well as its emphasis on lifetime consequences.

The MAST consists of 25 questions. Each question is weighted 0, 1, 2 or 5, and possible scores range from 0 to 53.[44,47]

The TWEAK is a screening tool for identifying women who are risky drinkers.[46] The acronym 'TWEAK' is derived from the five questions of which it is composed, two of which it shares with the CAGE (*Eye-opener* and *Cut down*). The other three questions are as follows. How many drinks does it take for you to feel 'high' or how many drinks can you hold (*Tolerance*)? Do friends or relatives *Worry* about your drinking? Has a friend or family member ever told you things you said or did while you were drinking that you cannot remember (*Amnesia*)? The tolerance question is given a score of 2 points for a positive answer, and the other questions are given a score of 1 point each.[41,47] Among 135 pregnant women who were surveyed as they waited for their first prenatal appointment, with a cut-off score of ≥ 2, the TWEAK had a sensitivity of 84% in detecting lifetime alcohol diagnoses, 92% in detecting risk-drinking and 87% in detecting current alcohol consumption.[46]

The T-ACE consists of four questions, three from the TWEAK (*Tolerance, Cut down* and *Eye-opener*) and one from the CAGE (*Annoyed*). The T-ACE is scored in the same way as the TWEAK.[47] When used in the prenatal detection of risk-drinking in gravid women, the T-ACE correctly identified 69% of the risk drinkers,[41,42] and in other studies of screening for risk-drinking in pregnant women, the sensitivity was in the range 60–89% and the specificity was in the range 80–86%, depending on whether tolerance was defined as needing 3 drinks to get high or 5 drinks to get high.[41]

Pregnant women often under report their alcohol use because of fear of stigma attached to pregnant women who drink.[50] The T-ACE and the TWEAK both contain a question about tolerance that helps to compensate for underestimation.[47] One limitation of the MAST is that it is often criticized for being too long and difficult to score.[47] In one study comparing alcohol screening questionnaires with regard to their ability to detect prenatal drinking among 4743 African-American women who reported ever drinking and who attended an inner-city prenatal clinic, the TWEAK (with a cut-off point of 1 or 2) and T-ACE (with a cut-off point of 1 or 2) were more sensitive in detecting drinking than either the MAST (cut point of one or two) or the CAGE (cut-off point of 1 or 2), but somewhat less specific.[47] A recent critical review of a number of alcohol screening instruments in female patients who were not necessarily pregnant found that the TWEAK was an optimal questionnaire for identifying women with heavy drinking or alcohol abuse and dependence in racially mixed populations.[50] A limitation of all of these instruments is that none of them assess binge-drinking, which has been shown to have severe effects on the developing fetus.[1,16,22,51]

Screening can help to determine a woman's level of risk, which will aid the clinician in choosing the appropriate intervention and treatment. A pregnant woman who abstains from alcohol use is considered to be at low risk. Pregnant women who currently consume alcohol but do not have a history of alcohol abuse or dependence are more likely to be able to change their behavior with brief intervention,[8,52] and are considered to be at moderate risk. Pregnant women who currently consume alcohol and have a history of alcohol abuse or dependence may be less likely to change their behavior with brief intervention, and are considered to be at high risk.[8]

According to Redding and Selleck,[8] education, support through continued monitoring, and screening throughout the pregnancy should be provided for women at low risk. For women who appear to be at moderate risk, education is also recommended, but in addition the clinician should discuss with these women the dangers of prenatal drinking, and he or she should recommend abstinence. The clinician should also advise these women on ways to avoid situations that encourage alcohol use, draft short-term contracts, and schedule frequent visits to monitor their progress. In a short-term contract the patient might agree to abstain from alcohol until her next appointment, call her sponsor, physician or significant other if she has an urge to drink, go to Alcoholics Annoyous on a daily basis, agree to enter treatment if she uses alcohol, or engage in other behaviors and activities that are clinically appropriate and useful. The contract should be clinically specific to the individual woman and her circumstances, and both patient and physician should sign the contract. Such a contract makes both the agreed goals and the treatment plan explicit. It also makes explicit the next step in the treatment plan if the patient finds herself drinking in the interim. If she is unable to abstain from alcohol for 1 week, she should be referred for formal treatment. Women at high risk need to be confronted with the concern for a safe pregnancy and healthy outcome. They should also be referred for formal treatment and made aware of community treatment resources.[8]

As in any other medical context, a careful physical examination should include assessment of any signs of chronic alcohol dependence. These may include neurologic, gastrointestinal, dermatologic or other signs of chronic alcohol-related problems. However, many of these physical signs are manifested at a relatively late stage of dependence. The purpose of screening all women is to identify any drinking during pregnancy as well as detecting alcohol problems at the earliest possible stage. Therefore, the absence of physical manifestations of alcohol dependence should never preclude the screening of any individual woman.

As with any medical patient, elevated liver enzymes should heighten suspicion of problematic alcohol use, or another potential cause for this elevation should be sought. Only one liver enzyme is thought to be specific for alcohol-induced liver inflammation, namely gamma-gultamyl-transferase (GGT). Elevation of GGT activity would provide evidence of an alcohol use disorder. Recent research has indicated that measuring levels of carbohydrate-deficient transferrin (CDT) may be useful for detecting recent heavy drinking. CDT has been found to be superior to GGT for detecting relapse in male alcoholics,[53] and a combination of GGT and CDT may increase the sensitivity of detection of heavy drinking, especially in young women.[54] Finally, an increase in mean corpuscular volume (MCV) can be indicative of folic acid deficiency, which is sometimes seen in chronic alcoholism.

TREATMENT

If a woman has a pre-existing diagnosis of alcohol abuse or dependence and has been unable to discontinue her use of alcohol when pregnant, or if a new diagnosis of alcohol abuse or dependence is made during pregnancy, the patient should be referred for treatment to help her to discontinue alcohol use, to prevent relapse and to maintain abstinence.

It can be assumed that a woman who is consuming over 8 ounces of (absolute) alcohol (1 pint of liquor) daily has developed tolerance, but it is also possible to develop tolerance at lower levels of consumption.[12,55] Sudden cessation of drinking or a reduction in the amount that is consumed can precipitate withdrawal symptoms that can threaten both the mother and the fetus. Early symptoms of alcohol withdrawal generally occur 4–12 h after cessation of a reduction in consumption, but they can occur as late as 10 days after drinking.[12,56] These symptoms may include restlessness, tachycardia, sweating, tremulousness ('the shakes'), muscle tension, flushing and a sense of anxiety ('the jitters'). This can be followed by nausea, vomiting, anorexia and abdominal cramps. These symptoms usually peak 24–48 h after cessation of or reduction in alcohol consumption, and improve within 4–5 days. However, withdrawal may progress to the more severe symptoms of a major abstinence syndrome, which include increased tremulousness, agitation, sweating, grand mal seizures, delirium and hallucinations.[56] In some instances, a grand mal seizure may be the first sign of withdrawal.[12] Seizures usually develop 12–24 h after cessation of drinking, and one-third of those who have seizures develop delirium.[12,56] Symptoms of major abstinence syndrome should be treated as a medical emergency, and may require admission to an intensive-care unit.

In the case of a pregnant woman who is alcohol dependent and wishes to discontinue alcohol consumption or has already developed early warning signs of withdrawal, it is imperative that medical detoxification takes place on an inpatient unit with close medical supervision as well as collaboration with an obstetrician. This medical detoxification should include close observation of the medical and withdrawal status of the mother, as well as monitoring of the fetus.[12]

Most programs will treat pregnant alcohol-dependent women with benzodiazepines that have a relatively rapid rate of oral absorption and an intermediate duration of action, such as chlordiazepoxide (Librium) or diazepam (Valium), or with barbiturates (e.g. phenobarbital, seconal).[12] These are also potentially teratogenic, and the risks and benefits of their use require assessment as well as discussion with the patient. Disulfiram (Antabuse) is contraindicated during pregnancy as it has been associated with a number of malformations, including clubfoot, VACTERL syndrome (a pattern of congenital anomalies) and phocomelia of the lower extremities.[55]

Pregnant women who are admitted for a medical detoxification require a detailed health history including alcohol and other drug use, symptoms of other psychiatric disorders, and arrangements for prenatal care if none is already being provided. A comprehensive physical examination including weight, vital signs and an obstetrical evaluation is also necessary. Initial blood tests should include blood group, Rh factor determination, antibody screening, serologic testing for syphilis, hepatitis B and C screening, a complete blood count and indices, electrolytes and a magnesium blood level.[12] A purified protein derivative of tuberculin (PPD) test and antigen panel should be obtained. It is also appropriate to provide HIV-antibody counseling and testing. Other initial tests should include cervical cytology (unless this has been obtained in the previous 3 months), cervical culture for gonorrhea, a urine screen for urinary tract infection, protein and glucose, and a chlamydia screen. A baseline sonogram may also be obtained if appropriate,[12] as well as a maternal electrocardiogram (ECG). Urine or blood toxicology for other substances is also appropriate.

It can be helpful to obtain an initial blood alcohol concentration in order to determine the extent of intoxication at admission, a safe time to start medication, and the expected time when full withdrawal will begin. The usual rate of elimination of alcohol from a healthy alcohol-dependent person is 30 mg/dL/h, but this rate may increase during pregnancy. Continuous monitoring for the signs and symptoms of withdrawal should take place. It is particularly important to monitor all vital signs, including temperature, blood pressure and pulse.

There are a number of withdrawal protocols that can be followed. One typical withdrawal schedule uses chlordiazepoxide, 25–50 mg four times a day for the first 2 days, decreasing gradually to 10 mg four times a day for days 8–10.[12] In the case of elevated liver enzymes or liver disease, oxazepam can be substituted for chlordiazepoxide (50 mg of chlordiazepoxide are approximately equivalent to 30–60 mg of oxazepam). Continuous monitoring for signs of withdrawal must be continued throughout this period, and doses can be adjusted upward for continued elevation of blood pressure and pulse, or downward for over-sedation. It is also appropriate to monitor patients for delirium, psychosis, irritability and other increased autonomic reflexes (e.g. sweating, goosebumps). Other protocols using phenobarbital or diazepam are available.[12] In addition to medical detoxification, the patient should be given thiamine, folic acid, prenatal iron and vitamins. Fetal well-being (as indicated by fetal heart-tones, sonograms or non-stress tests) should be monitored as indicated and as appropriate for gestational age.[12]

During medical detoxification there are other non-pharmacologic interventions that can be helpful. These include helping the patient to maintain physical comfort, providing nutritional support, maintaining hydration, maintaining body temperature, encouraging sleep and rest, encouraging self-care, and providing positive reassurance.[12] When medical detoxification is completed, the patient should be discharged to aftercare to help her to maintain abstinence and to prevent relapse, as well as to provide prenatal care.

For those women who do not require medical detoxification because they are not physiologically dependent on alcohol, but who want to stop drinking and/or maintain abstinence from alcohol during pregnancy (and also those women who are being discharged from inpatient medical detoxification) a variety of different treatment settings may be appropriate, depending on the clinical circumstances. Treatment may include any combination of partial hospitalization, residential treatment, outpatient individual or group psychotherapy, family or couples therapy, or involvement in self-help groups.[56,57] The level and intensity of care will depend on the severity of the woman's alcohol problem, her level of motivation to abstain, the presence or absence of other psychiatric disorders, and the degree of social and community support. In some instances, women's recovery groups or women's self-help groups (Alcoholics Anonymous or Self-Management and Recovery Training – SMART Recovery) may be available and provide an additional source of support and reassurance for the pregnant woman who is in recovery. A full evaluation will help to determine what treatment or combination of treatments will be most helpful. Such an evaluation should include a complete alcohol history, including patterns of use, triggers to use, patterns of relapse, a history of successful abstinence in the past and treatment strategies that might have worked towards that end, a full psychiatric evaluation for co-existing psychiatric disorders (especially mood and anxiety disorders) and an assessment for any history of physical or sexual trauma in adulthood or childhood.[13,58]

After delivery, interventions and treatments that can help with recovery, abstinence and relapse prevention are especially important. Parenting can be very stressful, and parenting support groups, instruction in successful parenting, and attempts to increase social or community supports can all be crucial. These may promote better attachment between mother and infant, better caretaking and reduced stress, and they may also help to prevent relapse. It may also be important to help new mothers to identify their relapse triggers in this setting of new parenthood, and to develop alternate methods of coping.[57]

Women who give birth to a child with FAS or some other problem associated with prenatal alcohol exposure should be counseled about parenting. Many parents experience feelings of guilt. Often these mothers were inadequately parented themselves. They may not have grown up with a parental role model, and may therefore not know how to meet the basic needs of an infant. To make matters worse, a child with FAS or associated problems may be 'difficult', and this can contribute to feelings of rejection in the mother. Parents should be counseled and trained about parenting strategies for these children.[8]

BARRIERS TO TREATMENT

Only about 5–10% of pregnant women in need of substance abuse treatment actually receive professional treatment. One reason for this is that clinicians often fail to detect substance abuse among prenatal patients.[59] Physicians are less likely to diagnose women than men with drinking problems and they are also less likely to take an alcohol history from women. A national survey of 4756 physicians showed that only 19% of general medical physicians believed that they had good or excellent training in assisting problem drinkers.[51] When women do seek out treatment, they often encounter many problems, including a lack of insurance or financial resources to pay for treatment. In addition, many pregnant substance abusers do not have access to the necessary treatment services.[59] Many treatment programs do not admit pregnant women due to concerns about liability, and the few that do so often have long waiting-lists.[59,60] Residential treatment programs may also be impractical for pregnant women who already have dependent children. Mothers who are receiving public assistance may lose their income if they go into treatment and leave their children with someone else. Substance abuse or partial hospital day-treatment programs that have an associated child-care facility would help to eliminate this problem,[61] but very few of these exist nationally.

LEGAL IMPLICATIONS

Alcohol is a legal substance, and its widespread social acceptance makes it difficult to prevent its use. It has been proposed that pregnant women who abuse alcohol or other substances should be criminally prosecuted.[60] Currently there is not one state in the USA that has a statute specifically criminalizing substance abuse in pregnant women. However, over 200 pregnant substance abusers in 30 states have been criminally prosecuted for using alcohol or drugs during pregnancy.[62] One consequence of imposing criminal or civil sanctions on pregnant substance abusers is that these women may become even more reluctant to seek help, or may even seek pregnancy termination in order to avoid legal repercussions. Another problem is that prisons do not provide adequate health care for pregnant women. They lack the proper nutrition, prenatal diet and exercise that pregnant women need. In general, most experts believe that punitive approaches alone deter women from seeking prenatal care.[57] Moreover, punishment is an ineffective treatment for alcohol abuse or dependence.[60]

SUMMARY

Women are more vulnerable than men to the physical effects of alcohol, and alcohol abuse and dependence in women pose a risk of accelerated onset of negative physical and social consequences. In addition to the potential negative effects of excessive drinking in women, alcohol use during pregnancy results in a wide range of harmful effects on the exposed offspring. The resulting public health, social and economic consequences are quite severe, and include increased morbidity and mortality among the offspring, family stress and an increased need for long-term special education and medical services. These effects could be completely prevented by eliminating the consumption of alcohol during pregnancy. Given the scope of this well-documented problem, increased attention needs to be paid to education, screening, early intervention and treatment. Clinicians can play an important role by providing information and education for their women patients about the use of alcohol throughout the life cycle.

Acknowledgements

This work was supported by grants DA 00407 and DA 09400 from the National Institute on Drug Abuse, grant AA 11756 from the National Institute on Alcohol Abuse and Alcoholism, the Lilly Center for Women's Health Scholars in Medicine Fellowship, Harvard Medical School, and by the Dr. Ralph and Marian C. Falk Research Trust.

REFERENCES

1. Stratton K, Howe C, Battaglia F (eds). *Fetal alcohol syndrome: diagnosis, epidemiology, prevention, and treatment*. Washington, DC: National Academy Press, 1996.
2. Hawks SR. Fetal alcohol syndrome: implications for health education. *Journal of Health Education* 1993; **24**: 22–6.
3. National Institute on Alcohol Abuse and Alcoholism. *Ninth Special Report to the US Congress on Alcohol and Health*. Bethesda, MD: National Institutes of Health, 1997.

4. Finnegan LP, Kandall SR. Maternal and neonatal effects of alcohol and drugs. In: Lowinson JH, Pedro R, Millman RB (eds) *Substance abuse: a comprehensive textbook*, 2nd edn. Baltimore, MD: Williams and Wilkins, 1992: 628–56.

5. Abel EL, Sokol RJ. A revised conservative estimate of the incidence of FAS-related anomalies. *Alcoholism, Clinical and Experiment Research* 1991; **15**: 514–24.

6. Lewis DD, Woods SE. Fetal alcohol syndrome. *American Family Physician* 1994; **50**: 1025–32.

7. Substance Abuse and Mental Health Services Administration. *Substance use among women in the United States*. Rockville, MD: Department of Health and Human Services, 1997.

8. Redding BA, Selleck CS. Perinatal substance abuse: assessment and management of the pregnant woman and her children. *Nurse Practitioner Forum* 1993; **4**: 216–23.

9. Larroque B, Kaminski M. Prenatal alcohol exposure and development at preschool age: main results of a French study. *Alcoholism, Clinical and Experimental Research* 1998; **22**: 295–303.

10. Serdula M, Williamson DF, Kendrick JS, Anda RF, Byers T. Trends in alcohol consumption by pregnant women. *Journal of the American Medical Association* 1991; **265**: 876–9.

11. Smith IE, Lancaster JS, Moss-Wells S, Coles CD, Falek A. Identifying high-risk pregnant drinkers: biological and behavioral correlates of continuous heavy drinking during pregnancy. *Journal of Studies on Alcohol* 1987; **48**: 304–9.

12. Center for Substance Abuse Treatment. *Pregnant, substance-using women: treatment improvement protocol series*. Rockville, MD: US Department of Health and Human Services, 1993.

13. Greenfield S, O'Leary G. Gender differences in substance use disorders. In: Herrerra J (ed.) *Gender issues in psychiatry*. Washington, DC: American Psychiatric Press, 1998, 427–524.

14. Frezza M, DiPadova C, Pozzato G, Terpin M, Baraona E, Lieber CS. High blood alcohol levels in women: the role of decreased gastric alcohol dehydrogenase activity and first-pass metabolism. *New England Journal of Medicine* 1990; **322**: 95–9.

15. Piazza NJ, Vrbka JL, Yeager RD. Telescoping of alcoholism in women alcoholics. *International Journal of Addiction* 1989; **24**: 19–28.

16. Osborn JA, Harris SR, Weinberg J. Fetal alcohol syndrome: review of the literature with implications for physical therapists. *Physical Therapy* 1993; **73**: 599–607.

17. Appelbaum MG. Fetal alcohol syndrome: diagnosis, management, and prevention. *Nurse Practitioner* 1995; **20**: 24–36.

18. Substance Abuse and Mental Health Services Administration. *National household survey on drug abuse: main findings 1997*. Rockville, MD: Department of Health and Human Services, 1999.

19. National Institute on Alcohol Abuse and Alcoholism. Fetal alcohol syndrome. *Alcohol Alert* 1991; **13**: 1–5.

20. Stewart DE, Streiner D. Alcohol drinking in pregnancy. *General Hospital Psychiatry* 1994; **16**: 406–12.

21. Jacobson JL, Jacobson SW, Sokol RJ, Ager JW Jr. Relation of maternal age and pattern of pregnancy drinking to functionally significant cognitive deficit in infancy. *Alcoholism, Clinical and Experimental Research* 1998; **22**: 345–51.

22. Hannigan JH, Welch RA, Sokol RJ. Recognition of fetal alcohol syndrome and alcohol-related birth defects. In: Mendelson JH, Mello NK (eds) *Medical diagnosis and treatment of alcoholism*. New York: McGraw-Hill, Inc., 1992: 639–67.

23. Kline J, Shrout P, Stein Z, Susser M, Warburton D. Drinking during pregnancy and spontaneous abortion. *Lancet* 1980; **2**: 176–80.

24. Windham G, Von Behren J, Fenster L, Schaefer C, Swan S. Moderate maternal alcohol consumption and risk of spontaneous abortion. *Epidemiology* 1997; **8**: 509–14.

25. Lazzaroni F, Bonassi S, Magnani M *et al*. Moderate maternal drinking and outcome of pregnancy. *European Journal of Epidemiology* 1993; **9**: 599–606.

26. Faden V, Graubard B. Alcohol consumption during pregnancy and infant birth weight. *Annals of Epidemiology* 1994; **4**: 279–84.

27. Cavallo F, Russo R, Zotti C, Camerlengo A, Ruggenini A. Moderate alcohol consumption and spontaneous abortion. *Alcohol* 1995; **30**: 195–201.
28. Savitz D, Zhang J, Schwingl P, John E. Association of paternal alcohol use with gestational age and birth weight. *Teratology* 1992; **46**: 465–71.
29. Bayley N. *Bayley scales of infant development*. New York: Psychological Corporation, 1969.
30. Streissguth AP, Barr HM, Martin DC, Herman CS. Effects of maternal alcohol, nicotine and caffeine use during pregnancy on infant mental and motor development at eight months. *Alcoholism, Clinical and Experimental Research* 1980; **4**: 152–63.
31. National Organization on Fetal Alcohol Syndrome. *Fetal alcohol syndrome factsheet*.Washington, DC: Georgetown University School of Medicine and the National Organization on Fetal Alcohol Syndrome, 1996.
32. Goodwin DW. Alcohol: clinical aspects. In: Lowinson JH, Pedro R, Millman RB (eds) *Substance abuse: a comprehensive textbook*, 2nd edn. Baltimore, MD: Williams and Wilkins, 1992: 144–51.
33. Mendelson JH, Mello NK (eds). *Medical diagnosis and treatment of alcoholism*. New York: McGraw-Hill, Inc, 1992.
34. Committee on Substance Abuse and Committee on Children with Disabilities. Fetal alcohol syndrome and fetal alcohol effects. *Pediatrics* 1993; **91**: 1004–6.
35. Harris SR, MacKay LL, Osborn JA. Autistic behaviors in offspring of mothers abusing alcohol and other drugs: a series of case reports. *Alcoholism, Clinical and Experimental Research* 1995; **19**: 660–5.
36. Aronson M, Hagberg B. Neuropsychological disorders in children exposed to alcohol during pregnancy: a follow-up study of 24 children to alcoholic mothers in Göteborg, Sweden. *Alcoholism, Clinical and Experimental Research* 1998; **22**: 321–4.
37. Welty T, Canfield L, Selva K. Use of international classification of diseases coding to identify fetal alcohol syndrome: Indian health service facilities, 1981–1992. *Addictions Nursing* 1995; **7**: 49–51.
38. Steinhausen H-C, Spohr H-L. Long-term outcome of children with fetal alcohol syndrome: psychopathology, behavior, and intelligence. *Alcoholism, Clinical and Experimental Research* 1998; **22**: 334–8.
39. National Organization on Fetal Alcohol Syndrome. *Fetal alcohol syndrome selective curriculum guide: 9 April–4 June, 1997*. Washington, DC: Georgetown University School of Medicine and the National Organization on Fetal Alcohol Syndrome, 1997.
40. Weisner C, Schmidt L. Gender disparities in treatment for alcohol problems. *Journal of the American Medical Association* 1992; **268**: 1872–6.
41. Chan AW, Pristach EA, Welte JW, Russell M. Use of the TWEAK test in screening for alcoholism/heavy drinking in three populations. *Alcoholism, Clinical and Experimental Research* 1993; **17**: 1188–92.
42. Sokol R, Martier S, Ager J. The T-ACE questions: practical prenatal detection of risk drinking. *American Journal of Obstetrics and Gynecology* 1989; **160**: 863–70.
43. Mayfield D, McLeod G, Hall P. The CAGE questionnaire: validation of a new alcoholism screening instrument. *American Journal of Psychiatry* 1974; **131**: 1121–3.
44. Selzer ML The Michigan Alcoholism Screening Test: the quest for a new diagnostic instrument. *American Journal of Psychiatry* 1971; **127**: 1653–8.
45. Chang G, Goetz MA, Wilkins-Haug L, Berman S. Identifying prenatal alcohol use: screening instruments versus clinical predictors. *American Journal of Addiction* 1999; **8**: 87–93.
46. Chang G, Wilkins-Haug L, Berman S, Goetz MA. The TWEAK: application in a prenatal setting. *Journal of Studies on Alcohol* 1999; **60**: 306–9.
47. Russell M, Martier SS, Sokol RJ *et al.* Screening for pregnancy risk drinking. *Alcoholism, Clinical and Experimental Research* 1994; **18**: 1156–61.
48. Ewing J. Detecting alcoholism: the CAGE questionnaire. *Journal of the American Medical Association* 1984; **252**: 1905–7.

49. Smart R, Adlaf E, Knoke D. Use of the CAGE scale in a population survey of drinking. *Journal of Studies on Alcohol* 1991; **52**: 593–6.
50. Bradley KA, Boyd-Wickizer J, Powell SH, Burman ML. Alcohol screening questionnaires in women. *Journal of American Medical Association* 1998; **280**: 166–71.
51. Chang G. Primary care: detection of women with alcohol use disorders. *Harvard Review Psychiatry* 1997; **4**: 334–7.
52. Cox N. *Perinatal substance abuse: an intervention kit for providers.* Madison, WI: University of Wisconsin, 1991.
53. Schmidt LG, Schmidt K, Dufeu P, Ohse A, Rommelspacher H, Müller C. Superiority of carbohydrate-deficient transferrin to g-glutamyltransferase in detecting relapse in alcoholism. *American Journal of Psychiatry* 1997; **154**: 75–80.
54. Anton RF, Moak DH. Carbohydrate-deficient transferrin and g-glutamyltransferase as markers of heavy alcohol consumption: gender differences. *Alcoholism, Clinical and Experimental Research* 1994; **18**: 747–54.
55. Jessup M, Green J. Treatment of the pregnant alcohol-dependent woman. *Journal of Psychoactive Drugs* 1987; **19**: 193–203.
56. Greenfield SF, Weiss RD, Mirin SM. Psychoactive substance use disorders. In: Gelenberg AJ, Bassuk EL (eds) *The practitioner's guide to psychoactive drugs.* New York: Plenum Medical Book Company, 1997: 291–363.
57. Reed BG. Perinatal substance use. In: Galanter M, Kleber HD (eds) *Textbook of substance abuse treatment.* Washington, DC: American Psychiatric Press, Inc, 1999: 491–501.
58. Greenfield SF. Women and substance use disorders. In: Jensvold MF, Hamilton JA (eds) *Psychopharmacology of women: sex, gender, and hormonal considerations.* Washington, DC: American Psychiatric Press, Inc, 1996: 229–321.
59. Messer K, Clark K, Martin S. Characteristics associated with pregnant women's utilization of substance abuse treatment services. *American Journal of Drug and Alcohol Abuse* 1996; **22**: 403–22.
60. American Medical Association, Board of Trustee. Legal interventions during pregnancy: court-ordered medical treatments and legal penalties for potentially harmful behavior by pregnant women. *Journal of the American Medical Association* 1990; **264**: 2663–70.
61. Goldberg M. Substance abusing women: false stereotypes and real needs. *Social Work* 1995; **40**: 789–98.
62. Marshall MF, Nelson LJ. Update on criminal prosecution of substance-abusing pregnant women. *BioLaw* 1995; **2**: S17–19.

13

Treatment of substance abuse during pregnancy: an overview

BERTIS B. LITTLE AND KIMBERLY A. YONKERS

INTRODUCTION

Non-medical use of mood-altering substances in the USA is estimated to be as high as 70–90%.[1,2] A large group of women between 15 and 40 years of age abuse substances, and frequently conceive while using them.[3] More than 50% of pregnant substance abusers are unmarried, receive prenatal care, use cocaine, and are financially dependent on public assistance.[2,4] Detrimental risks exist for pregnant women and their unborn children who are exposed to substance abuse.[5] The most critical period for the induction of congenital anomalies is the first trimester (specifically the first 58 days post-conception), a time when most women do not know that they are pregnant. The fetal period of development is also a time of great vulnerability, and continued substance use during this period carries the risk of causing atypical development (i.e. certain congenital anomalies, growth retardation and neurobehavioral abnormalities).

COCAINE ABUSE DURING PREGNANCY

Cocaine use is widespread in Western society today as a result of an epidemic that began in the mid- to late 1970s, and now occurs in virtually every age, sex, racial and socio-economic subgroup. This rapid increase in use has been due in part to the initial perception by some, even in the scientific community, that cocaine was a relatively innocuous drug that did not cause addiction. Over time these views have been found to be fallacious – cocaine is addictive and harmful to human physiology. In the mid- to late 1980s, a relatively inexpensive and even more addictive form of cocaine known as 'crack' became available, which is the freebase form of the drug that can be smoked. The new drug increased the epidemic of cocaine use in Western nations. Five million Americans are daily cocaine users, and at least 20 million Americans use the drug once a month or more. At least 50% of these users are women of reproductive age.[6]

The use of cocaine is dangerous not only because of its addictive property for the mother, but also because of its potential to cause damage to unborn children who are exposed to the drug. Although the evidence is not conclusive, a growing scientific database suggests that cocaine use during pregnancy may have deleterious effects on the intrauterine development of the embryo and fetus, particularly with regard to the genitourinary tract.[7] Accordingly, cocaine is currently being considered by researchers as a possible human teratogen. In addition, there is the immediate social and economic cost of the increased maternal and neonatal morbidity and mortality associated with use of this drug during pregnancy. Cocaine is primarily metabolized via plasma cholinesterase to ecgonine methyl ester, a major active metabolite by the placenta.[8] Differences in plasma cholinesterase, activity that are genetically programmed can enhance the potential for toxicity due to cocaine.

Epidemiology

Studies of the prevalence of cocaine use indicate that there has been a 10- to 15-fold increase in its use since the early 1970s. Between 1970 and 1975, as few as 1% of the college and high-school-aged population reported using cocaine in the past year. By 1985, that figure had risen to 20%. One interesting aspect of these surveys was that women in the same cohort used cocaine approximately 30% more frequently than did their male counterparts. Thus the prevalence of cocaine use among women of reproductive age would appear to be at least as high, if not higher, than that among men of reproductive age.[6,9]

The first published study on the prevalence of cocaine use during pregnancy revealed a rate of 9.8% at one of the nation's largest hospitals.[10] The first nationwide survey of 36 hospitals found an average of 11% of women using cocaine during pregnancy, with the percentage ranging from 0.2% to 28%.[11] A study by Ostrea and colleagues[12] revealed that 31% of the infants born in a Detroit public hospital tested positive for cocaine when a meconium test was used, and Nair and colleagues[13] obtained the same results in Baltimore (31% of infants had been exposed to cocaine). In one study, an incredibly high rate of 48% in a San Francisco public hospital was reported.[14]

At Parkland Memorial Hospital in Dallas, the typical profile of a pregnant cocaine user is a woman aged 25–26 years with two living children, who has had an average of three to four abortions, about equally divided between miscarriages and elective terminations. Approximately 77% of pregnant cocaine abusers at this hospital use other drugs of abuse and/or alcohol.[15] In Dallas County, Texas, cocaine use during pregnancy is almost equally divided between white (40%) and black (55%) pregnant women, but only a small proportion of Hispanics (5%) use the drug. This pattern is subject to regional variation. For example, in New York City the ethnic distribution of pregnant cocaine abusers is evenly spread across all three racial groups. In Pittsburgh, pregnant cocaine users tend to be predominantly white,[16] while in one Atlanta hospital 63 of 500 women who presented consecutively for labor and delivery tested positive for cocaine metabolite in their urine, and all of them were either black or Hispanic.[17]

The socio-economic distribution of pregnant cocaine abusers appears to be weighted toward the lower end of the scale. However, statewide data from Texas indicate that the epidemic of cocaine use began in the middle to upper-middle classes and reached lower social strata as the drug's availability increased and its cost decreased. Moreover, there is no evidence for diminished cocaine use in the more affluent socio-economic strata over time.[18] It is important to realize that almost all of the available surveys of cocaine use during pregnancy tend to be based upon information from public and teaching hospitals from around the USA. One exception is a study by Chasnoff and colleagues,[19] which compared the prevalence of illicit drug use among women during pregnancy in a number of public hospitals with that among women in several private clinics. The investigators did not find any significant differences between the two groups of women with regards to drug use, irrespective of socio-economic background and ethnicity.

Maternal and embryofetal effects

Pharmacologically, cocaine acts upon human physiology via three independent systems, namely the dopaminergic system, beta-sympathetic system and direct vasoconstriction. Cocaine competes for dopaminergic receptors and inhibits the reuptake of serotonin, epinephrine and norepinephrine from synaptic cleft and postsynaptic dopamine receptors. It also precipitates the interneuronal release of catecholamines. The drug stimulates the sympathetic nervous system, producing tachycardia and physiological stimulation. By direct action of cocaine on the vasculature, profound vasoconstriction is produced, which is probably aggravated to a degree by the blocked reuptake of catecholamines. Monga and colleagues[20] have found that cocaine alters the placental production of prostaglandins in-vitro. Cocaine increases thromboxane production and decreases protacyclin production, thus increasing the ratio of thromboxane to prostacyclin production. This may be the main mechanism for the intense vasoconstriction and decreased uteroplacental blood flow associated with cocaine use. Cocaine's potent vasoconstricting properties, with concomitant stimulation of the sympathetic nervous system, produce an aggravated state of hypertension, which accounts for the plethora of adverse effects of the drug on the cardiovascular and neurovascular systems.[21]

One of the main adverse effects of cocaine abuse is addiction. The actions of cocaine on the vasculature precipitate a number of serious effects. Coronary artery vasospasm and arrhythmias occur even at very low doses of cocaine use.[22] Chronic cocaine use can lead to myocardial infarction, congestive heart failure, dilated cardiomyopathy or severe ischemic events in the heart or brain. In more severe situations, cocaine can aggravate vascular weakness and cause serious vascular accidents. Other vascular accidents precipitated by cocaine include intracerebral infarctions and hemorrhages that can cause permanent brain damage, seizures and ultimately death. Less severe effects include acute ischemic brain events.[21,23] Death from cocaine toxicity is usually preceded by hyperpyrexia, shock, unconsciousness and respiratory and cardiac depression, probably related to the potent local anesthetic actions of the drug. Chronic cocaine use is associated with epileptogenic seizures and cerebral atrophy, probably caused by ischemic insults – perhaps in addition to microvascular infarction or hemorrhage.[24]

Prenatal cocaine exposure is also associated with increased levels of adrenergic compounds.[25–27] Similar down-regulation of fetal adrenergic receptor-binding sites could result in disruption of the synaptic development of the fetal nervous system.

Cocaine's sympathomimetic action inhibits the reuptake of serotonin, epinephrine and norepinephrine at adrenergic nerve endings. Maternal–fetal physiologic effects are precipitated by the drug's action on the uteroplacental vasculature and myometrium. This tonic sympathetic stimulation results in acute maternal hypertension, which may lead to abruptio placentae. Premature rupture of membranes and preterm labor, uteroplacental insufficiency resulting from vasoconstriction, reduced birth weight, fetal growth retardation, and fetal intolerance of labor are associated with cocaine use in pregnancy.[28] Cocaine is also linked with embryofetal systemic vasoconstriction, resulting in cardiovascular, genitourinary, gastrointestinal and musculoskeletal anomalies as well as perinatal cerebrovascular accidents. Cocaine exerts strong effects on the cardiovascular system, and these effects would appear to be more profound during pregnancy.

Congenital anomalies

Cocaine abuse during pregnancy has been associated with numerous congenital anomalies. The most consistent association between cocaine use and fetal malformations involves the genitourinary tract. Additional reported abnormalities observed in cocaine-exposed infants include prune belly syndrome with urethral obstruction, bilateral cryptorchidism, absent digits 3 and 4 on the left hand in two infants, and hypospadias, female pseudohermaphroditism, hydronephrosis with ambiguous genitalia and absent uterus and ovaries, anal atresia, clubfoot, limb-body wall complex, limb deficiencies, secondary hypospadias, bilateral hydronephrosis and unilateral hydronephrosis with renal infarction of the contralateral kidney, and congenital heart disease.

Skull defects, exencephaly (stillborn), interparietal encephalocele and parietal bone defects without herniation of meninges or cerebral tissue have also been reported.

Head circumference was found to be reduced proportionately more than birth weight in one study of infants whose mothers used only cocaine during pregnancy, exhibiting a pattern of brain growth similar to that of infants whose mothers had used only alcohol during pregnancy.[29]

Facial defects that were observed in 10 of 11 infants exposed to cocaine in the antepartum period included blepharophimosis, ptosis and facial diplegia, unilateral oro-orbital cleft, Pierre–Robin anomaly, cleft palate, cleft lip and palate, skin tags and cutis aplasia.[30] All of the infants had major brain abnormalities, cavitations, holoproscencephaly and porencephaly.

In summary, most of the available evidence supports the view that cocaine has teratogenic potential as well as the ability to cause adverse fetal effects. The mechanisms of both the embryonic and fetal effects appear to be vascular disruption, hypoperfusion, hemorrhage and vascular occlusion, similar to the known effects of cocaine on adults.

It was suggested that a cocaine syndrome may occur, characterized by unusual facies similar to fetal alcohol syndrome.[31] However, in a case–control study of 50 infants who were chronically exposed to cocaine prenatally, no evidence of a syndrome was found.[32] Fetal growth retardation was the only significant finding in that study.

Cerebrovascular accidents

Perinatal complications (e.g. tachycardia, bradycardia, respiratory problems, jaundice, elevated bilirubin) are significantly increased among infants born to cocaine abusers.[33] Perinatal or newborn cerebrovascular accidents and resulting brain damage in fetuses and infants that have been exposed to cocaine *in utero* have been described in a number of reports.

Maternal cocaine use may cause major neuropathology of the fetus and newborn. The mechanisms of brain injury may be vascular accidents or ischemia, or a combination of these effects. An association between cocaine abuse and cerebral palsy is unclear at this time, but it seems reasonable to suspect such a link. Newborn infants exposed to cocaine *in utero* also appear to show significant neurobehavioral impairment in the neonatal period, including increased irritability, tremulousness and muscular rigidity.[34]

Developmental outcomes of exposed children

Only a limited number of studies have been published on the long-term effects of prenatal cocaine exposure on child development. Mental and psychomotor development at 2 years of age are delayed, and they score significantly lower on verbal reasoning than non-drug-exposed children. A limitation of these findings is that some mothers who used cocaine during pregnancy also used alcohol – a well-known cause of delayed mental and motor development and smaller head circumference.[35] Van Beveren and colleagues[36] evaluated cognitive performance, motor development and physical growth of cocaine-exposed children, and compared the results of the evaluations with those of non-drug-exposed children. To control for the often poor quality of the environment in which many drug-exposed children are living, adopted cocaine-exposed children and adopted non-drug-exposed children were also evaluated. All of the children in the four groups were 12 months old. Comparisons of the results of the tests revealed that the cocaine-exposed children, regardless of their living environments, demonstrated delays in all domains that were evaluated. In addition, no differences were found between the performance of the cocaine-exposed children living with their birth mothers and that of the adopted cocaine-exposed children. The researchers concluded that maternal cocaine use during pregnancy accounted for significant differences in cognitive, motor and physical developmental outcomes between cocaine-exposed and non-drug-exposed children at 12 months of age.

Small head circumference, found at birth in cocaine-exposed children, was again found in the 2-year-old cocaine-exposed children in the study by Chasnoff and colleagues[37] and in the 12-month-old children in the study by VanBeveren and colleagues.[36] It appears that cocaine-exposed children do not exhibit catch-up growth in head circumference during the first years of life. This finding may have important implications for intellectual development, since a number of studies have found a significant relationship between decreased head circumference and cognitive abilities.[38–40]

Language development of intrauterine cocaine-exposed children has been studied by several investigators. Angelilli and colleagues[41] found that children with language impairments identified in a clinical setting were significantly more likely to have been exposed to cocaine *in utero* than children who did not display any language delays. Nulman and colleagues[42] found, in a follow-up study of cocaine-exposed children, that although there were no differences in scores on intelligence tests between the cocaine-exposed children and a control group, the cocaine-exposed children scored significantly lower than the control children on language assessments.

Summary

In summary, the epidemic use of cocaine during pregnancy has resulted in serious adverse outcomes in the mother, fetus and newborn. The effects of use of cocaine are often compounded by frequent concomitant heavy use of other illicit drugs and alcohol. Many of the studies reviewed here were unable to partition the effects of abuse of many substances during pregnancy. A further problem is the self-reported nature of information about cocaine use, resulting in possible misclassification of patients into control vs. drug-exposed groups. It is likely that the adverse effects reported in association with cocaine use in pregnancy are due in part to selection biases, cocaine itself, the use of drugs that act independently of or interact with cocaine, poor health status, lack of prenatal care and other maternal characteristics. Women who use cocaine during pregnancy are at significant risk for no prenatal care, shorter gestations, premature rupture of membranes, premature labor and delivery, spontaneous abortions, abruptio placentae, decreased uterine blood flow and death. The fetuses of these women who use cocaine are growth-retarded or severely distressed, and have an increased mortality risk. Fetal and maternal cerebrovascular accidents, with attendant profound morbidity and mortality, occur in association with maternal cocaine use during pregnancy. Major congenital anomalies involving the brain, genitourinary tract, bowel, heart, limbs and face occur with significantly increased frequency among infants whose mothers used cocaine during gestation. Hence, cocaine use during pregnancy should be considered teratogenic and fetotoxic.

OPIATE ABUSE DURING PREGNANCY

Opiates, a class of drugs that have both sedative and narcotic effects, are derived from milky secretions of the opium poppy plant (*Papaver somniferum*). They are commonly used as medical treatment for moderate to severe pain, and their various constituents and derivatives include morphine, codeine, meperidine, paperavine, thebaine and heroin. These drugs act on opioid receptors, producing analgesia and euphoria. A serious withdrawal syndrome resulting from either prescribed or illicit chronic use can occur among both adults and infants who become addicted to these drugs. Although methadone is technically not an opioid, it will be discussed here because of its use as a medical alternative to heroin. Heroin and methadone both have a physiologically significant and recognized withdrawal syndrome.

Heroin

Heroin is available commercially as a narcotic analgesic in many countries, including the UK. In the USA it is a schedule I drug and cannot be prescribed for medical treatment. The abuse of heroin occurs worldwide, and most population studies have reported the prevalence of illicit heroin use to be in the range 2–5%.

The review of studies of heroin use during pregnancy in this section is limited to illicit use of the drug. In any discussion of the literature on the health effects of heroin use, it is important to realize that addicts often abuse other drugs, alcohol and cigarettes, and have poor nutritional and health status. It is also important to consider that the dosage and duration of heroin use and the trimesters of exposure are not usually known. A number of studies have found that the frequency of congenital anomalies is not higher among infants born to heroin-addicted mothers than would be expected among infants born to non-heroin-addicted mothers.

Pregnant heroin addicts and their offspring often develop severe infections related to intravenous drug use, such as hepatitis, syphilis and HIV. Birth weight and other measures of fetal growth (e.g. head circumference and birth length) have been consistently found to be decreased among infants born to heroin addicts. Intrauterine growth retardation, miscarriages, perinatal death and a variety of other perinatal complications have been observed at a high frequency in heroin-exposed infants and children. However, it was not possible to ascribe these effects purely to fetal heroin exposure because of the generally poor health of the mothers. Postnatal growth of these children appears to be normal in most cases, although head circumference seems to be smaller than that of children who were not exposed to heroin prenatally. Neonatal withdrawal symptoms have been observed in 40–80% of infants born to heroin-addicted women, and may appear shortly after birth or take from 6 to 10 days to develop. Withdrawal symptoms can be of prolonged duration, usually persisting for less than 3 weeks. The postnatal environment seems to be the major determinant of developmental progress, rather than prenatal exposure to heroin.[43]

Methadone

Methadone is a synthetic opiate narcotic that resembles propoxyphene structurally. Its principal medical use is as maintenance therapy for heroin addiction. It is also obtained illegally and abused on the street as a substitute for heroin. The studies reported below were of pregnant women on regimented-dose maintenance therapy who took methadone of known pharmacological purity.

The frequency of congenital anomalies was found not to be increased above the background rate in cohort studies and in clinical case studies of infants born to heroin-addicted women who were treated with methadone during pregnancy. A significantly higher rate of obstetrical complications, including prolonged rupture of membranes, breech presentations, abruptio pre-eclampsia and postpartum hemorrhage, was found among the methadone-dependent women. Intrauterine growth retardation, neonatal problems such as asphyxia neonatorum, transient tachypnea, aspiration pneumonia, congenital syphilis and jaundice were also observed with increased frequency in methadone-exposed infants. In addition, 70–90% of infants who were chronically exposed to methadone suffer from abstinence symptoms.

Opiate-exposed neonates were significantly more tremulous and more irritable, and exhibited less control over arm and leg movements than non-drug-exposed neonates. A significant depression of organizational responses to environmental stimuli, a lower excitability threshold and a reduced capacity to attend and react to noxious stimuli were observed in the drug-exposed newborns.[43]

Developmental outcomes of exposed children

Heroin- and methadone-exposed children scored lower than comparison groups on motor coordination, attention and focus, activity level and behavior tests. In long-term studies, no differences were found in measures of cognitive, social and emotional development between the methadone-exposed children and a control group of non-drug-exposed children. Notably, methadone-exposed children had more emotional disturbances and behavioral problems, such as aggression, anxiety and rejection.[43]

Summary

Habitual use of opiates during pregnancy does not increase the risk of congenital anomalies, but other adverse outcomes are increased in frequency. Abruptio placentae, neonatal withdrawal, preterm birth and fetal growth retardation are associated with the abuse of these substances during pregnancy. There are also differences in cognitive abilities, motor development and behavior between opiate-exposed children and non-drug-exposed children. However, maternal personality traits, degree of life stress, quality of the mother–child relationship and quality of the postnatal environment need to be taken into consideration in order to determine more accurately the delays and impairments that occur in the development of opiate-exposed children.

AMPHETAMINE ABUSE DURING PREGNANCY

Amphetamines (*d*-amphetamine) and methamphetamines are sympathomimetic agents that may be used medically during pregnancy, primarily as a treatment for narcolepsy, but also as central nervous system stimulants and anorectics. These drugs are also used illicitly as stimulants, and have a number of street names. No studies on the illicit use of amphetamines during pregnancy have been published, although medical use of the drug during pregnancy has been reported. Several factors complicate extrapolation of these results to illicit use or abuse. First, dose regimens in illicit use are not controlled, and probably involve much greater amounts than those used therapeutically. Secondly, the harmful impurities that may be present in illicit amphetamines or methamphetamines are unknown, because illegal laboratories have no quality control, and even lead oxides have been reported as contaminants of illicit amphetamines and methamphetamines. These drugs are known to be diluted with finely ground glass, quinine, talc, powdered sugar and a variety of other fine crystalline-looking white powders.

Congenital anomalies

Treatment of amphetamine abuse is similar to that of cocaine abuse (see Table 13.2). Pharmacologic treatment of amphetamine abuse is based on the theory of serotonin depletion with medications that increase the levels of this neurotransmitter.

Methamphetamine abuse during the first trimester was reported in four studies, but the findings were not consistent with regard to the types of congenital anomalies observed, and they conflict with data from large cohort studies and case–control studies. Thus any interpretation of the results is of no relevance for assessing the potential human teratogenicity of amphetamine use or abuse.

Methamphetamines are sympathomimetics with potent central nervous system stimulant properties, and they are prescribed medically to treat obesity and narcolepsy. Illegally produced methamphetamines are known as designer drugs because they are synthesized by methylating novel sites along the carbon chain and ring. Methamphetamines are also used to 'cut' or dilute other illicit drugs, particularly cocaine.

The frequency of congenital anomalies was not significantly increased in the studies that have been reported, nor was that of perinatal infant abnormalities or maternal pregnancy complications. There was a slight clinically non-significant but statistically significant reduction in birth weight in the methamphetamine-exposed group, but no other adverse pregnancy or neonatal outcomes were found.[44]

Developmental outcomes of exposed children

Children whose mothers took amphetamines during pregnancy were followed prospectively from birth in a study in Sweden.[45] At 4 years of age the children as a group had a significantly lower IQ (103) than a sampled control group (110) on standardized IQ tests. A high percentage of the children also demonstrated behavioral problems or disturbances. The same group of children was evaluated at 8 years of age, and a significant correlation was found between the extent of prenatal amphetamine exposure and scores on psychometric tests, behavioral problems (specifically aggression) and general adjustment. The children who had been exposed to higher levels of the drug scored lower on the assessment than the children who had been less exposed.[46] At 10 years of age, more children (12%) attended one class below what is considered typical for their biological age (the normal figure in Sweden is less than

5%).[47] At 14–15 years old, these children performed at a similarly delayed level, with 15% performing at one or more grades below their chronological peers.[48]

Struthers and Hansen[49] evaluated 36 cocaine/amphetamine/methamphetamine-exposed children at 27 and 52 weeks of age with the Fagan Test of Infant Intelligence, and compared their scores with the scores of a group of non-drug-exposed children. The Fagan test is an assessment tool based on visual recognition memory. The test has been shown to have a significant predictive ability for later cognitive deficits in high-risk children. The amphetamine-exposed children scored significantly lower on developmental tests and IQ and demonstrated significantly more behavioral problems (including extreme activity, high distractibility and inability to concentrate) during the testing.

Summary

The medically supervised use of amphetamines and methamphetamines during pregnancy does not pose a significantly increased risk of congenital anomalies or maternal–fetal complications. However, increased risks cannot be ruled out.

ABUSE OF HALLUCINOGENS DURING PREGNANCY

Psychedelic drugs produce visual hallucinations by disruption of higher central nervous system functioning. Some hallucinogens are actually functional analogs of neurotransmitters. For example, LSD resembles serotonin, and it is thought that it may exert its hallucinogenic effect by displacing this neurotransmitter. In general, tolerance of hallucinogens develops quickly, and the chronic user will increase the dose rapidly over the course of the drug's use to maintain the desired effects.[50]

Hallucinogens or psychedelic drugs are not nearly as popular as they were 30 to 40 years ago. Less than 2% of the population use psychedelic drugs, based on data that are not partitioned by sex, ethnicity or pregnancy status. In a study of pregnant women at a large urban hospital in Dallas, Texas, it was estimated that approximately 1% used psychedelic drugs (LSD, mescaline or psilocybin) during gestation.[51] There is no recognized withdrawal syndrome associated with the use of hallucinogens, and no medication is recommended to treat hallucinogen abstinence.

LSD

Lysergic acid amides (classically known as lysergic acid diethylamide or LSD) or lysergides are amine alkaloids that can only be obtained by chemical synthesis, and they have a variety of street names. Under medical supervision lysergide has been used to treat psychiatric illness. LSD stimulates the sympathetic nervous system, often producing increased heart rate and blood pressure and a rise in body temperature. LSD also has powerful hallucinogenic effects for which it is used recreationally.

Congenital anomalies have been reported among infants born to mothers who used LSD before or during pregnancy, but a causal relationship is highly unlikely because no consistent pattern of anomalies was found. Limb defects were noted most frequently among exposed infants, but the defect types were highly heterogeneous. There is no evidence that LSD is a human teratogen, although lifestyle practices attendant to drug abuse may be detrimental to intrauterine development. Julien[52] reported that the clinical data show that the incidence of deficits and impairments found in children of LSD users is not higher than that found in the offspring of the non-drug-using population.

Increased frequencies of chromosomal breakage in somatic cells of individuals who used LSD have been reported, but many other investigators have reported negative results. Chromosomal aberrations in somatic cells show no clinical correlation with the risk of congenital anomalies in the children of parents who have used LSD.[51]

Mescaline

Mescaline is a hallucinogenic alkaloid that is obtained from the peyote cactus *Lophophora williamsii*. Flattened dried seed pods from this plant, called 'buttons' or 'peyote,' are ingested for recreational use and in Native American rituals. Members of the Native American Church use mescaline legally in their ceremonies. Natural mescaline is often contaminated with strychnine. Mescaline may also be synthesized chemically. The effects of this drug are similar to the effects of LSD. No published studies of congenital anomalies in infants born to mothers who used mescaline during pregnancy are available.[51]

Psilocybin

Psilocybin is a naturally occurring hallucinogenic alkaloid found in several species of psyche-delic mushrooms belonging to the genus *Psilocin*. Psilocybin mushrooms are eaten as an illegal recreational drug, and the effects usually last from 6 to 8 hours. Ingestion of these hallucinogenic mushrooms has become a popular form of substance abuse among some adolescents and young adults.[53] The hallucinogenic effects of psilocybin ingestion include hallucinogenic visions, altered states of consciousness and a pronounced pyrogenic effect. No studies have been published on the frequency of congenital anomalies in the offspring of mothers who ingested psilocybin during pregnancy.[51]

Summary

The use of hallucinogens has not been well studied, and unknown risks may exist. It seems unlikely that the association of LSD with limb defects found in the offspring of LSD-using women, as reported in the 1960s, was causal or biologically plausible. The pyrogenic effects and concomitant use of other substances may be cause for concern, but this area has not yet been adequately studied.

OTHER SUBSTANCES OF ABUSE DURING PREGNANCY

Cannabinoids

It is estimated that approximately 12 million people in the USA use marijuana or its deriva-tives (hash, hash oil, Thai sticks, THC) regularly, and at least 50% of these are women of reproductive age. Approximately 3% of the population uses marijuana daily, and as many as 10–15% of Americans use the drug at least monthly.[54] Estimated prevalence rates of cannabi-noid use during pregnancy vary widely, ranging from 3% to more than 20% of gravidas.

Some studies have reported an increased frequency of preterm labor and other pregnancy complications in association with marijuana use, but other investigations have failed to confirm these observations. There is no recognized withdrawal syndrome among marijuana users, and no medication is indicated.

Significantly lowered birth weights have been reported among infants whose mothers used marijuana during pregnancy in some studies but not in others. It is likely that the discrepancies in findings between studies are due to confounding factors (e.g. drug potency, frequency of use, patterns of use, other substances used). The reductions in birth weight that were observed among infants born to women who used marijuana during pregnancy were not large enough to be clinically significant (50–100 g), and they parallel those observed for tobacco smoking. Among infants whose mothers smoked marijuana during pregnancy, the frequency of major congenital anomalies was not increased.[55]

Among infants whose mothers used marijuana close to the time of delivery, certain neonatal neurobehavioral abnormalities have been reported, including tremulousness and abnormal response to light and visual stimuli. Disturbances in sleep cycling, motility and arousal has been reported in infants and children whose mothers used marijuana during their pregnancies.[35]

The only medical risks that can reasonably be ascribed to marijuana use during pregnancy appear to be mild fetal growth retardation and maternal lung damage. Perhaps the greatest concern with regard to marijuana use during pregnancy should be the high probability that the woman may be using other more harmful substances of abuse (e.g. alcohol and/or cocaine). More research is needed to evaluate the long-term effects of intrauterine marijuana exposure on child sleep patterns and intellectual, language and behavioral development.

Inhalants (organic solvents)

Compared to other substances of abuse (e.g. cocaine, marijuana, tobacco), the use of inhalants during pregnancy is relatively infrequent. It has been estimated that 1% of women use inhalants during pregnancy, including toluene, spray paint, gasoline, freon and other substances. Women who use inhalants during pregnancy have been found to be primarily Hispanic or Native American. Abstinence from inhalant use is treated in a similar manner to alcohol dependence, with benzodiazepines and clonidine (see Table 13.2).

Dysmorphic features collectively referred to as 'fetal solvent syndrome' have been described among infants born to women who abused toluene, gasoline, benzene and other aromatic liquids. Prenatal growth retardation (low birth weight, microcephaly), facial dysmorphism (resembling fetal alcohol syndrome, FAS) and digital malformations (short phalanges, nail hypoplasia) characterize the syndrome. Importantly, women who use inhalants during pregnancy frequently also use other substances, including alcohol. It should be noted that normal occupational exposure to organic solvents cannot be compared to inhalant abuse because the doses encountered during occupational exposure are of a significantly lower magnitude.[56]

Solvent abuse during pregnancy endangers both the mother and the fetus. Severe maternal distal renal tubular acidosis and hyperchloremic metabolic acidosis may result. Premature labor should be anticipated, and will often follow toluene toxicity. Infant metabolic acidosis (arterial pH $\leq$ 7.0), respiratory difficulties and renal function abnormalities should be expected, compounded by the usual complications of prematurity.

Polysubstance abuse

The morbidity risk increases with the number of substances used and the frequency of their use. While not all substances of abuse cause congenital anomalies, abuse of any substance during pregnancy appears to be associated with fetal growth retardation and possibly with neurological dysfunctioning. Attendant risks include sexually transmitted diseases, hepatitis and undernutrition. Tobacco smoking is linked to lower birth weight and is possibly associated with prematurity. However, the risk of birth defects is apparently not increased among infants whose mothers smoked tobacco during pregnancy.[57] Tobacco smoking is highly prevalent among pregnant substance abusers, frequently approaching 100%.

Many other substances are used during pregnancy in addition to the ones discussed in this chapter, including street substitutes for heroin, sedatives, hypnotics and synthetic narcotics.[58]

DRUG OVERDOSES DURING PREGNANCY

Drug overdoses during pregnancy are frequently part of a suicide gesture or (less often) an attempt to induce abortion. None the less, overdoses are considered to represent acute abuse of substances. Quinine overdoses are nearly always associated with an attempt to induce abortion, whereas the vast majority of other overdoses represent suicide gestures.[59] In one large study of 162 pregnant women who were medically evaluated for poisoning, 86% of the cases were intentional overdoses, with 78% attempting suicide and 8% attempting to induce an abortion.[60] Maternal death associated with suicide gestures occurs in approximately 1% of gravid women, and more than 95% of suicide gestures involve ingestion of a combination of drugs.[61] Recently, in a study in New York City, suicide was identified as the cause of 13% of maternal deaths.[62]

Deliberate ingestion of potentially lethal doses of drugs during pregnancy raises concern about both maternal and fetal well-being. Evaluation of the gravida who has ingested potentially lethal doses of drugs and/or chemicals begins with an evaluation of the substances taken. If the patient is still conscious she will probably provide the most accurate report, because drug overdoses are for the most part premeditated. The patient will usually know approximately how much she took of which substances. If family members or significant others are present, they may be able to provide corroborative information (e.g. presence of medicine bottles etc.). Toxicology screens should be ordered as soon as possible to determine exactly what substances are present. However, a generalized treatment plan may be undertaken before the toxicology results are available.[59]

Treatment of cocaine use is usually with an anti-anxiolytic and an antidepressant, possibly with a clonidine adjuvant. Antidepressant therapy is based on the theory that the acute effects of cocaine abstinence are caused by serotonin depletion.

HIDDEN RISKS OF SUBSTANCE ABUSE

Impurities

All substances of abuse, even alcohol, may be either intentionally or unintentionally contaminated by certain impurities. 'Moonshine' may contain significant amounts of lead that may cause heavy metal poisoning in the mother and fetus. Drugs such as amphetamine and methamphetamine may contain impurities such as lead oxides.[63] During the extraction of cocaine paste from cocoa leaves, leaded gasoline is sometimes used as the solvent, resulting in lead contamination. During the illicit production of some drugs, such as phencyclepiperadine (PCP), cyanohydrin intermediate reactions are involved that may not be fully reacted in the final product. Cyanide may be present because illicit laboratories are usually crudely equipped for purification, with no quality control. Both lead and cyanide poisoning result from the use of substances produced in illicit laboratories. These toxic substances are known to be associated with significant maternal and fetal morbidity and mortality. Similarly, failure to complete the conversion of lysergic acid to lysergic acid diethylamide (LSD), or to purify the product, will result in lysergic acid toxicity, including peripheral neuropathy and progressive necrosis in humans and animals.[64] Drugs that are available as tablets or capsules (e.g. codeine, methadone, morphine, benzodiazepines, pentazocine) contain a significant amount of tablet/capsule base (normally more than 90%), which is usually microcrystalline cellulose. Tablet/capsule substances are dissolved in water for parenteral use, which results in a high potential for pulmonary emboli, placental infarcts and other maternal vascular blockages. Inhalants such as toluene and gasoline may also contain lead or nitriles that can cause toxicity. Even marijuana may contain dangerous vegetable contaminants such as nightshade, poison sumac, poison ivy and poison oak, all of which could cause serious pulmonary-cardiac morbidity or even death. In addition, herbicides (e.g. paraquat) and/or pesticides (e.g. chlordane) may be present in the marijuana itself as a result of treatment during the plant's growth, as there is no quality control of production practices.[65]

Other drugs and chemicals as dilutants

Illicit drugs are often intentionally 'cut' or diluted with other substances by dealers to increase their profits. Cocaine is commonly 'cut' with lidocaine, amphetamines or insert substances such as talcum or fine glass beads. Amphetamines are sometimes diluted with certain antihistamines or ephedrine. Heroin is cut with a very wide variety of compounds, ranging from confectioner's sugar to finely ground sawdust. These dilutants are probably not teratogenic, but may cause serious maternal and/or placental complications when used parenterally. Heroin has been cut with warfarin, and abuse of heroin so diluted during pregnancy was the cause of the warfarin embryopathy. Strychnine and arsenic are deliberately added to amphetamine, methamphetamine, cocaine, heroin and LSD to intensify their effects, although the 'intensification' is actually due to subclinical toxicity.[66] Whether the presence of additional compounds is intentional or unintentional, the potentially toxic or adverse effects of these additional compounds need to be considered when evaluating the teratogenic risk of substance use/abuse.

PSYCHIATRIC DISORDERS ASSOCIATED WITH SUBSTANCE ABUSE

For many drug abuse patients, mood disorders are a constant companion – an estimated 60% of substance abusers have a comorbid psychiatric condition. Among cocaine abusers, for example, depressive disorders are the most commonly diagnosed coexisting or comorbid conditions. The relationship between mood disorders and drug abuse in these patients is often complex and interconnected. Drug abuse patients may develop depression and as a result of the physical and psychological suffering caused by this mood disorder they may become drug dependent in an attempt to self-medicate.[5] For patients suffering from both drug abuse and mood disorders, the conditions once seemed impossible to untangle, but recent National Institute on Drug Abuse (NIDA) research suggests that treatment for the mood disorder alone can also have a positive effect on drug abuse treatment.[67]

One NIDA-supported study found that drug use declined among teenage drug-dependent patients who were being treated with a medication for bipolar disorder, a condition which is characterized by alternating periods of depression and mania. In a related study, chronic opiate-dependent adults reported less drug abuse when they were treated with the antidepressant imipramine for comorbid depression.[68]

CLINICAL EVALUATION

Medicolegal considerations

Substance abuse during pregnancy places legal and ethical obligations on the physician. First, it is necessary for the interview and history-taking process to be sufficiently detailed to discover information regarding the history and frequency of use of potentially dangerous substances. During routine psychiatric evaluation the nature and extent of the social or illicit substance use will be defined. If exposure did occur during gestation, the physician should take steps to find out as much as possible about the teratogenic and toxic potential of the substance or combination of substances. This should be determined in consultation with a specialist. The medicolegally correct action is to disclose fully to the patient the medically known risks posed by maternal substance abuse. The disclosure should be documented in the medical record in a clear and concise manner. The physician must emphasize to the patient that social or illicit substance use is contraindicated during pregnancy.[5] The risk–benefit ratio for substance abuse during pregnancy is *increased risk with no benefit*, and this should be documented in the medical record. Medical risks and treatment modalities for specific substances of abuse (with the exception of alcohol) are described in this chapter.

Patient consultation

Patients will often admit to 'trying' a substance of abuse during pregnancy, but they will rarely admit that they are addicted to it. Once some use is admitted, tandem approaches to the history-taking process are suggested. First, it is important to determine how the substance use varies between weekdays and weekends, because it is common for the user's pattern of use to differ greatly between these two time periods. The patient should be asked to describe her daily activities, including any substances used, from awakening to going to sleep on a normal weekday. Weekend activities and substance use should be assessed in a similar way. The second approach is to ask about substance use in particular. The patient should be asked when she begins drinking or using drugs during the course of a day, and the duration of such use. For example, does she use the substance as an 'eye-opener' in the morning?[69] In addition, an inquiry should be made about how much of the substance is used in an average day and approximately how much would be consumed in an hour's time. In combination with information about the weekly pattern (weekend vs. weekday), a semi-quantitative estimate of the amount and frequency of substance use can be made.

   However, estimates made by any method are notoriously low. Several standardized instruments are available to assess substance abuse.[5] The TWEAK was discussed in the previous chapter. With abuse of alcohol, the most extensively studied substance, crude risks of fetal alcohol syndrome can be assessed by average daily use. With other less well-researched substances, information on daily doses may only be of value for assessing the severity of maternal addiction. More severe dependencies are, of course, associated with more severe adverse effects. At the beginning of the counseling session, the physician should explain to the patient that the purpose of obtaining this personal and private information is to manage the pregnancy more safely and effectively, i.e. to give medical care that is more suited to the patient's specific needs. The patient should also be reassured that this information is confidential, like the remainder of the medical record, and that its confidentiality will be maintained.

Another important aspect of patient consultation is to provide information about substance use-associated pregnancy risks. It is important that this information should be as accurate and objective as possible. Exaggerations designed as 'scare' deterrents should be avoided because most substance users are aware of this commonly employed tactic, and their trust in the physician will then be eroded. The most ethical and legally sound approach is to provide information that may be verified directly by consulting the medical literature. Ultimately, the clinical recommendation will be that social and illicit substance use during pregnancy is contraindicated because of associated maternal and embryo–fetal risks. Virtually every substance of abuse crosses the placenta and reaches the unborn child.[70]

Patient evaluation

The pregnant substance user is a high-risk obstetric patient. Pregnant substance users are at increased risk for many complications, including sexually transmitted diseases (STDs), hepatitis, poor nutrition and bacterial endocarditis. Chronic use of substances of abuse is an indication for syphilis, gonorrhea, herpes, chlamdia, HIV and hepatitis testing. Women who use drugs parenterally are at greatest risk, not only for HIV but also for other STDs and hepatitis. Obvious drug injection sites on the upper forearm, called 'track marks,' indicate a serious substance use problem, but the injection sites are not usually obvious. For example, in one cohort of 122 gravid parenteral substance users, only one woman presented with forearm injection sites. The remaining 121 women used less obvious sites of injection, such as veins in the breasts, thighs, calves or ankles.[15]

Other possible signs of substance use during pregnancy include poor weight gain, new-onset 'spontaneously arising' heart murmur and hypertension. Most substances that are used recreationally are anorectics and may result in decreased weight gain during pregnancy. Heart murmurs appear to occur more frequently among women who are chronic substance users. They also occur frequently in association with bacterial endocarditis or a history of this disease. Chronic use of any illegal substances can induce hypertension in non-pregnant adults, although not all of them have been studied for hypertensive effects during pregnancy. Chronic use of cocaine, heroin and tobacco is known to be associated with hypertension during pregnancy.[15,71–73] Moreover, abruptio placentae or a history of this serious complication is also an indication that substance use may be a factor. The risk of severe abruptio placentae may be as high as 1–2% among substance abusers, compared to 0.1% (1 in 830) in the general population.[74] Stillbirth is often associated with substance use, and a history of stillbirths may, together with other risk factors, be a clue that substance use was a risk factor in the obstetrics history.

This chapter merely provides an overview of a broad subject area. Other resources should be consulted when planning the long-term treatment of substance-dependent pregnant women. A treatment program for the individual patient should be designed in consultation with a substance abuse professional. Two resources of primary interest are the American Society of Addiction Medicine's *Principles of Addiction Medicine*[75] and the American Psychiatric Association's *Textbook of Substance Abuse Treatment*.[76] Additional references that are of value in formulating a treatment plan include *Principles of Drug Addiction Treatment: A Research-Based Guide*[68] and *A Cognitive Behavioral Approach*.[67]

Table 13.1 *Selected scientifically based approaches to drug addiction treatment*

Approach	Alcohol	Amphetamines	Cocaine	Heroin	Inhalants	Marijuana	Cocaine + alcohol
Relapse prevention	+		+				
Supportive-expressive psychotherapy				+	+		
Individualized drug counseling	+				+		
Motivational enhancement therapy						+	
Behavioral therapy for adolescents	+	+	+	+	+	+	+
Multidimensional family therapy for adolescents	+	+	+	+	+	+	+
Multisystemic therapy	+	+	+	+	+	+	+
Community reinforcement approach plus vouchers				+			
Voucher based reinforcement therapy in methadone maintenance treatment			+		+		
Day treatment with abstinence contingencies and vouchers	+		+				
The matrix model	+	+	+	+	+	+	+

Source: Principles of Drug Addiction Treatment: A Research-Based Guide.[68]
+ technique has been used with this substance of abuse.

TRADITIONAL TREATMENT REGIMENS FOR NON-PREGNANT ADULTS

The NIDA classification of substance abuse treatment modalities is shown in Table 13.1. The majority of treatment programs have been developed for alcohol- or cocaine-dependent patients, and trials with other substances of abuse have not been conducted in many cases. Importantly, cognitive behavioral approaches are recommended for all substances of abuse. For pregnant women, the suitability of any substance abuse approach is enhanced by gender-specific program components.[5] Ideally, substance abuse treatment for pregnant women should be entirely gender-specific because urgent issues such as prenatal care, anticipation of mother–infant bonding and child-rearing practices will dominate care of the gravida. Much of the behavioral change that is targeted in substance abuse treatment will use the unborn child as a motivator for the patient to change her lifestyle. Hence, the more gender-specific the program of treatment, the greater the impact it can be expected to have on the expectant mother in substance abuse treatment.

Treatment of non-pregnant adults who have substance abuse problems normally involves withdrawing the patient from the substance. The exception to this is the use of opiates, for which methadone replacement/maintenance therapy is available. Various regimens are used to aid withdrawal. One frequently employed approach it to use a benzodiazepine. Another pharmacological strategy is to suppress the alpha-adrenergic action with drugs such as clonidine and to alleviate withdrawal symptoms, frequently with a benzodiazepine adjunct. These regimens are usually given in doses that are adjusted to the individual case in order to facilitate asymptomatic withdrawal, and the dose is gradually decreased over a period ranging from 10 days to 3–6 months.[69]

Substance addiction is a psychological phenomenon as well as a physical one, and both aspects must be addressed adequately in treatment protocols. Specialists in addiction psychology should be involved early on in therapy. Their recommendations may include private and/or group counseling, such as Narcotics Anonymous (NA) or Alcoholics Anonymous (AA). The physician should be supportive of these programs, because they have a relatively high success rate for participants and could thus be of great benefit to the patient.[69]

Alternative treatment programs for substance abuse exist, but very little has been reported about them in the scientific literature. Perhaps the most widely known 'alternative' technique for treating substance abuse is the religious community modality practiced by some groups. The 'sessions' are very similar to 'group therapy', and the structure is similar to the Twelve-Step method of Alcoholics Anonymous.[2,5]

OBSTETRICAL GOALS OF TREATMENT

Treatment during pregnancy is aimed to minimize maternal and fetal/infant morbidity and mortality (Table 13.2). MacGregor and colleagues[77] observed that the most important determinant of pregnancy outcome among substance abusers was prenatal care. Regular prenatal care was associated with better pregnancy outcomes, regardless of whether or not substance use was continued. This observation is important to obstetrical goals in the treatment of the gravid substance user.[5]

It is essential to weigh the attendant risks of continued substance use (e.g. maintenance) and the risks of withdrawal against the benefits of withdrawal (i.e. improved fetal growth). It has been recommended that withdrawal from heroin or methadone should not be attempted after 32 weeks of gestation because of the possible risk of abruptio placentae, preterm labor, premature rupture of membranes (PROM) or fetal death in more advanced pregnancies.

Table 13.2 *Pharmacologic detoxification and adjuvant therapies for substance abuse in pregnancy*

Substance of abuse	Detoxification	Adjuvant
Alcohol	Chlordiazepoxide, 25–100 mg PO q1h Diazepam Lorazepam Phenobarbital Haloperidol	Clonidine, 0.1–0.2 mg PO q8h
Amphetamine	Bromocriptine Amantidine Tricyclic antidepressants Lorazepam	
Cocaine	Diazepam* or Chlordiazepoxide, 25 mg PO qid × 6 days Bromocriptine Amantidine Tricyclic antidepressants Lorazepam	Doxepin, 25–50 mg PO bid
Heroin/Opioids	Methadone, 5–10 mg PO q4–6h 3 days Taper down 5 mg per day until dose is 10 mg/day, then taper down 2.5–5 mg/day Natrexone Naloxone	Clonidine, 0.1–0.2 mg PO q8h
Hallucinogens	None	
Inhalants	Chlordiazepoxide, 25–100 mg PO q1h Diazepam Lorazepam Phenobarbital Haloperidol	Clonidine, 0.1–0.2 mg PO q8h
Marijuana	None	

Source: Kasser *et a*.[69]
* Compiled from Miller.[78]

Withdrawal of the gravid patient from other substances is generally advocated, although no acceptable regimen is approved for use during pregnancy. As with non-pregnant adults, a benzodiazepine or a benzodiazepine together with a low-dose alpha-blocker regimen is used to assist pregnant women in withdrawal from a wide variety of substances (e.g. alcohol, cocaine, methamphetamine, amphetamine).[78] Some authors suggest the acute use of an antidepressant during cocaine or amphetamine withdrawal to treat the transient 'serotonin deficiency' which is thought to be induced by abuse of these stimulants.[78] The primary danger of the alpha-blockers or beta-blockers is maternal hypotension, possibly impeding placental perfusion. Therefore, only the minimal effective dose levels are used. Blood pressure and fetal heart rate should be monitored closely with this regimen, and Doppler flow studies may prove useful for monitoring umbilical blood flow in these patients.

DEPENDENCE DURING PREGNANCY

Substance abuse during pregnancy can be treated without the use of substances that are addictive. New approaches for detoxification have included drug combinations such as cloni-dine and naltrexone. Stine and Kosten[79] reported that a combination of these two drugs was successfully used for rapid opioid withdrawal as outpatient treatment. In addition, the combi-nation of naloxone with midazolam or methohexitone can be used for inpatient settings. Researchers have also found that this treatment can be used by switching to the partial opioid-receptor agonist buprenorphine for either heroin or methadone addiction. Limited experi-ence with clonidine transdermal patches has shown that these can be successfully applied to suppress the symptoms of withdrawal.[78] Low-dose nembutal as an adjunct may improve sleep. Importantly, the use of low-dose clonidine does not appear to be associated with adverse effects on the course of pregnancy.[80] Moreover, limited experience with this regimen indicates that it is effective and does not pose serious risks to advanced pregnancies (beyond 32 weeks). However, these are the results of uncontrolled, anecdotal studies, and only limited extrapolation is possible. In 1993, the Food and Drug Administration (FDA) approved a drug for the treatment of opioid dependence, namely levo-alpha-acetyl-methadol (LAAM). LAAM has a slower onset and a longer half-life than methadone. It is a pro-drug and therefore has a slower onset when administered intravenously than when given orally, thus reducing its potential for abuse.[81]

RISKS OF WITHDRAWAL AND MAINTENANCE

Some investigations have suggested that an increased frequency of fetal deaths and maternal morbidity is associated with opiate withdrawal, especially later in pregnancy.[82,83] However, the pregnancies reported in these case studies were complicated by other factors (e.g. hyperten-sion, syphilis and chorioamnionitis) in addition to heroin addiction that may have contributed to adverse pregnancy outcomes. Controlled withdrawal is recommended.[78]

The maintenance protocol most commonly employed for heroin-addicted gravidas is methadone, although the efficacy of this regimen is controversial.[84] Babies born to mothers on methadone, like those mothers on heroin, may experience withdrawal symptoms. With methadone, symptoms occur much later (i.e. at or after 1 week after birth) because methadone has a much longer half-life (30–40 h) than heroin (8–10 h). Importantly, withdrawal symptoms in methadone-exposed infants are physically more severe than those in heroin-exposed infants, with more seizures and a longer period of displaying withdrawal symptoms in the maintained group.[85] Fetal growth retardation has been found to be more severe among methadone-exposed infants than among heroin-exposed infants in one inves-tigation,[86] but not in other studies.[87,88]

SPECIFIC SOCIAL AND ILLICIT SUBSTANCES USED DURING PREGNANCY

Substance use during pregnancy has not been extensively enough investigated to assess fully the risks to the embryo/fetus and the possible untoward outcomes for the mother (Table 13.3). The available information is frequently confounded by a variety of factors (e.g. poor maternal health, lack of prenatal care, malnutrition, presence of infectious diseases, the use of several different substances). It is unusual for any substance user to take only one substance.

Table 13.3 *Summary of maternal effects of social and illicit substance use during pregnancy*

Substance	Abruption	CNS damage	ICH	Metabolic acidosis	Anorexia	Hepatic renal damage	Endocarditis with parenteral use
Alcohol	+	+	−	+	+	+	NA
Amphetamines	(+)	+	+	?	+	?	+
Cocaine*	+	+	+	?	+	+	+
Heroin	+	+	+	?	+	+	+
Inhalants	?	+	−	+	+	+	NA
LSD	?	+	−	?	+	?	NA
Marijuana	−	(−)	−	?	−	−	−
Methadone	+	+	−	?	+	+	+
Methamphetamine	(+)	+	?	?	+	?	+
Morphine	(+)	+	−	?	+	+	+

−, data inconclusive but suggestive of a negative finding;
+, data inconclusive but suggestive of a positive finding;
?, Unknown;
* Infarction/embolism;
Modified from Little *et al.*[15]

However, treatment of the predominant substance of abuse is frequently the best approach. Pharmacologic treatment of substance abuse during pregnancy is described in detail in *Principles of Addiction Medicine*,[75] which is published by the American Society of Addiction Medicine.

The goal of pharmacologic treatment of substance use is a substance-free state. The substances listed in Table 13.4 are not intended for chronic use. In fact, their chronic use may lead to chemical dependence on the medicine used to treat the substance abuse. It behooves the physician to establish this goal with the patient at the outset, and to allow a maintenance scenario to develop. This is a philosophical issue with some providers, but at least during pregnancy the goal is clearly to become substance free in order to achieve the best obstetrical outcome possible.[78]

Table 13.4 *Summary of embryo–fetal effects of social and illicit substance use during pregnancy*

Substance	Fetal growth rate	Congenital anomalies	Withdrawal syndrome	Perinatal morbidity	Other documented syndrome
Alcohol	+	+	+	+	+
Amphetamines	+	?(−)	+	+	−
Cocaine	+	+	+	+	?(+)
Heroin	+	−	+	+	−
Inhalants	+	+	?(−)	+	+
LSD	?	(−)	?(−)	?	?
Marijuana	+	−	−	+	−
Methadone	+	−	+	+	−
Methamphetamine	+	−	+	+	−
Morphine	+	(−)	+	+	−

−, data inconclusive but suggestive of a negative finding;
+, data inconclusive but suggestive of a positive finding;
?, Unknown;
Modified from Little *et al.*[15]

In general, the medications used to treat substance abuse are not known to be harmful to pregnant women or their fetuses. One class of medications of which there is suspicion is the benzodiazepines. This class of drugs has been suspected in the past of being teratogenic, but a balanced review of the data indicates that medications such as diazepam and chlordiazepoxide are very probably not associated with an increased risk of congenital anomalies.[89] An additional consideration is the timing of exposure of pregnant women to medication to treat substance abuse. The vast majority of pregnant women who present for substance abuse treatment will do so *after* the period of embryogenesis. Therefore, in most cases the issue of teratogenicity (i.e. inducing a birth defect with a medication) is a moot point because the organ systems and structures are already formed (see Chapter 3). The remaining issue concerns the fetal effects of medications used to treat substance abuse. Of the medications used to treat substance abuse, two of the drug categories listed in Table 13.4 have potential fetal effects. With the benzodiazepines, the risk of 'floppy infant syndrome' is significant if large doses of the drugs are taken near the time (within 3–7 days) of delivery. The symptoms are caused by withdrawal from the benzodiazepine, and may be treated with supportive therapy for lethargy, poor feeding and hypothermia.

Methadone is another medication that is used to treat substance abuse during pregnancy, and it may be associated with severe neonatal withdrawal symptoms. However, if the suggested tapering of the methadone dose is achieved before delivery, the neonate will probably remain symptom free. If the newborn infant exhibits withdrawal symptoms, they will require treatment with paragoric (tincture of morphine) to alleviate the symptoms until withdrawal is completed.

The other medications listed in Table 13.4 are not known to have any adverse effects on the second- and third-trimester fetus. However, no studies of naltrexone or naloxone have been reported, and the risk posed by the medication during pregnancy should be outweighed by the benefit before any medication is used for which there have been no studies of its use during pregnancy.

With regard to the specific effects of substance abuse during pregnancy, the two areas of interest are maternal and embryofetal effects. An overview of the maternal effects of substance abuse is given in Table 13.3, and the embryofetal effects of substance abuse are summarized in Table 13.4.

The need for services to assist pregnant substance users is being increasingly recognized, and programs now exist in most areas. Ideally, the pregnant substance user should be managed by an obstetrician in conjunction with a psychiatric treatment program designed to promote abstinence or at least to reduce the substance use. The medical positions of abstinence and treatment are clinically and legally appropriate.

REFERENCES

1. Rouse BA. Epidemiology of illicit and abused drugs in the general population, emergency department drug-related episodes, and arrestees. *Clinical Chemistry* 1996; **42**: 1330–6.
2. Gomberg EL. Social predicators of women's alcohol and drug use: implications for prevention and treatment. In: Graham AW, Schultz TK (eds) *ASAM principles of addiction medicine*, 2nd edn. Chevy Chase, MD: American Society of Addiction Medicine, Inc. Chevy Chase, Maryland 1998: 1191–9.
3. Finnegan LP. Perinatal morbidity and mortality in substance using families: effects and intervention strategies. *Bulletin on Narcotics* 1994; **46**: 19–43.
4. Slutsker L, Smith R, Higginson G, Fleming D. Recognizing illicit drug use by pregnant women: reports from Oregon birth attendants. *American Journal of Public Health* 1993; **83**: 61–4.

5. Blume SB. Understanding addictive disorders in women. In: Graham AW, Schultz TK (eds) *ASAM principles of addiction medicine*, 2nd edn. Chevy Chase, MD: American Society of Addiction Medicine, Inc. 1998: 1173–90.

6. Shikles JL. *Drug-exposed Infants: a generation at risk. Report to the Chairman, Committee on Finance, US Senate*. Washington, DC: US Government Printing Office, 1990.

7. Buehler BA, Conover B, Andres RL. Teratogenic potential of cocaine. *Seminars in Perinatology* 1996; **20**: 93.

8. Roe DA, Little BB, Bawdon RE, Gilstrap LC III. Metabolism of cocaine by human placentae: Implications for fetal exposure. *American Journal of Obstetrics and Gynecology* 1990; **163**: 713.

9. Kozel NJ, Adams EH. Epidemiology of drug abuse: an overview. *Science* 1986; **234**: 970–4.

10. Little BB, Snell LM, Palmore MK, Gilstrap LC III. Cocaine use in pregnant women in a large public hospital. *American Journal of Perinatology* 1988; **5**: 206–7.

11. Brody JE. Widespread abuse of drugs by pregnant women is found. *The New York Times* 1989; **137**: 1.

12. Ostrea EM, Brady M, Gause S *et al*. Drug-screening of newborns by meconium analysis: a large-scale, prospective epidemiological study. *Pediatrics* 1992; **89**: 107.

13. Nair P, Rothblum S, Hebel R. Neonatal outcome in infants with evidence of fetal exposure to opiates, cocaine, and cannabinoids. *Clinical Pediatrics* 1994; **33**: 280–5.

14. Osterloh JD, Lee BL. Urine drug screening in mothers and newborns. *Archives of Diseases in Childhood* 1989; **143**: 791–3.

15. Little BB, Gilstrap LC, Cunningham FG. Social and illicit substance use during pregnancy. In: Cunningham, McDonald, Gant (eds) *Williams' Obstetrics*, 18th edn. Norwalk, CT: Appleton and Lange, 1990.

16. Richardson GA, Day NL. Maternal and neonatal effects of moderate cocaine use during pregnancy. *Neurotoxicology and Teratology* 1991; **13**: 455–60.

17. Spear LP, Kirstein CL, Bell J *et al*. Effects of prenatal cocaine exposure on behavior during the early postnatal period. *Neurotoxicology and Teratology* 1991; **11**: 57–63.

18. Harlow KC. Patterns of rates of mortality from narcotics and cocaine overdose in Texas, 1976–87. *Public Health Reports* 1990; **105**: 455.

19. Chasnoff IJ, Landress HJ, Barrett ME. The prevalence of illicit-drug or alcohol use during pregnancy and discrepancies in mandatory reporting in Pinellas County, Florida. *New England Journal of Medical* 1990; **322**: 1202–6.

20. Monga M, Chmielowiec S, Andres RL, Troyer LR, Parisi VM. Cocaine alters placenta production of thromboxane and prostacyclin. *American Journal of Obstetrics and Gynecology* 1994; **171**: 965–9.

21. Jaffe JH. Drug addiction and drug abuse. In: Goodman A, Goodman L, Gilman AG (eds) *Goodman and Gilman's the pharmacological basis of therapeutics*. 8th edn. New York: Macmillan, 1990.

22. Lange RA, Cigarroa RG, Yancey CW *et al*. Cocaine-induced coronary-artery vasospasm. *New England Journal of Medicine* 1989; **321**: 1557–62.

23. Goodman Gilman A, Rall TW, Nies AS, Taylor A. *The pharmacological basis of therapeutics*. 8th edn. New York: Pergamon Press, 1990.

24. Pascual-Leone A, Dhuna A, Altafullah I, Anderson DC. Cocaine-induced seizures. *Neurology* 1990; **40**: 404–7.

25. Ostrea EM, Porter T, Balun J, Wardell JN, Bottoms S. Effect of chronic maternal addiction on placental drug metabolism. *Developmental Pharmacology and Therapeutics* 1989; **12**: 42.

26. Wang CH, Schnoll SH. Prenatal cocaine use associated with down-regulation of receptors in human placenta. *National Institute on Drug Abuse Research Monograph Series* 1987; **76**: 277.

27. Wang CH, Schnoll SH. Prenatal cocaine use associated with down-regulation of receptors in human placenta. *Neurotoxicology and Teratology* 1987; **9**: 301–4.

28. Little BB, Van Beveren TT, Gilstrap LC. Cocaine abuse during pregnancy. In: Gilstrap LC, Little BB (eds) *Drugs and pregnancy*. 2nd edn. London: Edward Arnold, 1998: 419–44.

29. Little BB, Snell LM. Brain growth among fetuses exposed to cocaine *in utero*: asymmetric growth retardation. *Obstetrics and Gynecology* 1991; **77**: 361–4.
30. Kobori JA, Ferriero DM, Golabi M. CNS and craniofacial anomalies in infants born to cocaine abusing mothers. *Clinical Research* 1989; **37**: 196 (abstract).
31. Fries MH, Kuller JA, Norton ME *et al.* Facial features of infants exposed to cocaine prenatally. *Teratology* 1993; **48**: 413–20.
32. Little BB, Wilson GN, Jackson G. Is there a cocaine syndrome? Dysmorphic and anthropometric assessment of infants exposed to cocaine. *Teratology* 1996; **54**: 145–9.
33. van de Bor M, Walther FJ, Ebrahimi M. Decreased cardiac output in infants of mothers who abused cocaine. *Pediatrics* 1990; **85**: 30–32.
34. Kandall SR. Treatment options for drug-exposed neonates. In: Graham AW, Schultz TK (eds) *ASAM principles of addiction medicine*, 2nd edn. Chevy Chase, MD: American Society of Addiction Medicine, Inc., 1998: 1211–22.
35. Hans SL. Developmental outcomes of prenatal exposure to alcohol and other drugs. In: Graham AW, Schultz TK (eds) *ASAM principles of addiction medicine*, 2nd edn. Chevy Chase, MD: American Society of Addiction Medicine, Inc., 1998: 1223–37.
36. Van Beveren TT, Little BB, Spence MJ. Effects of prenatal cocaine exposure and postnatal environment on child development. *American Journal of Human Biology* 2000; **12**: 417–28.
37. Chasnoff IJ, Griffith DR, Freier C *et al.* Cocaine/polydrug use in pregnancy: two-year follow-up. *Pediatrics* 1992; **89**: 284–9.
38. Ernhart CB, Marler MR, Morrow-Tlucak M. Size and cognitive development in the early preschool years. *Psychological Report* 1987; **61**: 103–6.
39. Gross SJ, Oehler JM, Eckerman CO. Head growth and developmental outcome in very-low-birth-weight infants. *Pediatrics* 1991; **71**: 70–5.
40. Hack M, Breslau N, Weissman B *et al.* Effects of very low birth weight and subnormal head size on cognitive abilities at school age. *New England Journal of Medicine* 1991; **325**: 231–7.
41. Angelilli ML, Fischer H, Delaney-Black V *et al.* History of *in utero* cocaine exposure in language-delayed children. *Clinical Pediatrics* 1994; **33**: 514–16.
42. Nulman I, Rovet J, Almann D *et al.* Neurodevelopment of adopted children exposed *in utero* to cocaine. *Canadian Medical Association Journal* 1994; **151**: 1591–7.
43. Little BB, Van Beveren TT, Gilstrap LC. Opiate abuse during pregnancy. In: Gilstrap LC, Little BB (eds) *Drugs and pregnancy*. 2nd edn. London: Edward Arnold, 1998: 449–56.
44. Little BB, Van Beveren TT, Gilstrap LC. Amphetamine abuse during pregnancy. In: Gilstrap LC, Little BB (eds) *Drugs and pregnancy*. 2nd edn. London: Edward Arnold, 1998: 405–12.
45. Billing L, Eriksson M, Steneroth G, Zetterstrom R. Pre-school children of amphetamine-addicted mothers. *Acta Paediatrica* 1985; **74**: 179.
46. Billing L, Eriksson M, Jonsson B, Steneroth G, Zetterstrom R. The influence of environmental factors on behavioral problems in 8–year-old children exposed to amphetamine during fetal life. *Child Abuse and Neglect* 1994; **18**: 3–9.
47. Eriksson M, Zetterstrom R. Amphetamine addiction during pregnancy: 10–year follow-up. *Acta Paediatrica* 1994; **404** (Supplement): 27–31.
48. Cernerud L, Eriksson M, Jonsson B, Steneroth G, Zetterstrom R. Amphetamine addiction during pregnancy: 14-year follow-up of growth and school performance. *Acta Paediatrica* 1996; **85**: 204–8.
49. Struthers JM, Hansen RL. Visual recognition memory in drug-exposed infants. *Journal of Developmental and Behavior Pediatrics* 1992; **13**: 108–11.
50. Carroll ME. PCP and hallucinogens. *Advances in Alcohol and Substance Abuse* 1990; **9**: 167–90.
51. Little BB, Van Beveren TT, Gilstrap LC. Use of hallucinogens during pregnancy. In: Gilstrap LC, Little BB (eds) *Drugs and pregnancy*. 2nd edn. London: Edward Arnold, 1998: 445–8.
52. Julien RM. *A primer of drug action*. New York: Freeman and Company, 1988.

53. Schwartz RH, Smith DE. Hallucinogenic mushrooms. *Clinical Pediatrics* 1988; **27**: 70–3.
54. National Institute on Drug Abuse. *National household survey on drug abuse*. Washington, DC: Government Printing Office, 1987.
55. Little BB, Van Beveren TT, Gilstrap LC. Cannabinoid use during pregnancy. In: Gilstrap LC, Little BB (eds) *Drugs and pregnancy*. 2nd edn. London: Edward Arnold, 1998: 413–18.
56. Little BB, Van Beveren TT, Gilstrap LC. Inhalant (organic solvent) abuse during pregnancy. In: Gilstrap LC, Little BB (eds) *Drugs and pregnancy*. 2nd edn. London: Edward Arnold, 1998: 457–62.
57. Little BB, Van Beveren TT, Gilstrap LC. Tobacco use in pregnancy. In: Gilstrap LC, Little BB (eds) *Drugs and pregnancy*. 2nd edn. London: Edward Arnold, 1998: 463–74.
58. Little BB, Van Beveren TT, Gilstrap LC. Other substances abuse during pregnancy. In: Gilstrap LC, Little BB (eds) *Drugs and pregnancy*. 2nd edn. London: Edward Arnold, 1998: 475–84.
59. Little BB, Gilstrap LC, Van Beveren TT. Drug overdoses during pregnancy. In: Gilstrap LC, Little BB (eds) *Drugs and pregnancy*. 2nd edn. London: Edward Arnold, 1998: 377–94.
60. Czeizel A, Szentesi I, Szekeres J, Glauber A, Bucski P, Molnar C. Pregnancy outcome and health conditions of offspring of self-poisoned pregnant women. *Acta Pediatrica* 1984; **25**: 209–36.
61. Rayburn W, Aronow R, Delaucy B, Hogan MJ. Drug overdose during pregnancy. An overview from a metropolitan poison control center. *Obstetrics and Gynecology* 1984; **64**: 611.
62. Dannenberg AL, Carter DM, Lawson HW, Ashton DM, Dorfman SF, Graham EH. Homicide and other injuries as causes of maternal death in New York City, 1987 through 1991. *American Journal of Obstetrics and Gynecology* 1995; **172**: 1557–64.
63. Allcott JV, Barnhart RA, Mooney LA. Acute lead poisoning in two users of illicit methamphetamine. *Journal of the American Medical Association* 1987; **258**: 510–11.
64. Rall TW, Schleifer LS. Oxytocin, prostaglandins, ergot alkaloids, and other agents. In: Goodman A, Goodman L, Gilman A (eds) *Goodman and Gilman's The pharmacological basis of therapeutics*, 6th edn. New York: Macmillan, 1985.
65. Klaassen CD. Nonmetallic environmental toxicants: air pollutants, solvents and vapors, and pesticides. In: Goodman A, Goodman L, and Gilman A (eds) *Goodman and Gilman's The pharmacological basis of therapeutics*, 6th edn. New York: Macmillan, 1985.
66. Little BB, Van Beveren TT, Gilstrap LC. Introduction to substance abuse. In: Gilstrap LC, Little BB (eds) *Drugs and pregnancy*, 2nd edn. London: Edward Arnold, 1998: 369–76.
67. Carroll KM. *A cognitive-behavioral approach: treating cocaine addiction*. Rockville, MD: National Institute on Drug Abuse, 1998: 1–127.
68. National Institute on Drug Abuse. *Principles of addiction treatment: a research based guide*. Rockville, MD: National Institute on Drug Abuse, 1999.
69. Kasser C, Geller A, Howell E, Wartenberg A. Detoxification: principles and protocols. In: Graham AW, Schultz TK (eds) *ASAM principles of addiction medicine*, 2nd edn. Checy Chase, MD: American Society of Addiction Medicine, Inc., 1998: 1–85.
70. Little BB, Van Beveren TT. Placental transfer of selected substances of abuse. *Seminars in Perinatology* 1996; **20**: 147–53.
71. Abel EL. Prenatal exposure to cannabis: a critical review of effect on growth, development, and behavior. *Behavioral Neurological Biology* 1980; **29**: 137–56.
72. Little BB, Snell LM, Klein VR, Gilstrap LC III. Cocaine abuse during pregnancy: maternal and fetal implications. *Obstetrics and Gynecology* 1989; **73**: 157–60.
73. Stillman RJ, Rosenberg MJ, Sachs BP. Smoking and reproduction. *Fertility and Sterility* 1986; **46**: 545–66.
74. Cunningham FG, MacDonald P, Gant N *et al*. *Williams' Obstetrics*, 20th edn. Norwalk, CT. Appleton and Lange, 1997.
75. Graham AW, Schultz TK (eds) *ASAM principles of addiction medicine*, 2nd edn. Chevy Chase, MD: American Society of Addiction Medicince, Inc., 1998.

76. Galanter M, Kleber HD. *American psychiatric textbook of substance abuse treatment*, 2nd edn. Washington, DC: American Psychiatric Press, 1999.
77. MacGregor SN, Keith LG, Bachicha JA, Chasnoff IJ. Cocaine abuse during pregnancy: correlation between prenatal care and perinatal outcome. *Obstetrics and Gynecology* 1989; **74**: 882.
78. Miller LJ. Treatment of the addicted woman in pregnancy. In: Graham AW, Schultz TK (eds) *ASAM principles of addiction medicine*, 2nd edn. Chevy Chase, MD: American Society of Addiction Medicine, Inc., 1998: 1199–209.
79. Stine SM, Kosten TR. Use of drug combinations in treatment of opioid withdrawal. *Journal of Clinical Psychopharmacology* 1992; **12**: 203–9.
80. Boutroy M-J. Fetal effects of maternally administered clonidine and angiotensin-converting enzyme inhibitors. *Developmental Pharmacology and Therapeutics* 1989; **13**: 199–204.
81. Rowe PM. Drug addiction: new therapies, old policies. *Lancet* 1993; **342**: 297.
82. Finnegan LP, Reeser DS, Connaughton JF. The effects of maternal drug dependence on neonatal mortality. *Drug and Alcohol Dependence* 1977; **2**: 131.
83. Rementeria JL, Nunag NN. Narcotic withdrawal in pregnancy: stillbirth incidence with a case report. *American Journal of Obstetrics and Gynecology* 1973; **116**: 1152–6.
84. Edelin KO, Gurganious L, Golar K, Oellerich D, Kyei-Aboagye K, Adel Hamid M. Methadone maintenance in pregnancy: consequences to care and outcome. *Obstetrics and Gynecology* 1988; **71**: 399–404.
85. Blinick G, Jerez E, Wallach RC. Methadone maintenance, pregnancy and progeny. *Journal of the American Medical Association* 1973; **30**: 477–9.
86. Wilson GS, Desmond MM, Verniaud WM. Early development of infants of heroin-addicted mothers. *Archives of Diseases in Childhood* 1973; **126**: 457.
87. Lifschitz MH, Wilson GS, Smith EO, Desmond MM. Fetal and postnatal growth of children born to narcotic-dependent women. *Journal of Pediatrics* 1983; **102**: 686–91.
88. Soepatimi S. Kinderen van verslaafde moeders (Children of addicted mothers). *Tijdschrift voor Bejaarden, Kraam and Ziekenverzorging* 1986; **4**: 103–8.
89. Friedman JM, Polifka JE. *Teratogenic effects of drugs*, 2nd edn. Baltimore, MD: Johns Hopkins University Press, 2000.

Index